The Cruciate Ligaments in Total Knee Arthroplasty

Alfred J. Tria Jr. • Giles R. Scuderi
Editors

The Cruciate Ligaments in Total Knee Arthroplasty

Design, Function and Rehabilitation

Springer

Editors
Alfred J. Tria Jr.
Orthopedic Surgery (Emeritus)
Rutgers-Robert Wood Johnson
Medical School
New Brunswick, NJ, USA

Giles R. Scuderi
Orthopaedic Surgery
Zucker School of Medicine at Hofstra/
Northwell
Hempstead, NY, USA

ISBN 978-3-031-75991-8 ISBN 978-3-031-75992-5 (eBook)
https://doi.org/10.1007/978-3-031-75992-5

This Springer imprint is published by the registered company Springer Nature Switzerland AG
The registered company address is: Gewerbestrasse 11, 6330 Cham, Switzerland

Through our academic pursuits for over four decades, we have had the opportunity to train and mentor numerous residents, fellows and surgeons. As our legacy, we are hopeful that they will pickup the baton and continue to influence the world of knee surgery. This book is dedicated to all of them.

Giles R. Scuderi, MD, Alfred J. Tria, Jr., MD

Foreword

It gives me great pleasure to be asked to write a foreword for the upcoming textbook entitled *The Cruciate Ligaments in Total Knee Arthroplasty: Design, Function, and Rehabilitation* to be edited by my good friends Gil Scuderi and Fred Tria.

This book has brought together many of my friends and colleagues from around the world of Knee Arthroplasty and I am proud to see them here, especially my dear old friend Peter Walker whose seminal engineering work allowed John Insall and me to implant the first Total Condylar Prosthesis (TCP) at HSS in 1974. The TCP (which of course sacrificed both cruciate ligaments) became the basis of the modern total knee design.

Indeed, I see the guiding influence of John Insall himself in the organization and authorship of this book. I daresay John would be pleased if not a little skeptical with how things have evolved in knee arthroplasty.

I will keep my opinions on these new designs to myself.

I am quite sure this textbook will become the foundational knowledge of knee design in years to come.

Hospital for Special Surgery
New York, NY, USA

Chitranjan S. Ranawat

Preface

This text represents our fifteenth passage together. Our fellowships with Dr. John N. Insall were our initial common bond and fostered a lifelong friendship. We have been fortunate to have honed our academic careers in The Knee Society and cultivated so many wonderful relationships with many of the authors who have contributed to this text. Our colleague, mentor, and friend, Dr. Chitranjan Ranawat, was kind enough to author the foreword to this text. As an internationally acclaimed surgeon, we are extremely grateful to him for his time and thoughts.

The text is centered on the cruciate ligaments that have challenged knee designers from the very beginning. With contributions from numerous expert authors, the history is reviewed, and the basics of anatomy and kinematics are presented. The total knee designs section discusses all the present-day prostheses with historical background. The surgical techniques consider the varying approaches with their advantages and limitations. The rehabilitation section ties the postoperative recovery program to each knee design. The results section compares the different prostheses and concludes with some considerations for the future.

The final answer for the cruciates and total knee arthroplasty is not yet completed; but, we do hope that this text will provide further insight into the direction of the changing paradigm.

New Brunswick, NJ, USA — Alfred J. Tria Jr
Hempstead, NY, USA — Giles R. Scuderi

Contents

Contributors

Zuhdi E. Abdo Lenox Hill Hospital/Northwell Health, New Hyde Park, NY, USA

Mohamed F. Albana Zucker School of Medicine at Hofstra/Northwell, Hempstead, NY, USA

David Backstein, MD, MEd, FRCSC Hospital for Special Surgery at NCH, Naples, FL, USA

Sandeep S. Bains LifeBridge Health, Sinai Hospital of Baltimore, Rubin Institute for Advanced Orthopedics, Baltimore, MD, USA

Todd E. Bertrand JIS Orthopedics, LLC, New Albany, OH, USA

Jason A. Bryman Colorado Joint Replacement, AdventHealth Porter, Denver, CO, USA

Antonia F. Chen Department of Orthopedic Surgery, Brigham and Women's Hospital, Harvard Medical School, Boston, MA, USA

Ryan Cheng Hospital for Special Surgery, New York, NY, USA

Adult Reconstruction and Joint Replacement Service, Hospital for Special Surgery, New York, NY, USA

Robert Wood Johnson Medical School, Rutgers University, New Brunswick, NJ, USA

Ronald E. Delanois LifeBridge Health, Sinai Hospital of Baltimore, Rubin Institute for Advanced Orthopedics, Baltimore, MD, USA

Douglas A. Dennis Colorado Joint Replacement, AdventHealth Porter, Denver, CO, USA

Department of Biomedical Engineering, University of Tennessee, Knoxville, TN, USA

Department of Biomedical Engineering, University of Denver, Denver, CO, USA

Department of Orthopaedics, University of Colorado Health School of Medicine, Aurora, CO, USA

Gabrielle Dituri Hospital for Special Surgery Florida, West Palm Beach, FL, USA

Seper Ekhtiari, MD, MSc, FRCSC Granovsky Gluskin Division of Orthopaedics, Sinai Health, Department of Surgery, University of Toronto, Toronto, ON, Canada

Division of Orthopaedic Surgery, Department of Surgery, McMaster University, Hamilton, ON, Canada

Jonathan R. Franco Department of Orthopedic Surgery, Brigham and Women's Hospital, Harvard Medical School, Boston, MA, USA

Tony K. George University Orthopaedic Associates, Somerset, NJ, USA

Steven B. Haas Hospital for Special Surgery, New York, NY, USA

Emilio D. Hernandez, MD Granovsky Gluskin Division of Orthopaedics, Sinai Health, Department of Surgery, University of Toronto, Toronto, ON, Canada

Stephen M. Howell Department of Biomedical Engineering, University of California at Davis, Davis, CA, USA

Peter P. Hsiue Hospital for Special Surgery, New York, NY, USA

Maury L. Hull Department of Biomedical Engineering, University of California at Davis, Davis, CA, USA

Department of Mechanical Engineering, University of California at Davis, Davis, CA, USA

Department of Orthopaedic Surgery, University of California at Davis, Davis, CA, USA

Faraz Jamal JFK Johnson Rehabilitation Institute, Edison, NJ, USA

Ebony James Hospital for Special Surgery Florida, West Palm Beach, FL, USA

Reza Katanbaf LifeBridge Health, Sinai Hospital of Baltimore, Rubin Institute for Advanced Orthopedics, Baltimore, MD, USA

Richard D. Komistek Department of Biomedical Engineering, University of Tennessee, Knoxville, TN, USA

Tsun Law Hospital for Special Surgery Florida, West Palm Beach, FL, USA

Adolph V. Lombardi Jr JIS Orthopedics, LLC, New Albany, OH, USA

David J. Mayman Adult Reconstruction and Joint Replacement Service, Hospital for Special Surgery, New York, NY, USA

Patricia R. Melvin JIS Orthopedics, LLC, New Albany, OH, USA

Michael A. Mont LifeBridge Health, Sinai Hospital of Baltimore, Rubin Institute for Advanced Orthopedics, Baltimore, MD, USA

Alexander J. Nedopil Department of Orthopaedic Surgery, König-Ludwig-Haus, University of Würzburg, Würzburg, Germany

Jeffrey A. O'Donnell Hospital for Special Surgery, New York, NY, USA

Martin Roche Hospital for Special Surgery Florida, West Palm Beach, FL, USA

Lauren Sacco JFK Johnson Rehabilitation Institute, Edison, NJ, USA

Sahil A. Sanghavi Department of Arthroplasty, Sancheti Institute for Orthopaedics and Rehabilitation, Pune, India

Giles R. Scuderi Department of Orthopaedic Surgery, Zucker School of Medicine at Hofstra/Northwell, Hempstead, NY, USA

Tony S. Shen Adult Reconstruction and Joint Replacement Service, Hospital for Special Surgery, New York, NY, USA

Gabrielle N. Swartz LifeBridge Health, Sinai Hospital of Baltimore, Rubin Institute for Advanced Orthopedics, Baltimore, MD, USA

Alfred J. Tria Jr Department of Orthopedic Surgery (Emeritus), Rutgers-Robert Wood Johnson Medical School, New Brunswick, NJ, USA

Peter S. Walker NYU Langone Orthopedic Hospital, New York, NY, USA

NYU Tandon School of Engineering, Brooklyn, NY, USA

Jesse I. Wolfstadt, MD, MSc, FRCSC Granovsky Gluskin Division of Orthopaedics, Sinai Health, Department of Surgery, University of Toronto, Toronto, ON, Canada

Part I
Background

Chapter 1
The Evolution of Total Knee Replacements

Mohamed F. Albana and Giles R. Scuderi

Introduction

Historically, total knee arthroplasty (TKA) has been the most reliable surgical procedure for end-stage knee arthritis. Currently, the most used implants in primary TKAs are posterior stabilized (PS) and cruciate retaining (CR) prostheses. In the late 1960s and early 1970s, these two implants were being designed in parallel. Michael Freeman and John N. Insall had a close personal relationship that began in medical school at the Corpus Christie College in Cambridge, UK [1]. Freeman continued on to the London Hospital and Insall began his journey at the Hospital for Special Surgery (HSS) in 1965. Over the next three decades, the two constantly communicated their ideas and experiences in both the management of knee arthritis and the design of total knee arthroplasty.

The conception and design of the condylar total knee, consisting of a single femoral component covering both medial and lateral femoral condyles and a single tibial component covering both medial and lateral tibial plateaus, began between 1966 and 1968 and are largely attributed to Freeman and SAV Swanson, PhD [1]. Freeman's main concern was replacing arthritic knees with severe flexion deformities, while Swanson's main concern was wear of the polyethylene liner [2, 3]. Together, Freeman and Swanson established three parameters to simplify the knee mechanics and subsequent prosthesis design: (1) both cruciate ligaments are resected during reconstruction to facilitate deformity correction and maximize the implant bone contact area; (2) resection of both cruciate ligaments limited posterior femoral rollback allowing for a single sagittal radius of curvature for the femoral component; (3) the implant should sit flat on cancellous bone allowing for preservation of bone, increased contact area between at the bone–implant interface, and

M. F. Albana · G. R. Scuderi (✉)
Zucker School of Medicine at Hofstra/Northwell, Hempstead, NY, USA
e-mail: malbana@northwell.edu

A. J. Tria Jr., G. R. Scuderi (eds.), *The Cruciate Ligaments in Total Knee Arthroplasty*, https://doi.org/10.1007/978-3-031-75992-5_1

simplifying the surgical procedure [2, 3]. This lead to the production of the Freeman-Swanson total knee, which did not contain a tibial post for fear of increased stress on the bone–implant interface. Freeman quickly identified this as a flaw due to mediolateral instability with subsequent implant failure [2, 3]. This design did not incorporate an anterior femoral flange for patellar articulation as the patella was not routinely resurfaced. Despite a design adjustment in 1974 to include a femoral flange, manufacturing delays limited availability of the newly designed femoral component until December 1976 [4]. This new design was renamed the Imperial College London Hospital (ICLH) knee.

The ICLH knee progressively evolved to include a tibial post and a groove in the femoral component that articulated with both the tibia and a patellar polyethylene button. KM Samuelson worked with Freeman to develop this new implant, the Freeman-Samuelson knee, whose influence has remained in present day designs [1].

In 1970, Insall along with Chitranjan Ranawat, Alan Inglis, and Peter Walker established a working group that would bring forward significant innovation and influence the present day TKA. This working group developed an anatomic cemented TKA that preserved both cruciate ligaments and the duocondylar knee (Fig. 1.1) [1]. Although this was occurring at the same time as Freeman's innovation in London, the philosophy was quite different with an emphasis on maintaining both cruciate ligaments. The duocondylar was first implanted by Ranawat with Insall as first assistant in 1971 and led to several realizations postoperatively: (1) replacing the patellofemoral compartment should be incorporated in future designs; (2) preservation of both cruciate ligaments limited correction of deformities; (3) fixation of separate tibial components, which the duocondylar knee had, was not as secure as a single tibial component [5].

The limitations of the duocondylar knee led to the development of the Total Condylar (TC) prosthesis (Fig. 1.2), which was the first functionally designed prosthesis that sacrificed both cruciate ligaments, and the duopatellar prosthesis, which preserved the PCL (Fig. 1.3). The TC prosthesis boasted a trough in the anterior femoral flange and a resurfaced polyethylene patellar button, resection of both

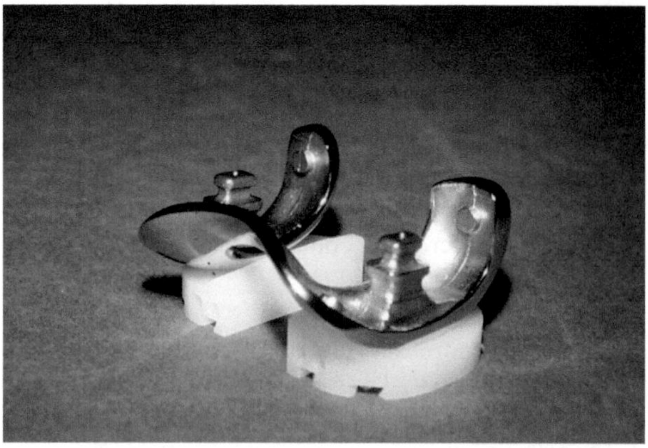

Fig. 1.1 Duocondylar prosthesis

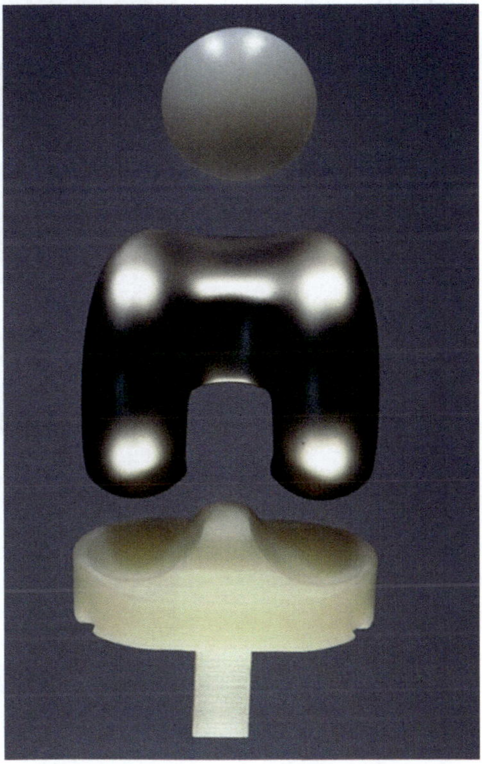

Fig. 1.2 Total condylar prosthesis

cruciate ligaments allowing for deformity correction, and a symmetric anatomic bicondylar design addressing the major limitations of the duocondylar knee [1]. The first TC knee was implanted by Insall in 1974. Concerns about tibial loosening due to the highly conforming femoral and tibial components were addressed by designing a single tibial polyethylene component with an added tibial peg that allowed for torsional stability [6]. Subsequent improvements on the total condylar prostheses incorporated a cam on the femoral component and a post on the tibial component. This provided mediolateral stability and allowed for femoral rollback in place of the sacrificed posterior cruciate ligament [1].

Posterior Stabilized

Insall and Walker would make further modifications to the TC knee to address two predictable consequences of cruciate resection [7–10]. The first was flexion instability leading to an anterior shifting of the femur on the tibial polyethylene. The second was the limited knee flexion obtained with the TC knee, which allowed an average of 90 degrees of flexion [10]. Both consequences were corrected with the advent of

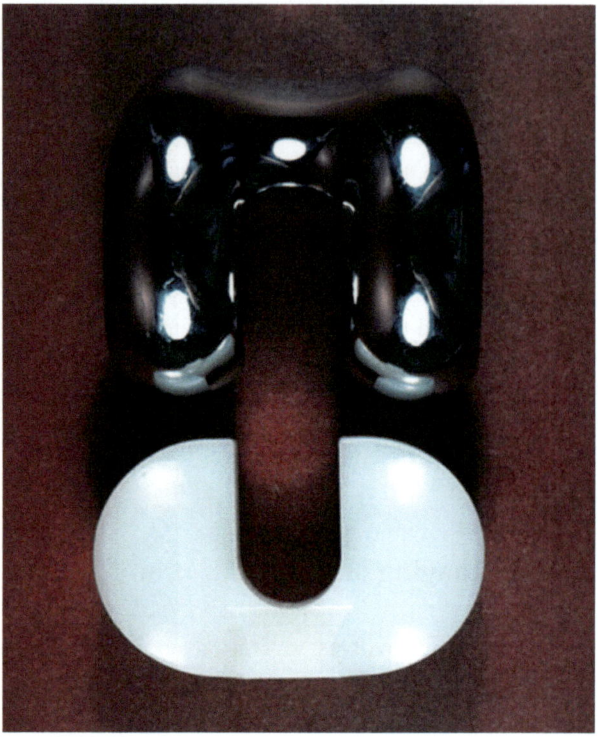
Fig. 1.3 Duopatellar prosthesis

the central tibial post. The tibial post acted to block hyperextension and prevented anterior displacement of the femur in flexion by incorporating posterior femoral roll back [11, 12]. This new design, called the Total Condylar Prosthesis II (TCP II), was short-lived due to early loosening. Following the failure of the TCP II, Insall began collaborating with a bioengineer, Albert Burstein, to produce the Insall-Burstein I (IB I) (Fig. 1.4). The IB I was introduced in 1978 and would act as the benchmark for all future posterior cruciate-substituting designs [13].

The IB I design contained a dished all-polyethylene tibial component with a tibial post-femoral cam mechanism that allowed for femoral rollback and increased ROM [11]. Shortly thereafter, laboratory studies demonstrated that metal-backed components transmitted loads from the prosthesis to the bone better than polyethylene alone [14]. By 1980, Insall was exclusively implanting IB I with a metal-backed tibial component, which demonstrated tremendous clinical performance and survivorship data for nearly a decade to follow [15–19]. In 1988, the IB II prosthesis was introduced to the market. This new iteration featured a modular tibial tray with the ability to add both augments and stem extensions to the core prosthesis (Fig. 1.5) [11]. While the IB II featured improvements in the tibial components, the NexGen Legacy Posterior Stabilized Knee Prosthesis (LPS) (Zimmer, Warsaw, IN), introduced in the mid-1990s, focused on the femoral component. The LPS prosthesis offered side-specific femoral components with a raised lateral femoral flange and a

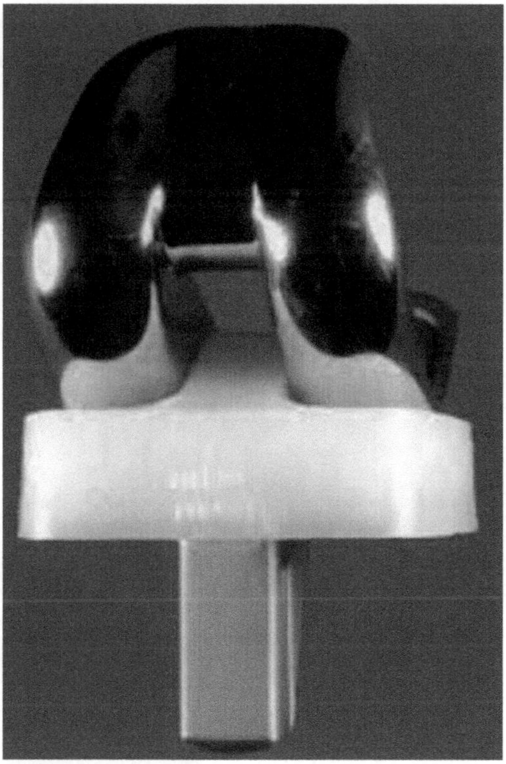

Fig. 1.4 Insall-Burstein I

deeper trochlear recess for optimal patellar tracking [11]. More recently, these devices evolved into the widely used Persona PS prosthesis (Zimmer Biomet, Warsaw, IN) with moderate sagittal and coronal plane conformity (Fig. 1.6). Further modifications including increased size options for better soft tissue balancing and, eventually, press-fit designs maintained the groundbreaking advances originally introduced with the IB I and IB II prostheses.

Cruciate Retaining

In the early 1970s, Phil Wilson, Jr., who was serving as the surgeon and chief of HSS at the time, encouraged Ranawat to concentrate on the duopatellar design while Insall was focuses on the total condylar prosthesis [1]. Ranawat drew from his experience in total hip arthroplasty fixation and convinced Walker to design similar stem fixation for the TC and duopatellar prostheses to improve torsional fixation [1]. The final peg geometry was incorporated into both prostheses in 1974 drawing from the Charnley hip stem fixation and biomechanical knee simulator tests carried out by Walker [1].

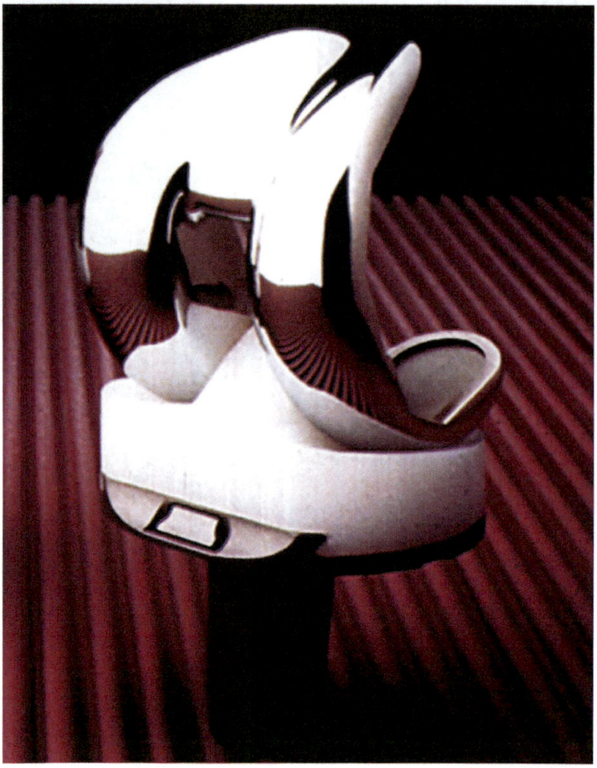

Fig. 1.5 Insall-Burstein II prosthesis

As discussed above, the duopatellar prosthesis preserved the posterior cruciate ligament in hopes of maintaining posterior femoral rollback allowing for increased passive knee range of motion. Insall reported his experience using the total condylar knee prosthesis in 125 consecutive knees with an average age of 68.2 years and noted patients had an average range of motion of 94° [75°–125°] [8]. A year later, Ewald et al. published their findings on kinematic total knee arthroplasties, which consisted of preserving the posterior cruciate ligament. In their review of 124 consecutive knees with an average age of 76 years old, the average range of motion 106° [93°–119°] [20]. The proponents of cruciate retaining designs touted this preservation of range of motion, particularly as it translated to improved maintenance of activities of daily living [21, 22]. Furthermore, a 10-year survival analysis comparing the cruciate retaining design to the total condylar knee demonstrated similar clinical and radiographic success rates [23]. In light of similar survival rates, greater range of motion, and reduced shear forces at the bone–prosthesis–cement interface [24] with a retained posterior cruciate ligament, the philosophy of posterior cruciate retention established itself as a reasonable alternative to the traditional cruciate resection approach.

The duopatellar prosthesis, the first cruciate preserving design, was implanted at HSS in 1974 and continued until 1976. In 1974, Ranawat and Walker introduced

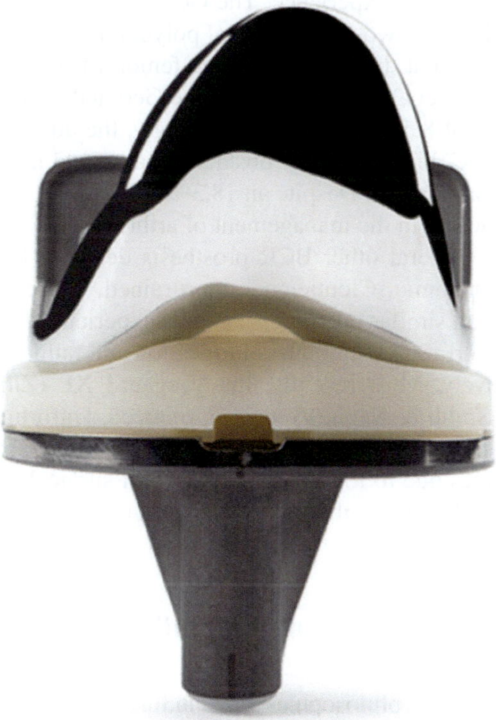

Fig. 1.6 Persona PS prosthesis

both the duopatellar and TC prostheses to the surgeons in Boston, where the posterior cruciate sparing approach would thrive. In 1975, Peter Walker left HSS to work with Clement Sledge and Fred Ewald on further developing the duopatellar design. Although the results of the duopatellar prosthesis demonstrated excellent outcomes, Ranawat and Inglis, who remained at HSS, determined that the results were no better than the TC prosthesis [1] and the power of deformity correction with excision of the posterior cruciate ligament was too valuable leading to the abandonment of duopatellar prosthesis and the preservation of the posterior cruciate ligament at HSS [1].

Bi-cruciate Retaining Designs

The bi-cruciate retaining (BCR) designs experienced a span of popularity early in the 1970s. The theory of preserving both cruciate ligaments for a more anatomic knee replacement was appealing to many, but the initial designs did not demonstrate longevity. The first BCR prosthesis was the polycentric TKA, which had failure rate as high as 34% at 10-year follow-up [25]. These early failures were attributed to surgeon inexperience. The Geomedic BCR TKA was the next generation and consisted of two separate tibial polyethylene components and a single femoral component that did not include the femoral trochlea or a patellar button. In a review by Riley et al., 71 patients had the Geomedic TKA implanted with a minimum follow-up of 8.5 years [26]. Interestingly, the authors accepted that there were "unavoidable" biomechanical obstacles that would inevitably lead to the failure of the tibial components. Despite an 18.3% failure rate, the authors deemed the prosthesis satisfactory in the management of arthritis.

Several other BCR prosthesis designs (Kodama-Yamamoto Mark II, Townley Anatomic, Cloutier non-constrained, Search TKA, Hermes 2C) were developed with similar outcomes. Patients experienced predictable pain relief and function in short term with high complication and failure rates, particularly 10-year postoperatively. Most recently, the Vangaurd XP (Zimmer Biomet) and the Journey XR (Smith & Nephew) were introduced. Unfortunately, these designs did not provide any better outcomes than the initial BCR prostheses, demonstrating high failure rates due to loosening and difficult surgical execution [25]. Given these reports in the literature, the BCR TKA designs have yet to gain popularity.

Gender and Cultural Influence

The two philosophies surrounding total condylar knee replacement drove innovation in the field of total knee replacement that are seen in today's prosthetic designs. The advocates for a functional approach created a posterior cruciate-substituting design using a cam and post mechanism. Excising the posterior cruciate ligament allowed for correction of significant deformity. The advocates for an anatomic design preserved the posterior cruciate ligament and took advantage of the natural kinematics of the knee to maximize knee range of motion and limit strain at the bone–prosthesis–cement interface. Most design innovations were made by the 1980s with future innovations focusing on advantages and disadvantages of modularity and optimizing polyethylene composition to limit wear.

While CR and PS surface replacement prostheses provided terrific pain relief and functional outcomes, some patient populations found limitations due to an inability to achieve greater degrees of flexion. Certain Asian populations require extreme degrees of flexion for both religious and cultural rituals. This prompted the development of prostheses designed to achieve flexion of up to 155°. Some of the modifications incorporated in these high-flexion designs include improved posterior condylar geometry leading to increased contact area in high flexion, modification to the anterior aspect of the polyethylene insert to limit impingement in high degrees of flexion, and an improved cam-post design to limit the risk of knee dislocation in high flexion [27–29]. Zimmer released the first high-flexion design in 2001 introducing the NexGen Legacy Posterior Stabilizing (LPS) Flex Fixed Bearing Knee and a cruciate retaining version (CR-Flex) in 2003. Other companies, including Depuy and Smith & Nephew released their version of a high-flexion prosthesis later that decade. While the initial drive to introduce these designs to the market was to accommodate a small subset of patients, the modifications made to allow for high flexion would be carried over to all future prostheses, including the Persona (Zimmer Biomet) and Attune (Depuy, Warsaw, IN), eliminating the distinction between standard and high-flexion designs. Despite the theoretical advantage of high-flexion designs, the literature does not support increased range of motion with these implants in both Asian and Western patients [28, 30, 31].

Similar to the needed high-flexion requirements for some patients, increased awareness surrounding variations among genders [32, 33], races [34], and ethnicities [35, 36] drove further innovation. These realizations led to the development of gender-specific prostheses which incorporated changes particularly to the femoral component. The main changes included adjustments to the mediolateral and anteroposterior dimensions and orientation and thickness of the anterior femoral flange. While historically 60% of TKA cases are performed on women [37, 38], there was a natural shift to accommodate this larger market share to provide a greater fit for most TKA cases performed. Two early adopters of these differences were Zimmer introducing their Gender Solutions High-Flex Knee, and Stryker (Stryker Orthopaedics, Mahwah, NJ), introducing their Triathalon Knee System. Zimmer made their modifications based on a computed tomography study looking at 800 femurs [39]. Stryker based on their femoral component changes on the anthropomorphic data looking at 337 knees, 209 of which were female [35]. Just as the high-flexion designs would be incorporated in all prostheses that followed their introduction, gender prostheses would be incorporated in designs to follow eliminating the need for separate product lines.

Polyethylene Advancements

Early fixed bearing prostheses struggled to balance the conflicting mechanical fixation needed for longevity of the total knee replacement with the physiologic requirements needed for normal knee function. The existing systems were faced with either compromised wear resistance or risk early loosening due to mechanical constraints [40]. The advent of low contact stress (LCS) mobile bearing devices aimed to mitigate this conundrum by allowing for the tibial insert to freely rotate within the tibial baseplate, thereby limiting the transfer of stress to the bone–cement–prosthesis interface. Unfortunately, no differences in clinical outcomes or implant survivorship were found between the fixed bearing and mobile bearing prostheses [41–43].

This led to the development of the ultra-congruent (UC) tibial polyethylene inserts. The UC tibial inserts are characterized by a higher anterior wall and deeper trough compared to the PS inserts, intended to prevent anterior subluxation of the tibia in deep knee flexion [44, 45]. This congruence increases the tibiofemoral surface contact area, hypothesized to reduce stress force transmission to the bone–implant interface. Many retrospective reviews would soon follow comparing the UC TKA to the PS or CR designs. Several variables including range of motion, clinical scores, radiographic results, patient satisfaction, revision, and complication rates were assessed. Interestingly, none of the studies identified a significant difference in any of the variables assessed, demonstrating comparable outcomes between insert designs [44–50].

As the general understanding or normal knee kinematics became more widely understood, a clear shift in prosthetic design logic began to emerge. The understanding that the medial compartment, composed of a larger medial femoral condyle with a congruent medial tibial plateau and fixed medial meniscus, experiences less rollback compared to the lateral compartment drove the development of medial-congruent (MC) tibial inserts. The idea was to replicate the native knee anatomy to allow for a more stable medial compartment contact point [51]. This pivoting around the medial joint is relatively fixed while the lateral joint rotates around the medial center of rotation [52]. Several companies incorporated this concept in their designs dubbing them "medial congruent," "medial dished," or "medial stabilizing" depending on the company. A major difference between the two groups of MC prostheses is whether the medial condyle has a single radius of curvature or multi-radius of curvature in the sagittal plane. In the single radius TKA, the constant radius of curvature leads to isometric tension on the superficial medial collateral ligament throughout knee range of motion [53]. The multi-radius TKA designs, also referred to as a "J-curve," have a larger radius of curvature anterior and a smaller radius of curvature more posterior allowing increased flexion and femoral rollback [54, 55].

Conclusion

Since the early 1970s, tremendous advances in TKA prosthesis design have been made following two main philosophies: a functional approach created by PCL substitution and an anatomic approach created by PCL preservation. Although posterior stabilized prostheses composed nearly 53% of all implanted prostheses in 2012, this number has dropped to 38.9% in 2022. The cruciate retaining designs demonstrated the opposite effect experiencing a consistent and substantial increase in implantation from 43.5% in 2012 to 56.1% in 2022 [56]. As the anthropomorphic differences between gender and ethnicities were better understood, innovation in femoral component design and size options flooded the market. The hopes of providing improved knee flexion and better fit in the mediolateral and anteroposterior dimensions of the femur as well as a mobile bearing tibial insert were introduced to limit stress transmission to the bone–implant–cement interface. These innovations would be incorporated in all prosthesis designs to follow. A trend toward replicating native knee kinematics led to the development of the ultra-congruent and medial-congruent tibial inserts. With better understanding of native knee kinematics and soft tissue tensioning, the future will experience continued design modifications that improve patient outcomes.

References

1. Robinson RP. The early innovators of today's resurfacing condylar knees. J Arthroplasty. 2005;20(1 Suppl 1):2–26.
2. Freeman MA, Swanson SA, Todd RC. Total replacement of the knee design considerations and early clinical results. Acta Orthop Belg. 1973;39(1):181–202.
3. Freeman MA, Swanson SA, Todd RC. Total replacement of the knee using the Freeman-Swanson knee prosthesis. Clin Orthop Relat Res. 1973;(94):153–170.
4. Freeman MA, Todd RC, Bamert P, Day WH. ICLH arthroplasty of the knee: 1968–1977. J Bone Joint Surg Br. 1978;60-B(3):339–44.
5. Ranawat CS, Shine JJ. Duo-condylar total knee arthroplasty. Clin Orthop Relat Res 1973;(94):185–195.
6. Walker PS, Ranawat C, Insall J. Fixation of the tibial components of condylar replacement knee prostheses. J Biomech. 1976;9(4):269–75.
7. Walker PS, Shoji H. Development of a stabilizing knee prosthesis employing physiological principles. Clin Orthop Relat Res. 1973;(94):222–233.
8. Insall JN, Hood RW, Flawn LB, Sullivan DJ. The total condylar knee prosthesis in gonarthrosis. A five to nine-year follow-up of the first one hundred consecutive replacements. J Bone Joint Surg Am. 1983;65(5):619–28.
9. Insall JN, Kelly M. The total condylar prosthesis. Clin Orthop Relat Res. 1986;(205):43–48.
10. Insall J, Scott WN, Ranawat CS. The total condylar knee prosthesis. A report of two hundred and twenty cases. J Bone Joint Surg Am. 1979;61(2):173–80.
11. Scuderi GR, Scott WN, Tchejeyan GH. The Insall legacy in total knee arthroplasty. Clin Orthop Relat Res. 2001;(392):3–14.
12. Insall JN, Thompson FM, Brause BD. Two-stage reimplantation for the salvage of infected total knee arthroplasty. J Bone Joint Surg Am. 1983;65(8):1087–98.
13. Insall JN, Lachiewicz PF, Burstein AH. The posterior stabilized condylar prosthesis: a modification of the total condylar design. Two to four-year clinical experience. J Bone Joint Surg Am. 1982;64(9):1317–23.
14. Bartel DL, Burstein AH, Santavicca EA, Insall JN. Performance of the tibial component in total knee replacement. J Bone Joint Surg Am. 1982;64(7):1026–33.
15. Colizza WA, Insall JN, Scuderi GR. The posterior stabilized total knee prosthesis. Assessment of polyethylene damage and osteolysis after a ten-year-minimum follow-up. J Bone Joint Surg Am. 1995;77(11):1713–20.
16. Scuderi GR, Insall JN, Haas SB, Becker-Fluegel MW, Windsor RE. Inlay autogeneic bone grafting of tibial defects in primary total knee arthroplasty. Clin Orthop Relat Res. 1989;(248):93–97.
17. Scuderi GR, Insall JN. The posterior stabilized knee prosthesis. Orthop Clin North Am. 1989;20(1):71–8.
18. Scuderi GR, Insall JN, Windsor RE, Moran MC. Survivorship of cemented knee replacements. J Bone Joint Surg Br. 1989;71(5):798–803.
19. Stern SH, Insall JN. Posterior stabilized prosthesis. Results after follow-up of nine to twelve years. J Bone Joint Surg Am. 1992;74(7):980–6.
20. Ewald FC, Jacobs MA, Miegel RE, Walker PS, Poss R, Sledge CB. Kinematic total knee replacement. J Bone Joint Surg Am. 1984;66(7):1032–40.
21. Andriacchi TP, Andersson GB, Fermier RW, Stern D, Galante JO. A study of lower-limb mechanics during stair-climbing. J Bone Joint Surg Am. 1980;62(5):749–57.
22. Andriacchi TP, Galante JO, Fermier RW. The influence of total knee-replacement design on walking and stair-climbing. J Bone Joint Surg Am. 1982;64(9):1328–35.
23. Ritter MA, Campbell E, Faris PM, Keating EM. Long-term survival analysis of the posterior cruciate condylar total knee arthroplasty. A 10-year evaluation. J Arthroplasty. 1989;4(4):293–6.
24. Andriacchi TP, Galante JO. Retention of the posterior cruciate in total knee arthroplasty. J Arthroplasty. 1988;3 Suppl:S13–9.

25. De Mulder J, Berger P, Vandenneucker H. Bicruciate retaining total knee arthroplasty: results throughout history. Acta Orthop Belg. 2021;87(1):73–83.
26. Riley D, Woodyard JE. Long-term results of geomedic total knee replacement. J Bone Joint Surg Br. 1985;67(4):548–50.
27. Argenson JNA, Scuderi GR, Komistek RD, Scott WN, Kelly MA, Aubaniac JM. In vivo kinematic evaluation and design considerations related to high flexion in total knee arthroplasty. J Biomech. 2005;38(2):277–84.
28. McCalden RW, MacDonald SJ, Bourne RB, Marr JT. A randomized controlled trial comparing "high-flex" vs "standard" posterior cruciate substituting polyethylene tibial inserts in total knee arthroplasty. J Arthroplasty. 2009;24(6 Suppl):33–8.
29. Ranawat AS, Gupta SK, Ranawat CS. The P.F.C. sigma RP-F total knee arthroplasty: designed for improved performance. Orthopedics. 2006;29(9 Suppl):S28–9.
30. Seon JK, Park SJ, Lee KB, Yoon TR, Kozanek M, Song EK. Range of motion in total knee arthroplasty: a prospective comparison of high-flexion and standard cruciate-retaining designs. J Bone Joint Surg Am. 2009;91(3):672–9.
31. Nutton RW, van der Linden ML, Rowe PJ, Gaston P, Wade FA. A prospective randomised double-blind study of functional outcome and range of flexion following total knee replacement with the NexGen standard and high flexion components. J Bone Joint Surg Br. 2008;90(1):37–42.
32. Booth RE. Sex and the total knee: gender-sensitive designs. Orthopedics. 2006;29(9):836–8.
33. Greene KA. Gender-specific design in total knee arthroplasty. J Arthroplasty. 2007;22(7 Suppl 3):27–31.
34. Lonner JH, Jasko JG, Thomas BS. Anthropomorphic differences between the distal femora of men and women. Clin Orthop Relat Res. 2008;466(11):2724–9.
35. Hitt K, Shurman JR, Greene K, McCarthy J, Moskal J, Hoeman T, et al. Anthropometric measurements of the human knee: correlation to the sizing of current knee arthroplasty systems. J Bone Joint Surg Am. 2003;85-A Suppl 4:115–22.
36. Kwak DS, Surendran S, Pengatteeri YH, Park SE, Choi KN, Gopinathan P, et al. Morphometry of the proximal tibia to design the tibial component of total knee arthroplasty for the Korean population. Knee. 2007;14(4):295–300.
37. Rand JA, Ilstrup DM. Survivorship analysis of total knee arthroplasty. Cumulative rates of survival of 9200 total knee arthroplasties. J Bone Joint Surg Am. 1991;73(3):397–409.
38. Font-Rodriguez DE, Scuderi GR, Insall JN. Survivorship of cemented total knee arthroplasty. Clin Orthop. 1997;(345):79–86.
39. Mahfouz M, Booth R, Argenson J, et al. Analysis of variation of adult femora using sex-specific statistical atlases. Presented at: computer methods in biomechanics and biomedical engineering conference Antibes, France; 2006.
40. Buechel FF, Pappas MJ. The New Jersey low-contact-stress knee replacement system: biomechanical rationale and review of the first 123 cemented cases. Arch Orthop Trauma Surg Arch (1978). 1986;105(4):197–204.
41. Bistolfi A, Massazza G, Lee GC, Deledda D, Berchialla P, Crova M. Comparison of fixed and mobile-bearing total knee arthroplasty at a mean follow-up of 116 months. J Bone Joint Surg Am. 2013;95(12):e83.
42. Jacobs W, Anderson P, Limbeek J, Wymenga A. Mobile bearing vs fixed bearing prostheses for total knee arthroplasty for post-operative functional status in patients with osteoarthritis and rheumatoid arthritis. Cochrane Database Syst Rev. 2004;(2):CD003130.
43. Van der Bracht H, Van Maele G, Verdonk P, Almqvist KF, Verdonk R, Freeman M. Is there any superiority in the clinical outcome of mobile-bearing knee prosthesis designs compared to fixed-bearing total knee prosthesis designs in the treatment of osteoarthritis of the knee joint? A review of the literature. Knee Surg Sports Traumatol Arthrosc. 2010;18(3):367–74.
44. Laskin RS, Maruyama Y, Villaneuva M, Bourne R. Deep-dish congruent tibial component use in total knee arthroplasty: a randomized prospective study. Clin Orthop Relat Res. 2000;(380):36–44.

45. Hofmann AA, Tkach TK, Evanich CJ, Camargo MP. Posterior stabilization in total knee arthroplasty with use of an ultracongruent polyethylene insert. J Arthroplasty. 2000;15(5):576–83.
46. Chavoix JB. Functionality and safety of an ultra-congruent rotating platform knee prosthesis at 5.6 years: more than 5- year follow-up of the e.motion ((®)) UC-TKA. Open Orthop J. 2013;7:152–7.
47. Argenson JN, Boisgard S, Parratte S, Descamps S, Bercovy M, Bonnevialle P, et al. Survival analysis of total knee arthroplasty at a minimum 10 years' follow-up: a multicenter French nationwide study including 846 cases. Orthop Traumatol Surg Res. 2013;99(4):385–90.
48. Ko YB, Jang EC, Park SM, Kim SH, Kwak YH, Lee HJ. No difference in clinical and radiologic outcomes after total knee arthroplasty with a new ultra-congruent mobile bearing system and rotating platform mobile bearing systems after minimum 5-year follow-up. J Arthroplasty. 2015;30(3):379–83.
49. Peters CL, Mulkey P, Erickson J, Anderson MB, Pelt CE. Comparison of total knee arthroplasty with highly congruent anterior-stabilized bearings versus a cruciate-retaining design. Clin Orthop. 2014;472(1):175–80.
50. Uvehammer J, Kärrholm J, Regnér L, Carlsson L, Herberts P. Concave versus posterior-stabilized tibial joint surface in total knee arthroplasty: randomized evaluation of 47 knees. J Arthroplasty. 2001;16(1):25–32.
51. Komistek RD, Dennis DA, Mahfouz M. In vivo fluoroscopic analysis of the normal human knee. Clin Orthop Relat Res. 2003;(410):69–81.
52. Sabatini L, Risitano S, Parisi G, Tosto F, Indelli PF, Atzori F, et al. Medial pivot in total knee arthroplasty: literature review and our first experience. Clin Med Insights Arthritis Musculoskelet Disord. 2018;11:1179544117751431.
53. Shimizu N, Tomita T, Yamazaki T, Yoshikawa H, Sugamoto K. In vivo movement of femoral flexion axis of a single-radius total knee arthroplasty. J Arthroplasty. 2014;29(12):2407–11.
54. Iwaki H, Pinskerova V, Freeman MA. Tibiofemoral movement 1: the shapes and relative movements of the femur and tibia in the unloaded cadaver knee. J Bone Joint Surg Br. 2000;82(8):1189–95.
55. Ng JWG, Bloch BV, James PJ. Sagittal radius of curvature, trochlea design and ultracongruent insert in total knee arthroplasty. EFORT Open Rev. 2019;4(8):519–24.
56. American Joint Replacement Registry (AJRR): 2023 annual report. Rosemont: American Academy of Orthopaedic Surgeons (AAOS); 2023.

Part II
Basics

Chapter 2
Anatomy: Cruciate Ligaments and Knee Surfaces

Alfred J. Tria Jr and Giles R. Scuderi

Introduction

The cruciate ligaments interact with the surface anatomy of the femur and tibia to guide the knee throughout the range of motion. They influence the patellar tracking, the flexion/extension balance, and the screw home mechanism.

The Cruciate Ligaments

The cruciate ligaments appear embryologically at the fourth to the sixth week of gestation and are extra synovial from the initial development [1]. The anterior cruciate ligament (ACL) originates from the medial aspect of the lateral femoral condyle wall and inserts onto the tibial plateau lateral to the anterior tibial spine (Fig. 2.1) [2, 3]. While some authors have recognized three ACL bundles, most anatomic dissections and surgical approaches consider the ACL as a two bundle ligament [4–7]. The anteromedial bundle originates from the anterior aspect of the lateral femoral condyle and inserts onto the tibial plateau surface lateral to the medial tibial spine [8, 9]. The fibers become tight at 90 degrees of flexion. The posterolateral bundle originates posteriorly on the lateral femoral condyle and inserts posterior to the anterior bundle and lateral to the anterior tibial spine. The posterolateral bundle is tightest in full extension. The footprint of the ACL on the femoral condyle is vertical when the knee is in full extension and becomes more horizontal as the knee flexes beyond 90°

A. J. Tria Jr (✉)
Rutgers-Robert Wood Johnson Medical School, New Brunswick, NJ, USA

G. R. Scuderi
Zucker School of Medicine at Hofstra/Northwell, Hempstead, NY, USA

A. J. Tria Jr., G. R. Scuderi (eds.), *The Cruciate Ligaments in Total Knee Arthroplasty*, https://doi.org/10.1007/978-3-031-75992-5_2

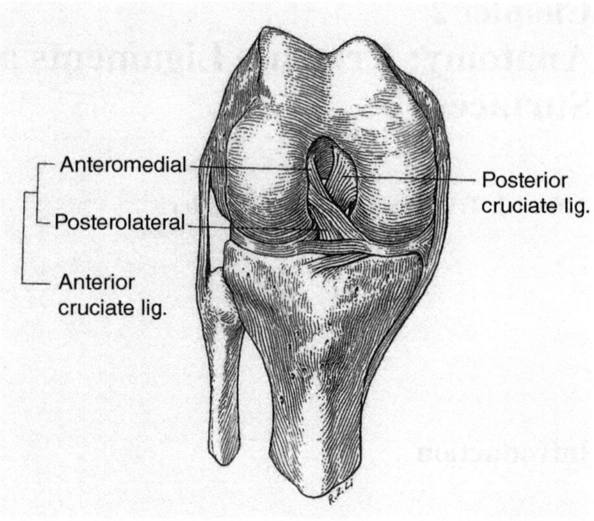

Fig. 2.1 The anatomy of the cruciate ligaments of the knee (with permission from AJ Tria from **An Illustrated Guide to The Knee**, Fig. 1–17, page 10, Churchill Livingstone, New York, 1992)

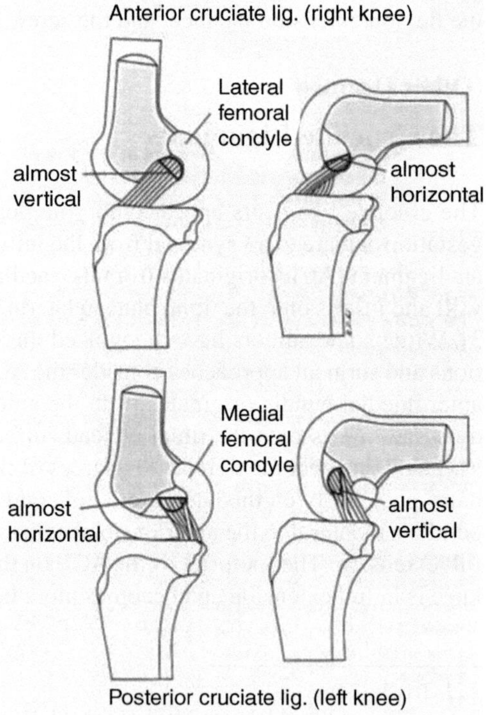

Fig. 2.2 The footprints of the ACL and the PCL (with permission from AJ Tria from **An Illustrated Guide to The Knee**, Fig. 1–19, page 11, Churchill Livingstone, New York, 1992)

(Fig. 2.2) [10, 11]. As the knee flexes, the insertion angle of the ACL into the tibial surface becomes more acute and improves the efficiency of the ligament preventing anterior translation [12]. During flexion, the anteromedial bundle lengthens and the posterolateral bundle shortens. The cross-sectional area also increases from proximal to distal [13].

The posterior cruciate ligament (PCL) originates from the lateral aspect of the medial femoral condyle and inserts into the posterior intercondylar fossa of the tibial plateau 1 cm below the articular surface (Fig. 2.1) [14, 15]. The PCL also consists of two bundles [16]. The anterolateral bundle forms the bulk of the ligament and is tightest in flexion. The posteromedial bundle is smaller and is tightest in full extension. The footprint of the PCL is opposite that of the ACL and is horizontal in full extension and becomes more vertical as the knee flexes beyond 90° (Fig. 2.2) [10, 11]. The PCL fibers become more vertical in flexion and have less effect upon anterior translation while assuming a greater effect in preventing posterior tibial motion. The ligament of Humphrey lies anterior to the PCL and connects the posterior horn of the lateral meniscus to the medial femoral condyle. The ligament of Wrisberg is posterior to the PCL and follows a similar course from the lateral meniscus to the medial femoral condyle [17, 18].

The cruciate ligaments are intraarticular but extrasynovial [1]. The blood supply to the ligaments is from a branch of the middle genicular artery that arises just distal to the superior genicular artery at a right angle closer to the lateral femoral condyle than the medial (Fig. 2.3) [19, 20]. The vessels travel along the synovial membrane but do not originate from the boney attachments of the ligament. The blood supply is more generous to the PCL than the ACL. Thus, the ACL is more susceptible to vascular insufficiency than the PCL. The ACL vascularity decreases significantly

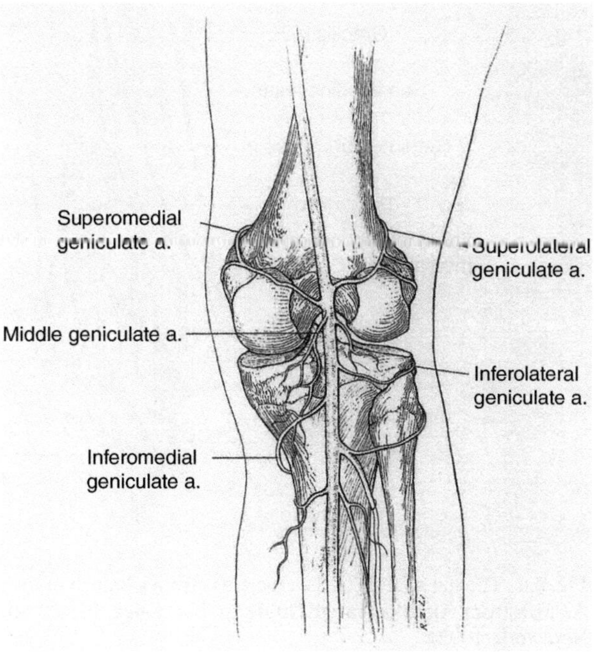

Fig. 2.3 The cruciate ligaments receive their blood supply from a branch of the middle geniculate artery (with permission from AJ Tria from **An Illustrated Guide to The Knee**, Fig. 1–38, page 25, Churchill Livingstone, New York, 1992)

from proximal to its distal insertion on the tibia. An area approximately 5–10 mm proximal to the ACL tibial insertion is almost avascular [21].

The innervation is from a branch of the posterior tibial nerve tracks along the synovial covering in association with the vasculature (Fig. 2.4). There are four types of nerve receptors: Ruffini receptors, Vater–Pacini receptors, Golgi-like tension receptors, and free-nerve endings. These receptors respond to stretching, tension, rapid movements, and pain. They can account for the proprioception thought to be associated with ACL/PCL function. Afferent nerve fibers may interact with the muscles about the knee to protect the ligament [22]. Rupture of the ACL/PCL results in a compromise of proprioception and muscle balance interaction.

The collateral ligaments are the main restraints to varus (lateral collateral ligament, LCL) and valgus (medial collateral ligament, MCL) stress (Figs. 2.5 and 2.6). The MCL originates from the adductor tubercle of the medial femoral condyle and inserts in a fan-like shape along the medial aspect of the tibial metaphysis. The ligament consists of two distinct layers. The deep layer has attachments to the medial meniscus while the superficial layer courses from the femoral condyle directly to the tibial metaphysis. The LCL originates from the lateral femoral condyle slightly posterior to the midline and superior to the insertion of the popliteus tendon and inserts into the posterior aspect of the fibular head. Rotary injuries to the knee often result in complex tears that can involve one or both cruciate ligaments along with a collateral ligament.

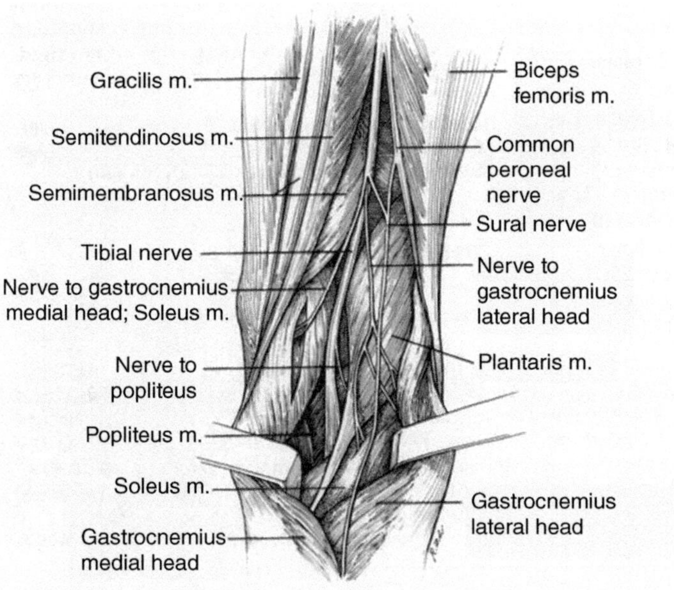

Fig. 2.4 The innervation of the cruciate is from a branch of the tibial nerve (with permission from AJ Tria from **An Illustrated Guide to The Knee**, Fig. 1–40, page 26, Churchill Livingstone, New York, 1992)

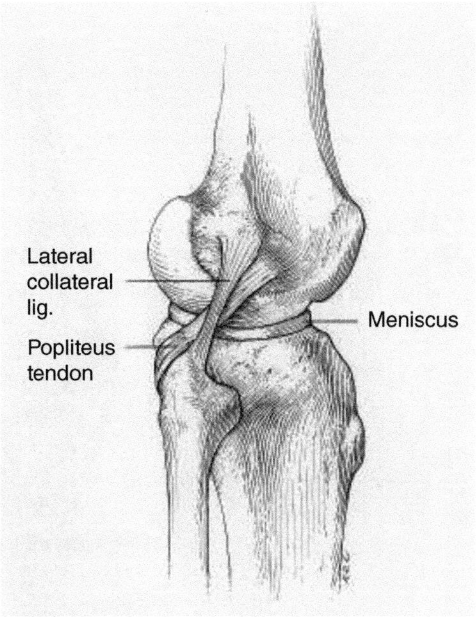

Fig. 2.5 The lateral collateral ligament with the relationship to the popliteus tendon (with permission from AJ Tria from **An Illustrated Guide to The Knee**, Fig. 1–26, page 16, Churchill Livingstone, New York, 1992)

Surface Anatomy

There is little constraint between the tibial and femoral surfaces allowing the ligaments to control the complex rotational motion of the joint. The femoral condyles are asymmetric with an intercondylar divergence angle of 28° (Fig. 2.7). The medial condyle is larger than the lateral condyle in the antero-posterior plane. The lateral condyle distal surface is slightly flattened and has an indent on the lateral edge. The sulcus of the femur can vary in its angle from 10 to 40° accommodating the motion of the patella. The medial condyle is circular posterior but not anteriorly. The lateral condyle is flatter on the leading surface.

The tibial condyles are also asymmetric with a concave medial surface and a convex lateral surface (Fig. 2.8). The medial tibial plateau is longer in the antero-posterior plane than the lateral but there is greater motion in this same plane on the lateral surface with more of a ball-in-socket motion medially [23]. The differential motion on the medial and lateral sides contributes to the screw home mechanism. The tibial spines contribute to stability between the femur and the tibia in the coronal plane.

The patella (Fig. 2.9) has seven facets that articulate with the trochlea of the femur throughout the range of motion. The tracking is influenced by several factors including the relationship of the femur and the tibia, the extensor mechanism, and the patellofemoral ligaments.

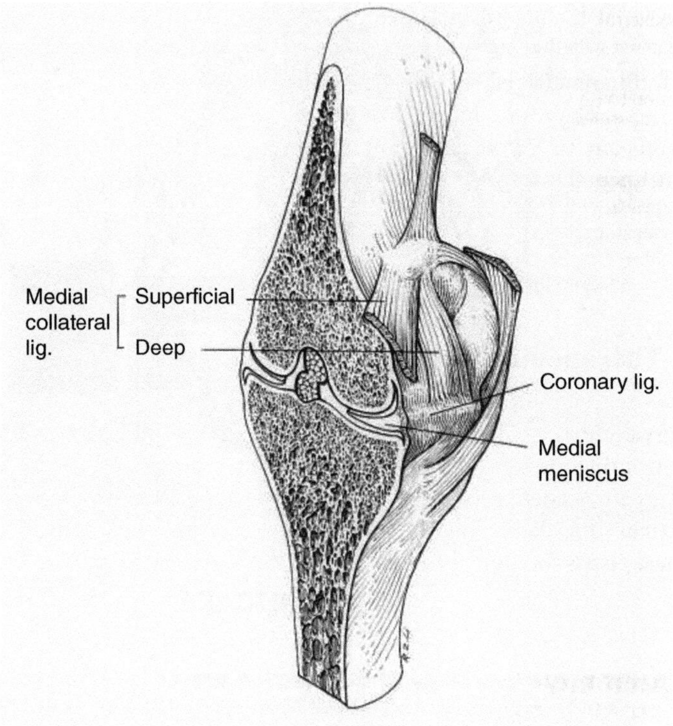

Fig. 2.6 The deep and superficial layers of the MCL with the deep attachments to the medial meniscus (with permission from AJ Tria from **An Illustrated Guide to The Knee**, Fig. 1–24, page 15, Churchill Livingstone, New York, 1992)

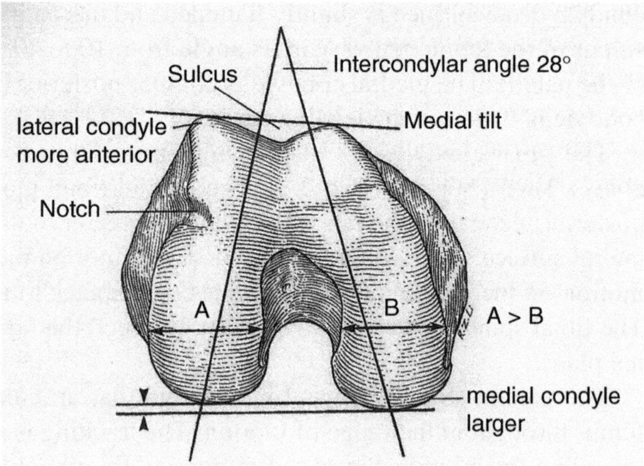

Fig. 2.7 The distal femoral surfaces with the 28 degree intercondylar angle and the lateral condyle notch (with permission from AJ Tria from **An Illustrated Guide to The Knee**, Fig. 1–7, page 5, Churchill Livingstone, New York, 1992)

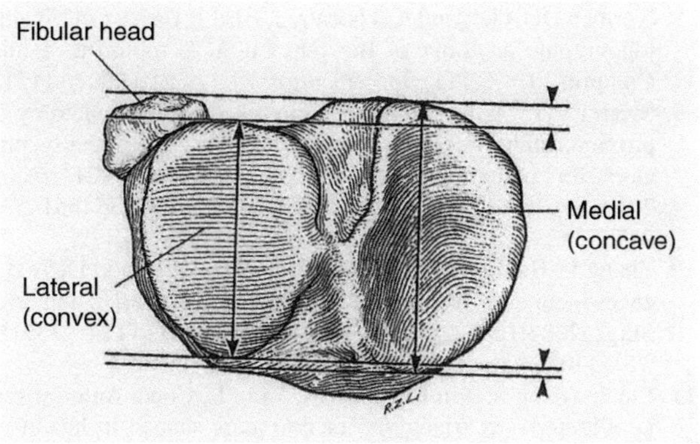

Fig. 2.8 The tibial surfaces are concave medially and convex laterally (with permission from AJ Tria from **An Illustrated Guide to The Knee**, Fig. 1–10, page 6, Churchill Livingstone, New York, 1992)

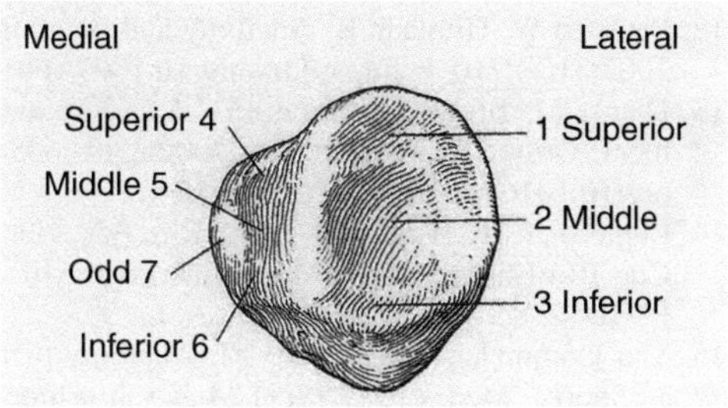

Fig. 2.9 The patellar facets (with permission from AJ Tria from **An Illustrated Guide to The Knee**, Fig. 1–13, page 7, Churchill Livingstone, New York, 1992)

References

1. Ellison AE, Berg EE. Embryology, anatomy, and function of the anterior cruciate ligament. Orthop Clin North Am. 1985;16(1):3–14. PMID: 3969275.
2. Girgis FG, Marshall JL, Monajem A. The cruciate ligaments of the knee joint. Anatomical, functional, and experimental analysis. Clin Orthop Relat Res. 1975;(106):216–31. https://doi.org/10.1097/00003086-197501000-00033. PMID: 1126079.
3. Duthon VB, Barea C, Abrassart S, Fasel JH, Fritschy D, Ménétrey J. Anatomy of the anterior cruciate ligament. Knee Surg Sports Traumatol Arthrosc. 2005;14:204. https://doi.org/10.1007/s00167-005-0679-9.
4. Otsubo H, Shino K, Suzuki D, Kamiya T, Suzuki T, Watanabe K, Fujimiya M, Iwahashi T, Yamashita T. The arrangement and the attachment areas of the three ACL bundles. Knee Surg Sports Traumatol Arthrosc. 2012;20(1):127–34. https://doi.org/10.1007/s00167-011-1576-z. Epub 2011 Jun 22. PMID: 21695467.
5. Petersen W, Zantop T. Anatomy of the anterior cruciate ligament with regard to its two bundles. Clin Orthop Relat Res. 2007;454:35–47. https://doi.org/10.1097/BLO.0b013e31802b4a59. PMID: 17075382. Review.
6. Giuliani JR, Kilcoyne KG, Rue JP. Anterior cruciate anatomy: a review of the antero-medial and postero-lateral bundles. J Knee Surg. 2009;22(2):148–54. https://doi.org/10.1055/s-0030-1247742. PMID: 19476182. Review.
7. Amis AA. The functions of the fibre bundles of the anterior cruciate ligament in anterior drawer, rotational laxity, and the pivot shift. Knee Surg Sports Traumatol Arthrosc. 2012;20(4):613–20. https://doi.org/10.1007/s00167-011-1864-7. Epub 2012 Jan 26. PMID: 22278656. Review.

8. Norman DG, Getgood A, Thornby J, Bird J, Turley GA, Spalding T, Williams MA. Quantitative topographic anatomy of the femoral ACL footprint: a micro-CT analysis. Med Biol Eng Comput. 2014;52(11):985–95. https://doi.org/10.1007/s11517-014-1196-0. Epub 2014 Sep 26.
9. Swami VG, Mabee M, Hui C, Jaremko JL. MRI anatomy of the tibial ACL attachment and proximal epiphysis in a large population of skeletally immature knees: reference parameters for planning anatomic physeal-sparing ACL reconstruction. Am J Sports Med. 2014;42(7):1644–51. https://doi.org/10.1177/0363546514530293. Epub 2014 Apr 22. PMID: 24755252.
10. Zhang L, Huang T, Li C, Xing X, Zou D, Dimitriou D, Tsai TY, Li P. Race and gender differences in anterior ligament femoral footprint location and orientation: a 3D MRI study. Orthop Surg. 2024;16(1):216–26. https://doi.org/10.1111/os.13918. Epub 2023 Nov 12. PMID: 37953405.
11. Lin J, Zhang S, Xin E, Liang M, Yang L, Chen. Anterior cruciate ligament femoral footprint is oblong-ovate, triangular, or two tears shaped in healthy young adults: three dimensional MRI analysis. J Knee Surg Sports Traumatol Arthrosc. 2023;31(12):5514–23. https://doi.org/10.1007/s00167-023-07606-6. Epub 2023 Oct 12.PMID: 37828405.
12. Petersen W, Tillmann B. Anatomy and function of the anterior cruciate ligament. Orthopade. 2002;31(8):710–8. https://doi.org/10.1007/s00132-002-0330-0. PMID: 12426749.
13. Dienst M, Burks RT, Greis PE. Anatomy and biomechanics of the anterior cruciate ligament. Orthop Clin North Am. 2002;33(4):605–20, v. PMID: 12528904. Review. https://doi.org/10.1016/s0030-5898(02)00010-x.
14. Logterman SL, Wydra FB, Frank RM. Posterior cruciate ligament: anatomy and biomechanics. Curr Rev Musculoskelet Med. 2018;11(3):510–4. https://doi.org/10.1007/s12178-018-9492-1. PMID: 29855794.
15. Van Dommelen BA, Fowler PJ. Anatomy of the posterior cruciate ligament: a review. Am J Sports Med. 1989;17(1):24–9. https://doi.org/10.1177/036354658901700104. PMID: 2648873.
16. Pache S, Aman ZS, Kennedy M, Nakama GY, Moatshe G, Ziegler C, LaPrade RF. Posterior Cruciate ligament: Current concepts review. Arch Bone Jt Surg. 2018;6(1):8–18. PMID: 29430489. Review.
17. Pękala PA, Rosa MA, Łazarz DP, Pękala JR, Baginski A, Gobbi A, Mann MR, Tomaszewski KA, LaPrade RF. Clinical anatomy of the menisco-femoral ligament of Humphrey: an original MRI study, meta-analysis, and systematic review. Orthop J Sports Med. 2021;9(2):2325967120973192. https://doi.org/10.1177/2325967120973192. eCollection 2021 Feb. PMID: 33748296. Review.
18. Knapik DM, Salata MJ, Voos JE, Greis PE, Karns MR. Role of the meniscofemoral ligaments in the stability of the posterolateral meniscus root after injury in the ACL deficient knee. JBJS Rev. 2020;8(1):e0071. https://doi.org/10.2106/JBJS.RVW.19.00071. PMID: 32105238. Review.
19. Petersen W, Tillmann B. Blood and lymph supply to the posterior cruciate ligament: a cadaver study. Knee Surg Sports Traumatol Arthrosc. 1999;7(1):42–50. https://doi.org/10.1007/s001670050119. PMID: 10024962.
20. Arnoczky SP. Blood supply to the anterior cruciate ligament and supporting structures. Orthop Clin North Am. 1985;16(1):15–28. PMID: 3969274.
21. Lin KM, Vermeijden HD, Klinger CE, Lazaro LE, Rodeo SA, Dyke JP, Helfet DL, DiFelice GS. Differential regional perfusion of the human anterior cruciate ligament: quantitative magnetic resonance assessment. J Exp Orthop. 2022;9(1):50. https://doi.org/10.1186/s40634-022-00486-8. PMID: 35635616.
22. Kennedy JC, Alexander IJ, Hayes KC. Nerve supply of the human knee and its functional importance. Am J Sports Med. 1982;10:329–35.
23. Victor JMK. Chapter 3. Biomechanics of the knee and alignment. In: Scuderi GR, Tria AJ, editors. The knee: a comprehensive review. New Jersey: World Scientific Publishing; 2010. p. 37–67.

Chapter 3
Kinematics of the Knee

Peter S. Walker

Introduction

In a 1947 report presented to the USA National Research Council by Professor HD Eberhardt from the University of California, entitled "Fundamental Studies of Human Locomotion," the importance of motions other than flexion–extension was emphasized. It was stated that "Transverse rotations, which refer to angular displacements of the various bony segments about their longitudinal axes, are an important factor in the ease and rhythm of walking. Relative transverse rotation of the tibia with respect to the femur averages 9°." This work was targeted to the development of artificial limbs. In the countless studies of knee kinematics since that time, it has been recognized that while the principal motion between the femur and the tibia is flexion–extension, a complete description of motion involves 3 rotations and 3 displacements. There are several ways in which motion can be described, ranging from a complete three-dimensional description to a single displacement value as in an anterior drawer test. Moreover, there are considerable differences in the motion values between individuals, varying with age, body type, gender, and other factors.

There have been many techniques used for measuring motion. Gait analysis has been used from early times. This field has included the measurement of ground-to-foot forces, as well as the angular values of limb segments, and highlighted left-right differences. Sensors have been attached at points in the body, including in the sole of the shoe. Standardized tests have been devised such as Timed-up-and-Go. Fluoroscopic imaging in conjunction with computer modelling has been used to obtain accurate three-dimensional models of the knee geometry and the motion in

P. S. Walker (✉)
NYU Langone Orthopedic Hospital, New York, NY, USA

NYU Tandon School of Engineering, Brooklyn, NY, USA

A. J. Tria Jr., G. R. Scuderi (eds.), *The Cruciate Ligaments in Total Knee Arthroplasty*, https://doi.org/10.1007/978-3-031-75992-5_3

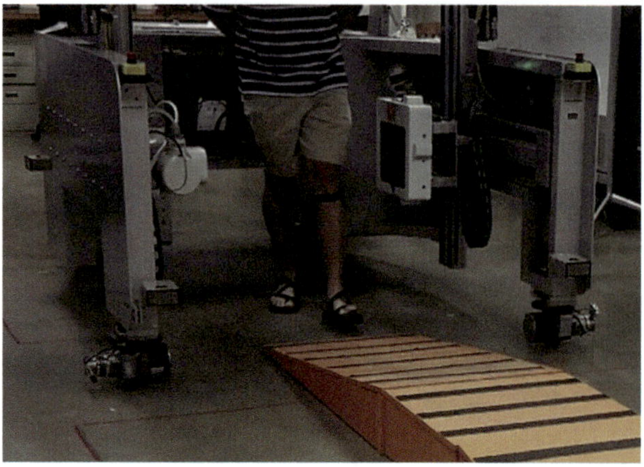

Fig. 3.1 A patient being tested with a mobile fluoroscopic unit to determine three-dimensional kinematic patterns of the knee [1]

various functions. Mobile fluoro units (Fig. 3.1) have recently been developed, greatly expanding the scope of the tests. In the laboratory, studies on knee specimens have enabled the functions of the various structures including ligaments to be studied. Such studies have used both simple and sophisticated test machines to study the kinematics of implanted artificial knees. Ligament behavior, laxity, and muscle actions have been measured. Finally, steady progress has been made in computer modelling, using real-life data for validation and enhancement. Patient-specific models have been created, and analyses carried out on different types of total knee and activity.

In considering kinematics, a key question is what is the ideal kinematic goal for an artificial knee? Should it closely reproduce the kinematics of the normal knee under a range of activities? Are there any negative consequences if all of the nuances of normal kinematics are not reproduced? In order to produce normal kinematics, do the bearing surfaces of the artificial knee have to closely resemble those of the patient's intact knee? Do all of the ligaments, particularly the cruciates, have to be retained? With this approach, how accurately do the bearing surfaces have to be reproduced, and what surgical alignment is needed to allow the ligaments to perform as normal? Given the technical difficulties of accomplishing such an ideal, is the best approach to design the total knee components so that they can reproduce the functions of both the bearing surfaces and the cruciate ligaments, in other words, resect the cruciates and rely entirely on the bearing surfaces? Would such an approach result in a greater degree of reliability, with fewer postoperative problems such as instability? However, is it possible to design an artificial knee which will closely reproduce the kinematics of the normal intact knee? These issues will be discussed in this chapter, based on the evidence of numerous laboratory and clinical studies which have been carried over many years.

Methods for Describing and Evaluating Knee Motion

The classical way in engineering of describing relative position and motion between two bodies is to define an xyz Cartesian axis system based on landmarks in each body. Choosing one body as fixed, the position of the moving body is first defined by x,y,z displacements of its origin, so that they coincide with the origin of the fixed body. Then the moving axes are rotated into registration with the fixed axes, by three successive rotations. The order of the rotations is important; a different order will result in different values for each angle. The definition of the axes in each body is also important in that different axis locations will lead to different values for the displacements and rotations.

Recognizing these complexities, Grood and Suntay [2] proposed a simplified system which could be closely related to clinical definitions of angles and displacements (Fig. 3.2). The starting point was, as above, to define a Cartesian axis system fixed in each body, namely the femur and the tibia. For the femur, the axes were the mechanical axis joining the center of the femoral head and the center of the distal femur, a perpendicular transverse axis parallel to the posterior femoral condyles, and an anterior-posterior axis mutually perpendicular to the other two. For the tibia, the axes were the mechanical axis (coincident to the anatomic axis), a transverse

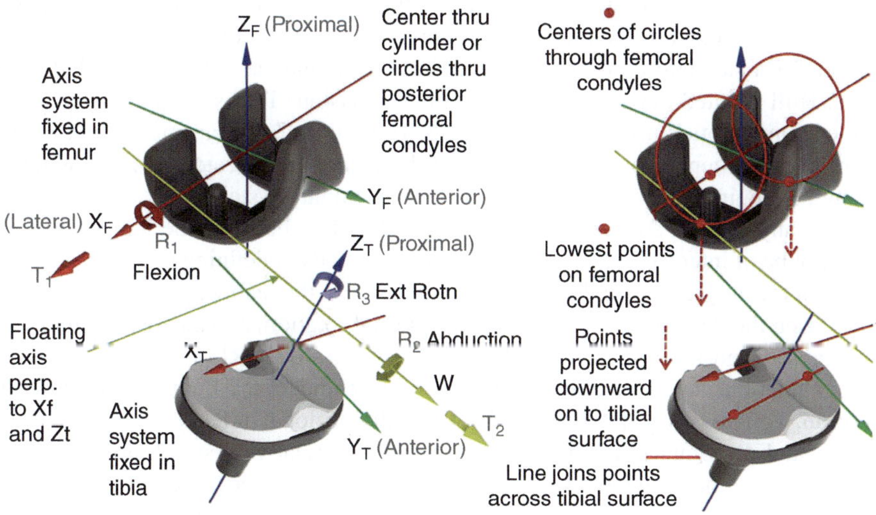

Fig. 3.2 Methods for defining axes in the femur and tibia, and the positions and motion between them. Left figure, definition of Grood–Suntay system [2]. Fixed axes defined in femur and tibia as shown. Flexion–extension about Xf axis (cylindrical or circular axis). Internal–external rotation about Zt (anatomic axis of tibia or perpendicular at center of tibial component). Varus–valgus about floating axis. Right figure, definitions suitable for fluoroscopy or lab tests. Circles through lateral and medial femoral condyles. The centers or the lowest points on circles, projected down along Zt axis on to tibial surface. Points are joined with a line. Multiple lines can be superimposed to describe a range of flexion during an activity. (Figure adapted from [3])

axis bisecting the proximal tibial profile, and a mutually perpendicular axis. However rather than defining angles as described above, a simpler system was defined; flexion–extension was defined as rotation of the tibia about the transverse femoral axis, internal–external rotation was defined as rotation of the femur about the longitudinal axis of the tibia, and varus–valgus rotation was about a mutually perpendicular line to the two previous axes. In this system, the rotation values were independent of each other. Displacements were related to the origins of the femur and tibia.

However, Hull [4] pointed out that to produce valid results, the axes in each body should be related to the functional axes of the motion. If not, crosstalk will occur, meaning that there will be displacements determined for the motion which are a result of incorrectly placed axes, rather than being valid motions themselves. As an example, the axis of flexion–extension occurs about a line joining the centers of the circles of the lateral and medial condyles; the axis of internal–external rotation is about a vertical axis through the medial side of the tibia. Axes in the femur and tibia which are displaced from these functional axes will result in displacements of the tibia and femur which are misleading. For example, if the vertical tibial axis is central in the tibia, it will result in AP displacements on the medial side, whereas in a normal knee, the medial contact is close to being constant. This requirement, that axes fixed in the femur and tibia should align with the functional axes, can be applied to the healthy intact knee, but even then, the functional axes are not constant through the motion, but will change during the flexion range. Furthermore after the implantation of an artificial knee, the functional axis in the tibia may well be in the center for a standard type of total knee, but on the medial side for a medial pivot type. Hull pointed out these aspects in his discussion. That said, studies of three-dimensional motion involving 6 parameters of motion, 3 displacements, and 3 rotations should attempt to define the axes in the locations indicated by Hull, whether using the engineering definitions, or the Grood–Suntay system.

In many studies, some of the 6 degrees of freedom between the femur and tibia may not be of interest. In this case, simplified methods of defining motion have been used. In recent years, with the advent of fluoroscopy, the main parameters of interest have been the flexion angle, the internal–external rotation, and the displacements in the anterior–posterior directions [1, 3, 5–7]. Generally, MRI or CT models of the femur and tibia have been obtained. For successive images in a fluoroscopic recorded motion, software has determined the three-dimensional orientation of the distal femur and proximal tibial. The flexion angle was relatively simple to specify. In addition, the images enabled a transverse axis in the femur to be defined. For the intact knee, two definitions have been used to describe the kinematics. Firstly, a transverse axis has been placed through the centers of the lateral and medial circles of the distal femoral condyles. Secondly, a transverse axis has been placed through the lowest points on the femoral condyles, the lowest points being defined in relation to the longitudinal axis in the tibia. This is not strictly a fixed axis in the femur, but a reference line which changes with each flexion angle. A third variant has been a line joining the centers of the lateral and medial contact areas on the tibia. This transverse axis has then been projected on to the proximal surface of the tibial plateau for visualization and analysis. These methods have been applied to both the intact knee, as well as to total knee replacement. All three definitions of the transverse axis have been shown to produce similar results, except at the extremes of motion, or when an artificial knee has tibial surfaces which are in close conformity with the femur. In addition, for an intact knee, defining the centers of the contact area is not simple due to the deformation of the surfaces and the presence of the menisci.

Laxity is one measurement of knee motion, which has been studied extensively due to its significance [8–14]. Laxity can be defined as the displacements and rotations which occur between the femur and tibia when displacing forces or moments are applied. The AP drawer test is a simple clinical example of laxity. In this test, with the femur fixed, a known force is applied to the tibia in both anterior and posterior directions. The displacements are measured, and the values can be compared with those of a healthy opposite knee. One question which arises when carrying out the test is whether the femur or tibia should be allowed to rotate. In other words, whether other degrees of freedom should be constrained or unconstrained. If the latter, laxity values will in general be larger. In vivo, such tests have been carried out with sophisticated measuring equipment, where linear forces and torques have been applied at different flexion angles, and in some cases true displacements and rotations measured radiographically. In the laboratory, elaborate test equipment, sometimes robotic, has been used for laxity testing.

An extremely important test condition is whether or not an axial force is applied to the knee when carrying out the laxity test. If there is no force applied, the knee is essentially "loose" and the boundaries of the measurements will be determined primarily by the ligaments (Fig. 3.3). On the other hand, on the application of a compressive force directed along the mechanical axis of the tibia, the displacements and

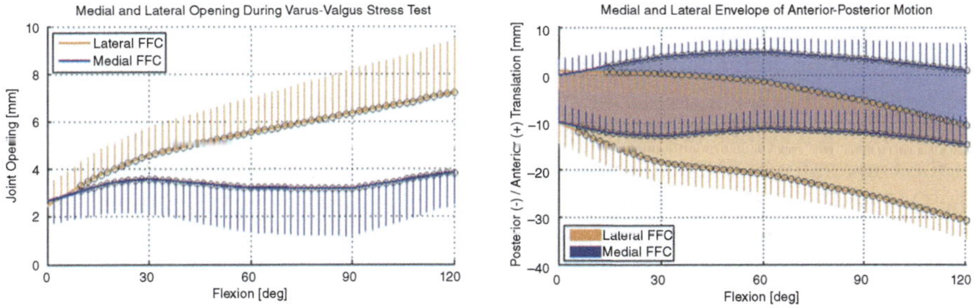

Fig. 3.3 Laxity testing of 54 knee specimens using a Kuka robot. Vertical bars = 1 SD. Circles = significant difference lateral/medial. Left: Medial and lateral joint opening for 11 Nm varus and valgus moments, 44 N compressive force. Medial, almost constant opening for flexion range. Lateral increasing opening with flexion angle. Right: Envelope of anterior–posterior (AP) motion of medial and lateral flexion facet centers (Centers of the circles thru the posterior lateral and medial femoral condyles). AP force 100 N. Minimum laxity values at 0 degrees flexion. Gradual increase to 15 degrees flexion. Then almost constant till 120 degrees flexion. Lateral laxity is 26% higher than medial. Medial laxity range remains in same AP position. Lateral laxity range steadily displaces posteriorly with flexion [8]

rotations in the laxity test will be greatly reduced. This is an important concept that the shape of the bearing surfaces, whether of the intact knee, or an artificial knee, is configured so as to carry a significant part of the applied shear or torque forces. In other words, while the ligaments, including the cruciates, may well still be tensed and contributing to equilibrate the applied forces, a large part of the applied forces are being resisted by the bearing surfaces. The higher the axial compressive force, the more the bearing surface resist shear and torque. The consequence of this phenomenon is that the bearing surfaces can be designed to resist all of the shear and torque, which is normally carried by the cruciates. However, this is not to say that all of the functions of the cruciates, such as inducing rotations in certain flexion ranges, can be replaced by the bearing surfaces of the artificial knee, at least not with simple curvatures as in conventional designs. However, when conducting laxity tests, the degrees of freedom other than anterior–posterior and internal–external should be unconstrained, and the measuring system should ideally measure all of the six degrees of freedom.

In an effort to standardize laxity testing for total knees, the American Society for Testing and Materials (ASTM) developed a test entitled Determination of TKR Constraint, known as ASTM 1223 [13]. The test involves applying cyclic loading to the total knee specimen and recording the force-deflection curves. These consist of a hysteresis loop, which reflect the constraints between the femoral and tibial components, the friction between the sliding surfaces, and the viscoelastic property of the polyethylene. The standard is currently being revised (Haider H, personal communication) to more specifically define the characteristics of the curves on a comparative basis between different designs, as an indicator of use with and without cruciates, and to identify positive or negative characteristics which can be used in the design process.

While the majority of the kinematic studies of the knee relate to the femoral-tibial joint, the patella-femoral joint must be considered also. The quadriceps muscle and the patella itself can be considered to be the engine of the knee, where any malfunction or deficiency in kinematics could significantly affect efficiency and performance. Early studies of the patella concentrated on the contact areas with the femur during a complete flexion range. Experiments were carried out in the 1990s at the University of Oxford, resulting in a new type of test rig eponomously called the Oxford Knee Rig. A flexing moment across the knee was balanced by a force in the quadriceps. The initial basic design was developed to a system where the entire leg was simulated with joints at the hip and ankle, each joint having appropriate degrees of freedom. A mechanism flexed and extended the leg with quadriceps action, in a crouching action. Knee simulating machines based on this principle have been widely used to study total knee constructs, knee specimens, or specimens with total knees implanted. The advantage of such testing is that ligaments and muscle actions, as well as the patella-femoral joint, are included.

More recent studies of the patella have focused on the application to a total knee [15–17]. These studies highlighted the tilt angle of the patella in the sagittal plane, and the patella tilt about its own longitudinal axis (Fig. 3.4). With the use of fluoroscopy, such angles have been coalesced to form the basis for a study of patella

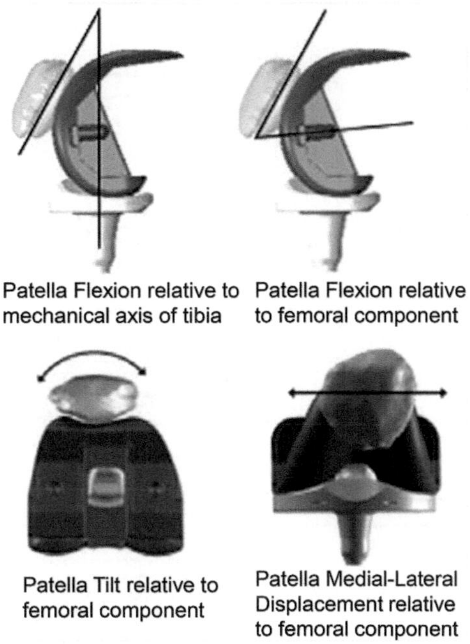

Fig. 3.4 High speed stereoradiography was used to measure the kinematics of the patella in knee extension and lunge activities. Four of the parameters used to describe the motion are shown in this figure [17]

mechanics related to total knee replacement, where the tracking of a dome and an anatomic patella were compared [17]. While various differences were found in the angles, an important finding was that the anatomic design provided significantly more extension strength than the dome. Another study pointed out that most femoral components were designed for mechanical alignment, which included a particular angle and geometry for the patella flange design [16]. However, an increasing number of knees are now implanted using kinematic alignment. In this case, the patella flange becomes angled incorrectly, and the groove becomes medialized. Tracking simulation showed the problems that this could cause including excess tensions on the lateral retinaculum of the quadriceps.

Properties of the Cruciate Ligaments and Implications

Both the anterior and posterior cruciate ligaments consist of two bundles, which loosen and tighten at different angles of flexion (Fig. 3.5) [15]. Due to their orientation, their principal role is in controlling the anterior–posterior position of the femur on the tibia. However, because they are angulated on the transverse plane, they can also exert forces which cause axial rotation of the femur on the tibia about a vertical axis. In the stance phase of a number of activities, the highest shear forces occurred in a posterior direction on the tibia, such that the PCL would be tensed. The magnitudes of the forces were up to approximately 300 Newtons in several activities, but

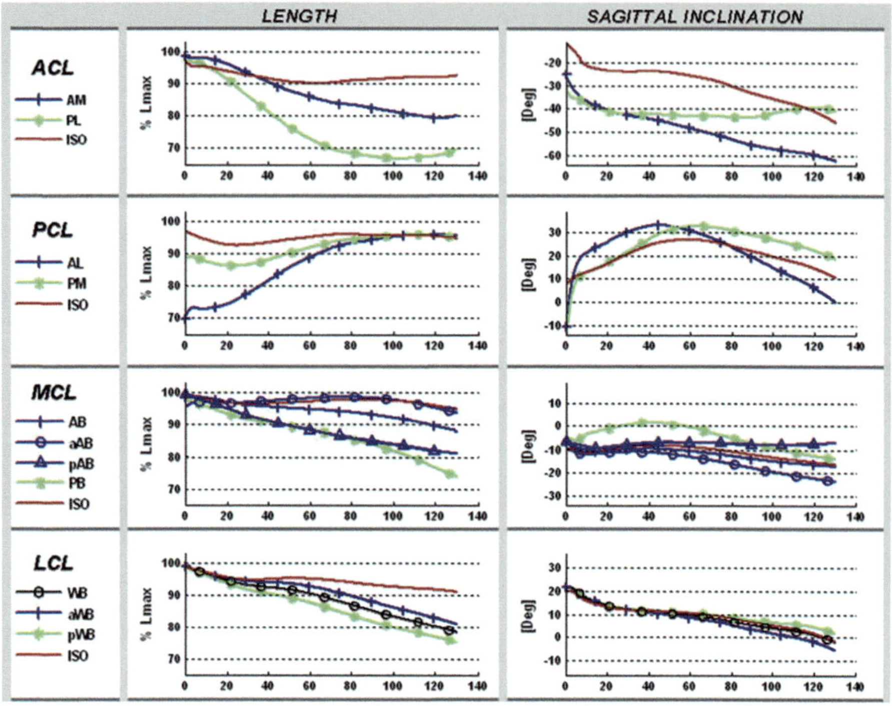

Fig. 3.5 Fiber lengths of the 4 major ligaments during flexion of the knee from 0 to 130 degrees. Results are average of 10 knee specimens. Attachments digitized. *ACL* anterior cruciate, *AM* anteromedial band, *PL* posterolateral band, *ISO* isometric fiber, *PCL* posterior cruciate, *AL* anterolateral band, *PM* posteromedial band, *ISO* isometric fiber, *MCL* medial collateral, *LCL* lateral collateral. Overall, the ACL loosened during flexion, the PCL tightened. The MCL loosened slightly, the LCL loosened significantly. Cruciate inclinations indicate different effectiveness in AP direction. Collaterals were close to vertical throughout flexion, effective in VV but not in AP [15]

reached 700 Newtons in jogging [18]. Such forces can be considered in relation to the mechanical properties of the two bundles of the PCL [19, 20]. The average tensile strength of the anterolateral fibers was 1620 N, while the postero-medial fibers only reached 258 N. Which of the fibers would resist a posterior shear force would depend on their tightness at the particular angle of flexion [15, 21]. The higher the angle of flexion, the more would the anterior fibers be tighter and resist the force. The actual force necessary to resist a shear force needs to account for the angulation of the ligament to the horizontal. In the case of the PCL, considering it is angulated approximately 60° to the horizontal, the force in the ligament would be twice the shear force. In the case of jogging, this force would approach the tensile strength of the anterior fibers. Another factor is the elongation of the ligament in response to the force acting. For a typical stiffness of 300 N/mm and a shear force of 300 N acting posteriorly on the tibia, the necessary force in the ligament would be 600 N (due to the angulation), resulting in an elongation of 2 mm. However, the horizontal displacement of the femur itself would be close to 4 mm. Based on the neutral lengths of the ligament bands during a full flexion range, the posterior cruciate is more able to carry shear forces at higher flexion angles, and the opposite for the anterior cruciate [22–25].

Hence based on the structure of the PCL and the fact that it becomes more elongated with flexion, it can be proposed that its primary function is stabilizing the knee in the higher angles of flexion. Activities such as walking down stairs or down a slope come into this category. Another possibility is that it may play a role in the posterior displacement of the lateral condyle of the femur in high flexion. However, the PCL attaches on the inside of the medial femoral condyle as well as in the notch between the lateral and medial condyles. The latter, the anterolateral fibers, are the strongest and stiffest, and are at maximum tightness by about 90 degrees flexion. On the assumption that the medial condyle provides a stable pivot point, the anterolateral fibers could exert a sufficient moment about the medial side to induce posterior displacement of the lateral femoral condyle.

It can also be proposed that the ACL can provide a mirror image affect toward full extension [26]. For this ligament, all of the fibers are tightest toward full extension [15, 27]. In this case, the ACL could contribute to the so-called screw-home effect, where the lateral femoral condyle displaces anteriorly in full extension and hyperextension. Once again, the medial side can act as a stable pivot for that lateral condyle motion. There is evidence that the anterior tibial slope and the anterior horn of the medial meniscus provide the necessary stability to provide a pivot point (Fig. 3.6) [11].

Hence one model for cruciate function is that they produce anterior lateral femoral displacement in full extension, provide general anterior-posterior stability during the major flexion range, and then cause the lateral femoral condyle to displace posteriorly in high flexion. The net effect of the lateral condyle displacements is a progressive external rotation of the femur during flexion, such motion being aided by the shape of the femoral and tibial condylar surfaces and the menisci. This can be regarded as the neutral path of motion where the principal forces act across the

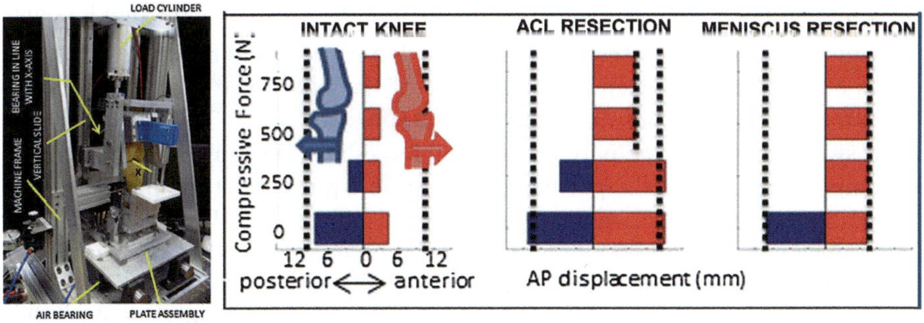

Fig. 3.6 Experiments on knee specimens showed that when an axial force of 250 N or more was applied to the knee in early flexion, the anterior-proximal tibial condyle shape and the menisci prevented posterior displacement of the tibia. Actual displacement values were higher than shown due to boundaries in the equipment preventing excess motions, indicated by dotted lines [11]

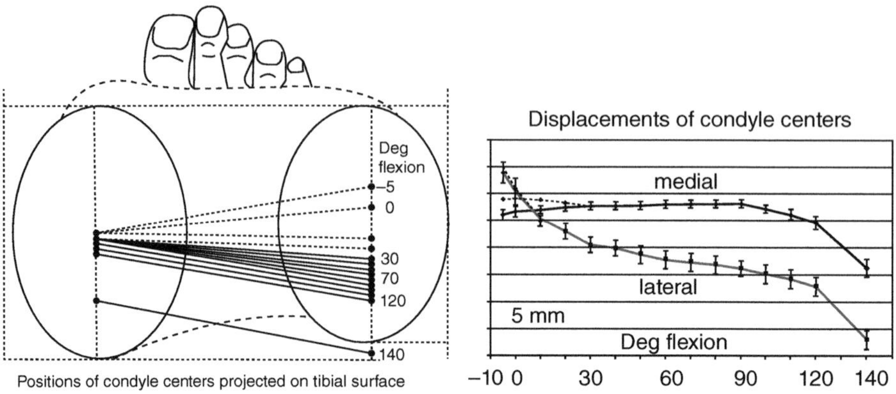

Fig. 3.7 Displacement of femoral condyle centers during loaded crouching down, recorded with MRI. Average of 10 knees. Small medial displacements except in high flexion. Lateral displacements highest in early flexion and late flexion. Close to a medial pivot action from 0 to 120 degrees flexion [28]

knee along the direction of the mechanical axis of the tibia, without any other shear or torque forces. This pattern of motion was demonstrated in MRI studies of the normal knee during a crouching action (Fig. 3.7) [28]. The same pattern has been reproduced using fluoroscopic methods [29].

In many studies, the compressive forces have been small, in which case the motion is determined by the boundaries exerted by the above structures. However for any given flexion angle, in a range of activities, both shear and torque are acting in addition to the axial compression. This combination of forces will produce motion which is different from the neutral path. Hence the basic model for knee motion requires elaboration due to the phenomenon of laxity. At a particular flexion angle, the relative position between the femur and the tibia can have a range of positions within the laxity boundaries. This means that for different activities, the paths of motion will be different, and there is no unique femoral-tibial position at a particular angle of flexion. Hence in describing knee motion, the input conditions need to be specified.

As indicated above, the neutral path of motion is defined to be where only axial forces are applied, and even here, the value of the axial force must be specified. When the force is zero (or small), that is termed passive motion. This motion applies to the swing phase of an activity where small forces are occurring. In active motion, the simplest case is where a specified axial force is applied. Most commonly, motion is specific to a particular activity such as level walking, stair climbing, and so on. For application to fluoroscopy and other measurement methods, a lunge or deep knee bend has been applied, with moderate compressive forces.

A further aspect of ligament behavior is the balancing procedure carried out during surgery. In this process, the looseness or tightness of the knee is measured over a full range of flexion. While balancing was usually carried out manually, in recent years quantitative methods have been developed. Instrumented sensors measuring either contact forces on the condyles [30], or the varus and varus gap openings have been developed. Some robotic systems incorporate the latter into the surgical process. It has been determined that the contact forces on each condyle are directly proportional to the tensions in the collateral ligaments [31, 32]. Furthermore, even small changes in the component placement of even 2 mm had major effects on balancing [33]. Based on the results, it can be determined if the bone cuts need modifying, if soft tissue releases are necessary, and what thickness of tibial insert is needed. However, there is still no consensus on the criteria for a "balanced knee." Equality of the lateral and medial forces or gaps continues to be the major goal, sometimes with allowing some lateral looseness in high flexion. The actual situation is that throughout a passive flexion range, the medial contact forces are higher than the lateral, the proportionate difference being greater at the higher flexion angles. Also, the contact forces toward extension are substantially higher than in the main flexion range [34]. One difficulty with the balancing procedure, however, is that the knee is in a passive state on the operating table, so that producing a controlled flexion–extension movement is subject to variations due to the inherent laxity of the knee. That said, balancing is expected to be important for several reasons. Tight regions of certain ligaments could produce discomfort during function. It has been discussed above that ligaments can generate high forces for only small elongations. On the other hand, looseness of ligaments could produce feelings of instability. In activity, during the swing phase, in a loose or imbalanced knee, the femoral-tibial relative position could be misaligned such that on heel strike, there could be geometric mismatch between the femoral and tibial surfaces, an area which needs further investigation.

Kinematics for Artificial Knees with Cruciate Retention

The ideal goal for a total knee is that all aspects of the kinematics are close to that of a normal anatomic knee. This would apply to the angles of flexion and ground-to-foot force patterns in a gait analysis, for walking, stair climbing, and descending, and other activities, laxity patterns in anterior–posterior and internal–external rotation; femoral-tibial contact point locations on the medial and lateral tibial plateaus for a range of activities; and angular and moment arm characteristics of the patella-femoral joint.

It would be expected that a unicompartmental knee would show close to normal kinematic values, because all cruciates are retained, the overall geometry of the joint is minimally altered, and the patella-femoral joint remains intact. In one study [35], unis and a bicruciate retaining design were compared with normal in a squatting activity (Fig. 3.8). In all designs, the position and displacement of the medial condyle remained constant within a few millimeters. However, on the lateral side, the posterior displacement with flexion was less the normal for the unis, and even less for the bicruciate design. There were also positional differences of the contacts for both implant types. Moreover, the high range of flexion for normal was not

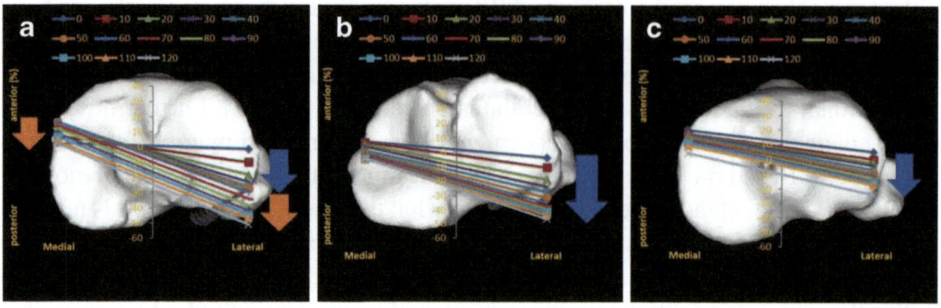

Fig. 3.8 Kinematic pathways during squatting motion. (**a**) Left, normal knee. (**b**) Center, Unicompartmental. (**c**) Right, bicruciate retaining. The patterns of displacements and axial rotation are closer to normal for the unicompartmental knee [35]

reproduced by the unis, with an even smaller range of flexion for the bicruciate design. Nevertheless, a bicruciate design was found to reproduce normal kinematics more closely than a CR design [36, 37].

Hence there is a question as to why the motion of the separate condyles with a unicompartmental knee where both cruciates are preserved does not closely resemble that of a normal intact knee. The lack of AP constraint on the medial side could be one explanation. However, another possibility is that the shape of the medial bearing surfaces together with the menisci is not reproduced. This would be especially the case in early and late flexion. The loss of flexion angle could be attributed to the reduced posterior displacement of the lateral femoral condyle, although other factors need to be considered. At this stage, it should be indicated that the selection of a uni knee will depend on intact cruciate ligaments, whereas in osteoarthritic knees overall, the ACL is intact and functional in only about 50% of cases [38].

There have been many studies using fluoroscopy on the motion of total knees with retention of both cruciate, or retention of only the PCL, some cited here [1, 3, 7, 17, 35, 36, 39]. With the advent of the mobile MRI units, level walking, and stair activities have been possible. When both cruciates have been retained, the motion has not been greatly different from unicompartmental, although still different from normal. Axial rotations have occurred near full extension and full flexion, but much less than for normal knees. There has generally been greater AP sliding medially, and less AP sliding lateral, compared with normal. This has resulted in less axial rotations, especially at the extremes of motion. In designs where only the posterior cruciate has been retained, an additional phenomenon has been measured, namely anterior sliding of the knee during early stance. This has been ascribed to the absence of the ACL, allowing the knee to slide posteriorly during the swing phase, such that in early stance there is a corrective anterior sliding. Some authors have termed this behavior "paradoxical motion" in that it does not match normal motion. Patella motion has been different from normal also, measured in terms of parameters such as patella angles and moment arms. Patella motion has been shown to be significantly affected by the surgical technique, notably between mechanical alignment versus kinematic alignment [16].

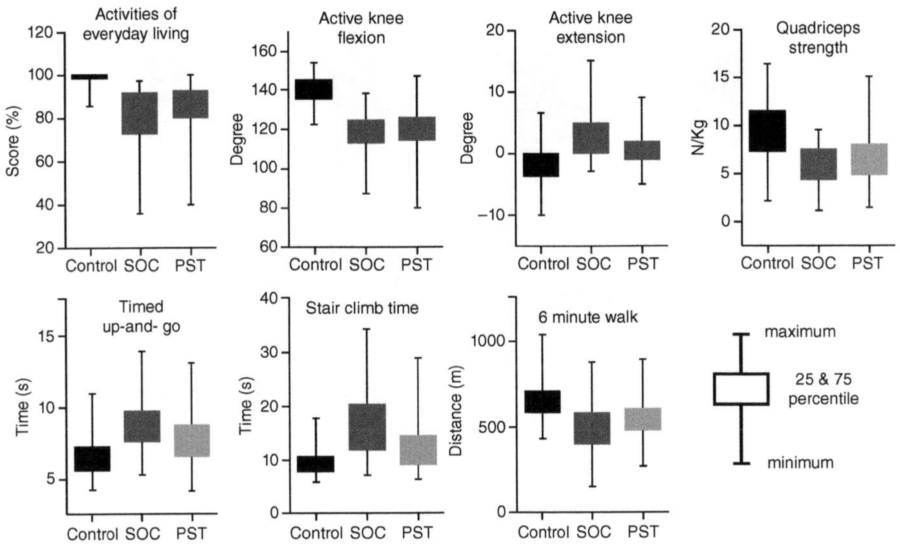

Fig. 3.9 Application of kinematic and functional parameters for evaluation of total knee. Three groups: age-matched normal controls (88), SOC standard-of-care rehab (40), PST progressive strengthening rehab (165). Performance at 1 year after total knee. Total knee did not match normal controls: main problem quadriceps weakness. PST better results in most tests [40]

Whatever the total knee design, there has been considerable variability of the motions between patients however. This can be ascribed to the inevitable variations in component placements, inexact match between the geometry of the implant and the patient's original anatomy, variations in the soft tissue properties, especially if ligament releases have been carried out, and the variations of muscle forces in activities. The type of rehabilitation can also make a difference to various postoperative kinematic performance parameters [40]. For example, patients who underwent a "progressive strengthening" program performed better than those with a conventional standard of care rehabilitation (Fig. 3.9). The main underlying reason was indicated to be quadriceps strength itself.

However, most of the above studies have been with total knee designs with symmetric medial-lateral geometries, which is completely different from normal. In symmetric designs, the lateral compartmental will be more constrained than normal, and the opposite for the medial compartment. This does not apply to medial pivot or medially constrained designs however. These are used both with and without the posterior cruciate ligament (Fig. 3.10) [41]. There is some data that such designs, particularly when the PCL is preserved, can show more normal motion patterns than the above-mentioned CR designs, but still not reproducing normal. These medial types of designs [42], will be discussed in the next section.

A further point in the kinematic performance after total knee is that the range of flexion has been much less than in normal knees. Various reasons have been cited for this problem, including tibial component slope, posterior condylar offset, tight

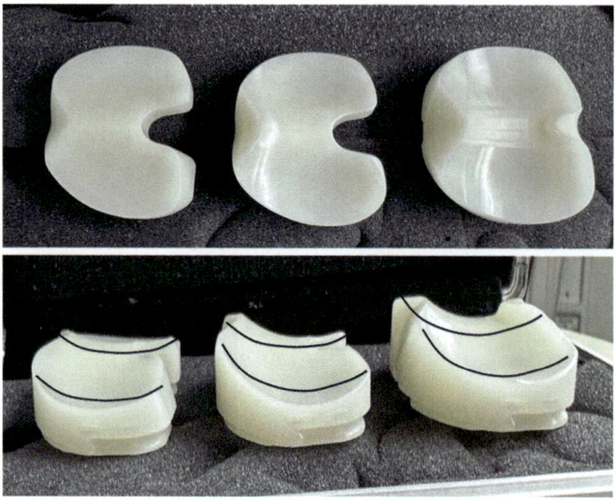

Fig. 3.10 Examples of tibial inserts widely used today. Left: Cruciate retaining. The radii in frontal and sagittal planes are much larger than the femoral component, allowing AP and rotational laxity. The PCL is retained. Center; Medially congruent. The medial radii are slightly larger than the femoral, allowing some laxity. The lateral radius is similar to the cruciate retaining. Retention of the PCL is optional. Right: ultra-congruent. Medial and lateral radii are the same, and similar to the medial side of the medially congruent. The PCL is not retained. (Photo from [41])

medial collateral structures, and the preoperative condition of the knee. However, further research is indicated on this aspect.

Cruciate Function Provided by Total Knee Bearing Surfaces

In the late 1960s and early 1970s when the very first artificial knees were being designed, there were two completely different approaches. The first seems the most obvious; replace the arthritic bearing surfaces with metal runners sliding on plastic tibial surfaces, and retain the remaining functional parts of the joint including the ligaments. This approach was first utilized by Gunston and Charnley at Wrightington Hospital in England, where rheumatoid arthritis without serious deformity was the problem to be addressed. At around the same time, Freeman and Swanson in London confronted the problem of severe OA with deformity. Hitherto, such cases had been treated with all-metal hinges. The Freeman-Swanson knee design consisted of a metal femoral roller in a plastic tibial trough. Both anterior–posterior displacement and internal–external rotation were constrained. This configuration replaced the major function of the cruciate, providing anterior-posterior stability, whereas axial rotation was not considered necessary. Perhaps the most sophisticated total knee design at that time, seen with today's lens, was the Leeds Knee designed by Seedhom in Leeds, England. It featured an anatomically shaped femoral component (similar to that of the MGH femoral condyle) and partially conforming tibial bearing surfaces, more conforming medially, while the cruciates were preserved. However, at that time, difficulties were encountered in both surgery and manufacture [43].

Meanwhile at the Hospital for Special Surgery, after using different condylar replacement designs, it was determined that the surgical technique could be simplified if the cruciates were resected and the bearing surfaces substituted for their function. Theoretical analysis showed that this could be achieved with partially conforming bearing surfaces [44] (Fig. 3.11) (Walker 1973). The design, called the Total Condylar, was based on studies of anatomic knee specimens, where the knee showed substantial AP and rotational laxity, but the laxity reduced substantially when axial force was applied, as in function. Partially conforming radii between the femoral and tibial surfaces provided close to anatomic values for the laxity and stability behavior of the anatomic knee. The above evolutionary steps in total knee design have been reviewed in detail [45].

Since that time, there have been several configurations which use a similar principle of providing stability by the condyles, the ultra-congruent being one of the first [39]. As with the Total Condylar, the shapes of the lateral and medial surfaces were similar. A further advancement, however, was made as the result of studies of the motion of the anatomic knee. Hitherto, it was widely accepted that during flexion, the lateral and medial condyles both moved posteriorly during flexion, which

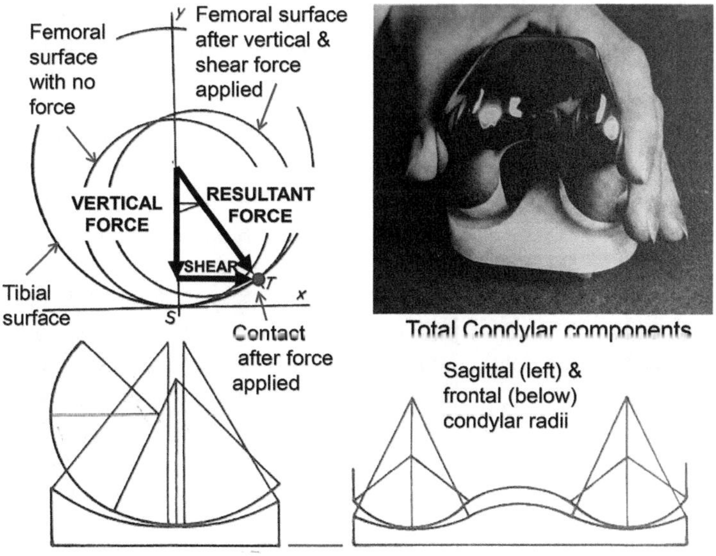

Fig. 3.11 Partially conforming condylar surfaces can sustain a shear force or a torque when there is an axial compressive force acting. The femoral condyles displace such that the reaction force is inclined to the vertical at the contact point. These displacements represent laxity, a characteristic of normal knees. With these bearing surfaces, the cruciate ligaments are not necessary to maintain stability. This principle was applied to the total condylar knee. Presented to the IMechE/BOA conference on Total Knee Replacement, London, September 1974 (Walker 1974) [44]

allowed for a high flexion angle. However Freeman, working with others including Tuke and Blaha, determined that the posterior displacement occurred primarily on the lateral side. On the medial side, while there were small anterior-posterior displacements at the extremes of flexion, in the major arc of flexion, the knee acted almost as a "medial pivot." This was consistent with the completely different shape between the lateral and medial bearing surfaces, as well as the shapes and mobility of the menisci. As a result of this work, and later studies showing a similar result, several "medial pivot" knees were designed, with limited AP laxity on the medial side. Fluoroscopic studies have shown that indeed these designs do pivot on the medial side during flexion, although generally, the degrees of rotation and the AP displacement on the lateral side have been smaller than in the normal intact knee.

A recent study [6] used mobile fluoroscopy to compare the kinematics of three different non-cruciate designs, all based on the same overall geometry; the GMK PS, ultra-congruent, and Sphere (a medial pivot) (Fig. 3.12). The activities tested were level walking, downhill walking, and stair descent. The AP displacements of the lateral and medial femoral centers, and the axial rotations were measured. In all activities, the medial displacements of the Sphere were 3 mm maximum even in the unloaded swing phases of the activities. These values were higher than in the other designs. This is easily explained by the almost complete conformity of the Sphere and the partial conformity of the other designs. On the lateral side, however, the Sphere showed the highest AP displacements under all conditions. This is explained by the flat surface of the Sphere's lateral tibial surface. In contrast, the other designs were symmetric medial-lateral, with partial femoral-tibial conformity. In all three designs, the AP sliding was highest in the swing phase, where there would be small

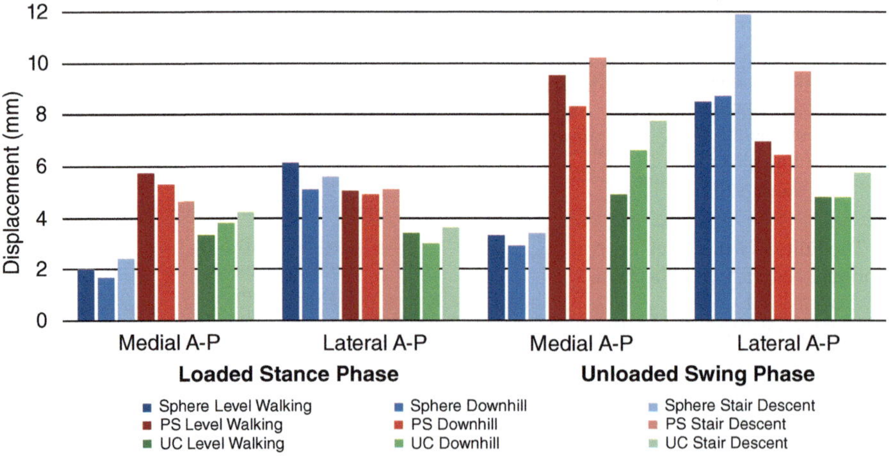

Fig. 3.12 Kinematic studies using dynamic videofluoroscopy. The bar graphs show the anterior–posterior displacements of the lateral and medial femoral condyles on the tibial surfaces for level walking, downhill walking and descent. Stance and swing phases are shown. The displacements for 3 different total knee designs are compared: GMK Sphere (a medial pivot with flat lateral tibial surface), a GMK posterior stabilized, and a GMK ultra-congruent symmetric lateral-medial [6]

axial forces. The PS showed higher AP sliding than the ultra-congruent. This was due to higher femoral-tibial conformity of the latter design. Also, in the PS, the added AP constraint of the PS only acts in high flexion. In another study [39], the AP motions were compared between UC and MC designs, for a sit to stand activity. The implants had the same CR type femoral components, and tibial baseplate, but the inserts were different. The mean medial AP displacements were 2–3 mm, for the lateral side, both 8 mm. This equality in displacements was surprising because of the asymmetric MC conformity and the symmetric UC conformity. This indicated that the motions were more affected by the activity itself rather than the insert conformities. In a recent review of medial pivot and medially congruent designs, Hodgeson et al. [42] concluded that "Medial pivot total knee arthroplasty implant designs (as well as medially congruent) function similar to that of the native knee with a relatively fixed medial center of rotation and a less conforming lateral compartment that follows an arcuate path." Nonetheless, other fluoroscopic studies have shown less axial rotation values than in the normal knee, even though the overall displacement and rotation patterns have been similar.

Conclusions Regarding Design and Kinematics

The kinematics of the normal knee has many facets, but can be regarded as the motion patterns of the femur, tibia, and patella, in multiple different functions. The motion is influenced by the complex shape of the bearing surfaces, including the menisci, and the ligaments. Variations in the motion patterns occur due to the laxity between the femur and the tibia. The control provided by the ligaments depends upon their geometry and mechanical properties. The tensions in the ligaments are very sensitive to their lengths.

There are numerous considerations regarding the selection of design types for total knee replacement. In general, the type of device is chosen depending on the severity of the arthritis. For this discussion, the major criterion will be the restoration of normal kinematics, on the assumption that this will produce the best functional result, and feel closest to normal to the patient. For mild osteoarthritis limited primarily to the medial side, a unicompartmental seems to produce results which are reasonably close to normal, although further improvements may still be possible. For the most severe cases, designs which provide adequate stability without preservation of the cruciates are apparently required. However, between these two extremes, there are several choices, which preserve both, one or neither of the cruciates.

If preservation of cruciate function is considered an advantage, then the design of the components and the surgical technique need to produce a geometry and kinematics which is closely matched to the patient. This is necessary because of the sensitivity of the ligament tensions to their length changes, where as little as 2 mm can produce major force differences. It has been proposed that this can be achieved by an optimization process using modelling and robotic surgery techniques [46].

The concept is that a computer model of the pre-arthritic condition of the patient's knee is generated based on a preoperative CT scan. The pre-diseased "normal" ligament length patterns are generated. In the computer, osteophytes are removed, and the total knee components are inserted using the robotic surgical technique (Fig. 3.13). The positions and sizes of the components are manipulated in computer software, to find the closest match to the normal ligament lengths. The surgery is then conducted robotically using the optimized data. This innovative approach has the advantage of being "personalised" to the individual patient, as well as being "optimised." However one limitation may be in the design of the components themselves; using present design configurations, how closely can normal kinematics actually be produced.

The alternate approach is that the bearing surfaces should substitute for the function of the cruciates. From data so far, designs where the medial side is fully or partially constrained in an AP direction, and the lateral side is relatively unconstrained, seem to provide kinematics which is reasonably close to normal. The advantage of this approach is that it is reproducible from knee to knee, and may have a certain degree of forgiveness in the accuracy of the component sizing and surgical placement. However, the disadvantage is that all knees would be given the same amount of constraint, whereas in reality there is a wide variation between patients. This could be solved by having components available with variations in the constraint.

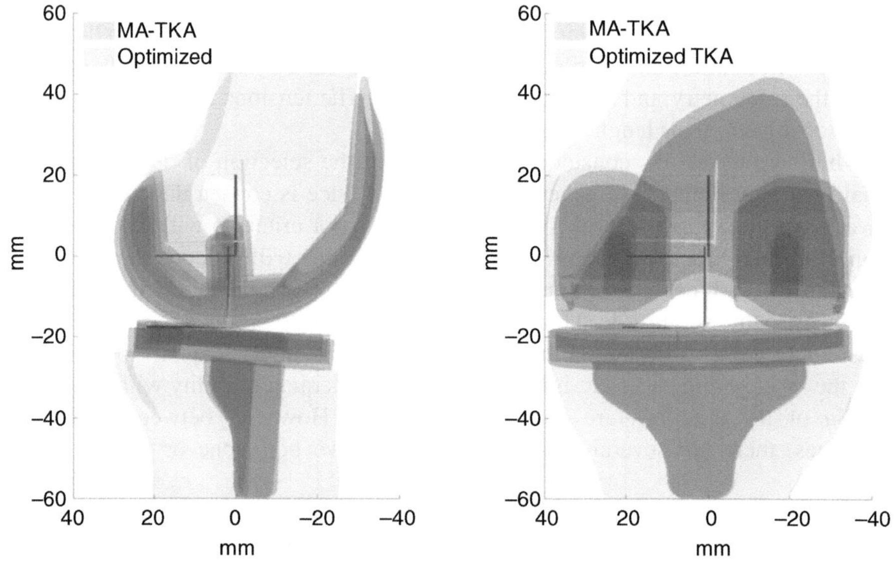

Fig. 3.13 Optimization of component position, for personalized surgery to the pre-arthritic state. After initial virtual component positions, multiple iterations of position to converge to the minimum difference between parameters of ligament lengths, tensions, and strains, with pre-diseased values [46]

Future kinematic studies, using many different parameters and techniques, will be pivotal in determining the best solutions.

References

1. Angerame MR, Holst DC, Jennings JM, Komistek RD, Dennis DA. Total knee arthroplasty kinematics. J Arthroplasty. 2019;34(10):2502–10. https://doi.org/10.1016/j.arth.2019.05.037.
2. Grood ES, Suntay WJ. A joint coordinate system for the clinical description of three-dimensional motions: application to the knee. J Biomech Eng. 1983;105(2):136–44. https://doi.org/10.1115/1.3138397.
3. Gray HA, Guan S, Young TJ, Dowsey MM, Choong PF, Pandy MG. Comparison of posterior-stabilized, cruciate-retaining, and medial-stabilized knee implant motion during gait. J Orthop Res. 2020;38(8):1753–68. https://doi.org/10.1002/jor.24613.
4. Hull ML. Coordinate system requirements to determine motions of the tibiofemoral joint free from kinematic crosstalk errors. J Biomech. 2020;109:109928. https://doi.org/10.1016/j.jbiomech.2020.109928.
5. Kour RY, Guan S, Dowsey MM, Choong PF, Pandy MG. Kinematic function of knee implant designs across a range of daily activities. J Orthop Res. 2022;41(6):1217–27. https://doi.org/10.1002/jor.25476.
6. Schütz P, Taylor WR, Postolka B, et al. Kinematic evaluation of the GMK sphere implant during gait activities: a dynamic videofluoroscopy study. J Orthop Res. 2019;37(11):2337–47. https://doi.org/10.1002/jor.24416.
7. Smith LA, Nachtrab J, LaCour M, Cates H, Freeman MG, Komistek RD. In vivo knee kinematics: how important are the roles of femoral geometry and the cruciate ligaments? J Arthroplasty. 2021;36(4):1445–54. https://doi.org/10.1016/j.arth.2020.10.020.
8. Bandi M, Siggelkow E, Mane AM, Sauerberg I, Wentorf F. Laxity characteristics of the medial and lateral compartment in normal female and male. Knees. Lecture presented at: Orthopedic Research Society 2015 annual meeting; 2015.
9. Boguszewski DV, Cheung EC, Joshi NB, Markolf KL, McAllister DR. Male-female differences in knee laxity and stiffness. Am J Sports Med. 2015;43(12):2982–7. https://doi.org/10.1177/0363546515608478.
10. Markolf KL, Feeley BT, Tejwani SG, Martin DE, McAllister DR. Changes in knee laxity and ligament force after sectioning the posteromedial bundle of the posterior cruciate ligament. Arthroscopy. 2006;22(10):1100–6. https://doi.org/10.1016/j.arthro.2006.05.018.
11. Reynolds RJ, Walker PS, Buza J. Mechanisms of anterior-posterior stability of the knee joint under load-bearing. J Biomech. 2017;57:39–45. https://doi.org/10.1016/j.jbiomech.2017.03.016.
12. Sekeitto AR, McGale JG, Montgomery LA, Vasarhelyi EM, Willing R, Lanting BA. Posterior-stabilized total knee arthroplasty kinematics and joint laxity: a hybrid biomechanical study. Arthroplasty. 2022;4(1):53. https://doi.org/10.1186/s42836-022-00153-4.
13. Walker PS, Hennessy D, Perez J, Rahman F, Zapata G, Bosco J. Achieving specified laxity in a noncruciate total knee: a laboratory design study. J Arthroplasty. 2024;39:S340. https://doi.org/10.1016/j.arth.2024.03.015.
14. Willing R, Moslemian A, Yamomo G, Wood T, Howard J, Lanting B. Condylar-stabilized TKR may not fully compensate for PCL-deficiency: an in vitro cadaver study. J Orthop Res. 2019;37(10):2172–81. https://doi.org/10.1002/jor.24392.
15. Belvedere C, Ensini A, Feliciangeli A, et al. Geometrical changes of knee ligaments and patellar tendon during passive flexion. J Biomech. 2012;45(11):1886–92. https://doi.org/10.1016/j.jbiomech.2012.05.029.

16. Hull ML, Simileysky A, Howell SM. Differences in trochlear morphology of a new femoral component designed for kinematic alignment from a mechanical alignment design. Bioengineering. 2024;11(1):62. https://doi.org/10.3390/bioengineering11010062.
17. Mannen EM, Ali AA, Dennis DA, Haas BD, Rullkoetter PJ, Shelburne KB. Influence of component geometry on patellar mechanics in posterior-stabilized rotating platform total knee arthroplasty. J Arthroplasty. 2019;34(5):974–80. https://doi.org/10.1016/j.arth.2019.01.013.
18. Bergmann G, Bender A, Graichen F, et al. Standardized loads acting in knee implants. PLoS One. 2014;9(1):e86035. https://doi.org/10.1371/journal.pone.0086035.
19. Amis AA, Bull AMJ, Gupte CM, Hijazi I, Race A, Robinson JR. Biomechanics of the PCL and related structures: posterolateral, posteromedial and meniscofemoral ligaments. Knee Surg Sports Traumatol Arthrosc. 2003;11(5):271–81. https://doi.org/10.1007/s00167-003-0410-7.
20. Race A, Amis AA. The mechanical properties of the two bundles of the human posterior cruciate ligament. J Biomech. 1994;27(1):13–24. https://doi.org/10.1016/0021-9290(94)90028-0.
21. Wright JO, Skelley NW, Schur RP, Castile RM, Lake SP, Brophy RH. Microstructural and mechanical properties of the posterior cruciate ligament. J Bone Joint Surg. 2016;98(19):1656–64. https://doi.org/10.2106/jbjs.16.00032.
22. Amiri S, Cooke TDV, Wyss UP. A multiple-bundle model to characterize the mechanical behavior of the cruciate ligaments. Knee. 2011;18(1):34–41. https://doi.org/10.1016/j.knee.2010.01.003.
23. Hosseini Nasab SH, List R, Oberhofer K, Fucentese SF, Snedeker JG, Taylor WR. Loading patterns of the posterior cruciate ligament in the healthy knee: a systematic review. PLoS One. 2016;11(11):e0167106. https://doi.org/10.1371/journal.pone.0167106.
24. Jones R, Nawana N, Pearcy M, et al. Mechanical properties of the human anterior cruciate ligament. Clin Biomech. 1995;10(7):339–44. https://doi.org/10.1016/0268-0033(95)98193-x.
25. Moslemian A, Sidhu R, Roessler P, et al. Influence of the posterior cruciate ligament on kinematics of the knee during experimentally simulated clinical tests and activities of daily living. J Biomech. 2021;115:110133. https://doi.org/10.1016/j.jbiomech.2020.110133.
26. Wu J-L, Hosseini A, Kozanek M, Gadikota HR, Gill TJ, Li G. Kinematics of the anterior cruciate ligament during gait. Am J Sports Med. 2010;38(7):1475–82. https://doi.org/10.1177/0363546510364240.
27. Smigielski R, Zdanowicz U, Drwięga M, Ciszek B, Williams A. The anatomy of the anterior cruciate ligament and its relevance to the technique of reconstruction. Bone Joint J. 2016;98-B(8):1020–6. https://doi.org/10.1302/0301-620x.98b8.37117.
28. Johal P, Williams A, Wragg P, Hunt D, Gedroyc W. Tibio-femoral movement in the living knee. A study of weight bearing and non-weight bearing knee kinematics using 'interventional' MRI. J Biomech. 2005;38(2):269–76. https://doi.org/10.1016/j.jbiomech.2004.02.008.
29. Dennis DA, Mahfouz MR, Komistek RD, Hoff W. In vivo determination of normal and anterior cruciate ligament-deficient knee kinematics. J Biomech. 2005;38:241–53. https://doi.org/10.1016/j.jbiomech.2004.02.042.
30. Gustke KA, Golladay GJ, Roche MW, Elson LC, Anderson CR. A targeted approach to ligament balancing using kinetic sensors. J Arthroplasty. 2017;32(7):2127–32. https://doi.org/10.1016/j.arth.2017.02.021.
31. Sanz-Pena I, Zapata GE, Verstraete MA, Meere PA, Walker PS. Relationship between ligament forces and contact forces in balancing at total knee surgery. J Arthroplasty. 2019;34(6):1261–6. https://doi.org/10.1016/j.arth.2019.02.016.
32. Wirekoh J, Parody N, Meere PA. Functional knee apparatus for the evaluation of ligamentous tensions on contact loads. Knee. 2022;39:227–38. https://doi.org/10.1016/j.knee.2021.08.004.
33. Zapata G, Sanz-Pena I, Verstraete M, Walker PS. Effects of femoral component placement on the balancing of a total knee at surgery. J Biomech. 2019;86:117–24. https://doi.org/10.1016/j.jbiomech.2019.01.056.
34. Verstraete MA, Meere PA, Salvadore G, Victor J, Walker PS. Contact forces in the tibiofemoral joint from soft tissue tensions: implications to soft tissue balancing in total knee arthroplasty. J Biomech. 2017;58:195–202. https://doi.org/10.1016/j.jbiomech.2017.05.008.

35. Kono K, Inui H, Tomita T, Yamazaki T, Taketomi S, Tanaka S. Bicruciate-retaining total knee arthroplasty reproduces in vivo kinematics of normal knees to a lower extent than unicompartmental knee arthroplasty. Knee Surg Sports Traumatol Arthrosc. 2020;28:3007–15. https://doi.org/10.1007/s00167-019-05754-2.
36. Digennaro V, Zambianchi F, Marcovigi A, Mugnai R, Fiacchi F, Catani F. Design and kinematics in total knee arthroplasty. Int Orthop. 2014;38(2):227–33. https://doi.org/10.1007/s00264-013-2245-2.
37. Nabeki S, Okada Y, Teramoto A, et al. The function of cruciate ligaments in bi-cruciate retaining total knee arthroplasty with asymmetrical design. Clin Biomech. 2023;107:106038. https://doi.org/10.1016/j.clinbiomech.2023.106038.
38. Roussi K, Saunders C, Ries C, Rolvien T, Boese CK. Anterior cruciate ligament intactness in osteoarthritic patients indicated for total knee arthroplasty: a systematic literature review and meta-analysis. Knee Surg Sports Traumatol Arthrosc. 2020;29(10):3458–66. https://doi.org/10.1007/s00167-020-06292-y.
39. Alesi D, Di Paolo S, Bragonzoni L, et al. No kinematical difference between ultra-congruent and medial-congruent total knee arthroplasty when implanted with mechanical alignment: an in vivo dynamic RSA study. Knee Surg Sports Traumatol Arthrosc. 2022;30(9):2975–9. https://doi.org/10.1007/s00167-022-07033-z.
40. Pozzi F, White DK, Snyder-Mackler L, Zeni JA. Restoring physical function after knee replacement: a cross sectional comparison of progressive strengthening vs standard physical therapy. Physiother Theory Pract. 2018;36(1):122–33. https://doi.org/10.1080/09593985.2018.1479475.
41. Movassaghi K, Patel A, Ghulam-Jelani Z, Levine BR. Modern total knee arthroplasty bearing designs and the role of the posterior cruciate ligament. Arthroplast Today. 2023;21:101130. https://doi.org/10.1016/j.artd.2023.101130.
42. Hodgeson SM, Soeno T, Mears SC, Stambough JB, Barnes CL, Stronach BM. The medial pivot design in total knee arthroplasty. Orthop Clin North Am. 2024;55(1):49–59. https://doi.org/10.1016/j.ocl.2023.06.007.
43. Chan SCN, Seedhom BB. 'Equivalent geometry' of the knee and the prediction of tensions along the cruciates: an experimental study. J Biomech. 1999;32(1):35–48. https://doi.org/10.1016/s0021-9290(98)00141-9.
44. Walker PS, Insall JN, Ranawat CS, Wang CJ, Masse Y. Joint laxity as a criterion for the design of condylar prostheses. Clin Orthop Relat Res. 2003;(410):5–12. https://doi.org/10.1097/01.blo.0000062382.79828.bc. Reprinted from Proceedings of IMechE and BOA conference on total knee replacement, London, September 1974.
45. Walker PS. The artificial knee: an ongoing evolution. Cham: Springer Nature Switzerland; 2020. https://doi.org/10.1007/978-3-030-38171-4.
46. Tzanetis P, Fluit R, de Souza K, Robertson S, Koopman B, Verdonschot N. Pre-planning the surgical target for optimal implant positioning in robotic assisted total knee arthroplasty. Bioengineering. 2023;10(5):543. https://doi.org/10.3390/bioengineering10050543.

Part III
Total Knee Designs with Respect to the Cruciate Ligaments

Chapter 4
The PCL-Sparing Total Knee Arthroplasty

Jonathan R. Franco and Antonia F. Chen

Introduction

Total knee arthroplasty (TKA) remains one of the most common surgical procedures performed globally, with an expected increase of 601% from 2005 to 2030 [1]. While there have been advancements in technology, implant design, and surgical technique, a consistently debated technical topic within the field is posterior cruciate ligament (PCL) sparing versus PCL substituting TKA.

The main functions of the PCL are to resist posterior translation of the tibia on the femur and facilitate femoral rollback in knee flexion [2, 3]. Cruciate-retaining (CR) implant designs work under the premise of a competent PCL to maintain the native function after TKA. However, given concerns over patients in whom the PCL was deemed incompetent or scenarios in which iatrogenic injury occurred, the need to replace the function of the PCL was in demand. Thus, posterior stabilized (PS) knees were introduced to substitute the function of the PCL through a cam-post mechanism.

Proponents of the CR design cite several advantages, including improved gait mechanics that mirror the natural function of the native knee, longer survival, avoidance of cam-post impingement, and decreased rates of aseptic loosening and lower fracture risk [4–7]. On the other hand, those that support the use of PS-TKA cite improved range of motion and femoral rollback, the ability to more effectively balance severe deformity, and increased stability in the absence or injury to the PCL [8–10]. The goal of this chapter is to explore the role of the PCL-sparing TKA and its implant design, surgical technique, and outcomes.

J. R. Franco (✉) · A. F. Chen
Department of Orthopedic Surgery, Brigham and Women's Hospital, Harvard Medical School, Boston, MA, USA
e-mail: Jfranco5@bwh.harvard.edu; afchen@bwh.harvard.edu

A. J. Tria Jr., G. R. Scuderi (eds.), *The Cruciate Ligaments in Total Knee Arthroplasty*, https://doi.org/10.1007/978-3-031-75992-5_4

Role of the PCL

The PCL is an intra-articular structure that consists of two bundles, the anterolateral and posteromedial bundle. As previously mentioned, the primary function of the PCL is to resist posterior translation of the tibia on the femur and facilitate femoral rollback in knee flexion [2, 3]. Additionally, biomechanical studies demonstrate that the PCL also acts as a secondary stabilizer to varus/valgus and external rotation of the knee in deep flexion [2]. The primary role of the respective bundles is associated with their biomechanical differences in vivo; the anterolateral bundle is tight during knee flexion and the posteromedial bundle is tight in knee extension [2, 11].

The native kinematics that facilitates knee flexion includes posterior translation of the femoral condyles, particularly the lateral femoral condyle, in the phenomenon of femoral rollback [12]. Femoral rollback allows for deep knee flexion, by avoiding impingement [3, 13, 14]. Resection of the anterior cruciate ligament (ACL) during TKA can hinder these normal biomechanics by allowing increased anterior translation of the femoral condyles on the tibia. The PCL, when under appropriate tension, acts to resist the anterior translation of the femoral condyles and aids in femoral rollback (Fig. 4.1).

Through its ability to facilitate femoral rollback, the PCL aids in increasing the quadriceps lever arm via lengthening of the extensor mechanism [13–15]. This provides a biomechanical advantage through increasing the moment arm and thereby decreasing the forces exerted on the patellofemoral joint [16, 17]. However, given the importance of the PCL on the kinematics of the knee, this provides an

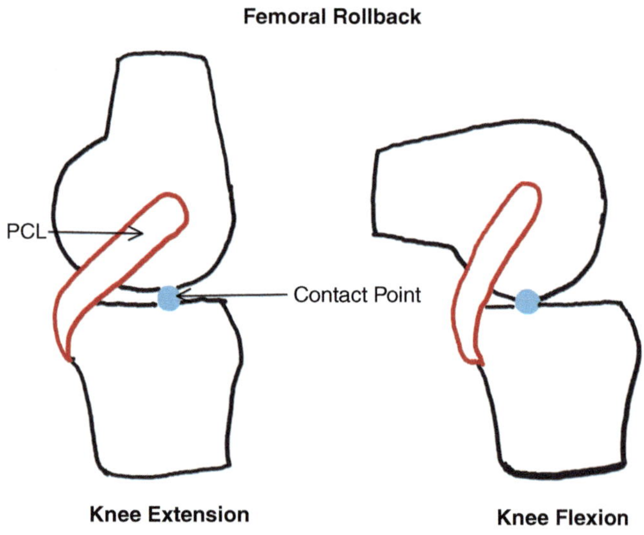

Fig. 4.1 Graphic illustration demonstrating femoral rollback, noted by the more posterior contact point between the femur and the tibia in knee flexion

opportunity for error during TKA with respect to improper tensioning. It may be difficult to restore native tension using soft tissue releases and bony resection to facilitate the above mechanical advantages, despite ACL resection. Additionally, proper tension remains a subjective measure. Nevertheless, studies have demonstrated that PCL tensioning alters joint biomechanics, stress, and patient-reported outcomes [18, 19].

Furthermore, studies assessing knee kinematics following PCL resection demonstrate significant impairments to normal motion, which suggest its importance in the native knee. Cromie et al., demonstrated that PCL resection doubled the anterior translation of the femur on the tibia, as well as increased the degree of flexion where femoral rollback was initiated [20]. More importantly, their study found that the cam-post mechanism on the PS-knee implant could not restore pre-PCL resection kinematics [20]. PCL resection is also associated with increased flexion and extension gap, with a greater impact on an increased flexion gap [21, 22].

Prosthesis Design

The PS total knee design was popularized given concerns around incompetency of the PCL in the arthritic knee and helped facilitate balancing within the extremes of knee deformity. The cam-post mechanism of the PS design was popularized in the United States with these concerns given the added stability to functionally replace the PCL. According to the American Joint Replacement Registry (AJRR), just under two-third of arthroplasty surgeons in the United States use PS implants [23]. This contrasts with the CR knee that is the most consistently used design in European countries [23].

In a CR-TKA design, the PCL plays a critical role in preventing anterior translation of the femur on the tibia by resisting the forces generated by the hamstring to pull the tibia posteriorly during knee flexion [3, 24]. In doing so, the PCL assists in producing femoral rollback, thereby preventing impingement in deep flexion, as well as increasing the moment arm and efficiency of the extensor mechanism [25, 26]. The CR-TKA polyethylene design contains a posterior cut out to facilitate the PCL to maintain its native anatomic position and facilitate the aforementioned functions.

It is not surprising that one of the major contraindications to CR-TKA would be an incompetent or attenuated PCL, given the lack of a cam-post mechanism to mimic this function. However, other commonly cited indications for surgeon decision to use a PS-TKA design include inflammatory arthritis, extensor mechanism deficiency, fixed knee flexion contractures, and significant coronal deformity [9, 27, 28]. Despite these early results suggesting better outcomes with PS-TKA over CR-TKA, several studies have since shown equivalency and/or non-inferiority with the use of modern CR designs in these scenarios. Recent literature has shown excellent long-term results with CR-TKA implants compared to PS designs when assessing patients with inflammatory arthritis, particularly rheumatoid arthritis [29, 30].

Similarly, several studies assessing the use of CR implants with significant varus or valgus deformity have demonstrated successful short- and long-term follow-up [31–33]. Specifically, Kubiak and colleagues (2008) found a 93% revision-free survivorship and no revisions for instability or loosening at a minimum of 10-year follow-up for CR implants in patients with a coronal plane deformity of 15 degrees or more [33].

Intraoperative Considerations

Though the basic tenets of TKA surgical approach and technique remain largely similar between cruciate-retaining and cruciate-substituting designs, subtle differences need to be considered intraoperatively. Following standard medial parapatellar approach and arthrotomy, it is crucial to objectively evaluate the integrity and competency of the PCL prior to moving forward with a CR design. As previously described, the PCL is critical to maintain the functional stability of the implant if there is no cam-post mechanism available. The PCL can be attenuated or deemed incompetent, especially in an arthritic knee. Similarly, consistent assessment of the integrity of the PCL throughout surgery is critical as iatrogenic injury is possible. Specifically, one must be critical during resection of the ACL as well as the posterior chamfer cuts on the femur.

The effects of PCL-sparing versus PCL resection on balancing flexion/extension gaps and anterior-posterior stability remain additional important surgical considerations. Studies suggest that resection of the PCL disproportionately opens the flexion gap approximately 2 mm more than the extension gap [34, 35]. Therefore, when performing a cruciate-retaining technique, the surgeon must consider the tension of the PCL. If sufficient release of the PCL is not performed, overtightening can lead to stiffness and impaired flexion post-operatively. The opposite remains true where too much resection can lead to an excessive flexion gap and instability. That being said, it is important to consider the amount of distal femoral resection when performing a CR-TKA. Specifically, since the PCL will remain intact, a smaller degree of flexion gap will be present intraoperatively. If the distal femur is over-resected, a significant mismatch may occur between the flexion and extension gap, which can pose a challenging intraoperative finding. Distal femoral augments or recession of the PCL may be needed in cases where upsizing the polyethylene leads significant stiffness in knee flexion.

Partial recession of the PCL is often performed intraoperatively in scenarios where the knee is balanced in extension, but tight in flexion. However, as previously mentioned, one significant challenge is difficulty in qualitatively assessing optimal PCL tensioning. Ritter et al., formerly described a technique of step-wise recession the PCL with intraoperative physical examination assessing anterior to posterior translation, superior tilting or posterior hinging of the tibial trial [36]. Others opt to increase the slope of the tibia when making their tibial resection to increase the flexion gap and loosen the tension on the PCL. However, a lack of reproducible and concrete data exist on appropriate tension of the PCL and remain an area of interest and future research.

Preoperative assessment of knee range of motion is valuable when deciding on implant choice. Specifically, one must consider the effects of advanced knee osteoarthritis with respect to preoperative knee flexion contracture. Severe knee flexion contracture, specifically over 20°, has been associated with a high rate of conversion to PS-TKA [9, 35]. In chronic knee flexion contracture, release of the posterior capsule and PCL is often necessary to obtain appropriate postoperative knee extension. Surgeons who use CR should be prepared for conversion to more constrained implants like a PS-TKA depending on a patient's comorbidities and deformity.

Clinical Results

Several randomized control trials and meta-analysis comparing PS versus CR designs demonstrated no evidence of superiority [37–41], citing that CR-TKA remains a viable option in patients with a competent PCL. Some recent studies have suggested modest improvements in knee flexion with PS-TKA, with no differences in patient-reported outcomes or clinical results [42–44]. That being said, several proposed advantages to the PCL-sparing technique exist within literature. Several international registry data as well as a recent meta-analysis by Kanna et al. have demonstrated a slight advantage for CR-TKA with respect to implant longevity, despite no differences in complication rates [45–47].

As previously mentioned, several of the most common proposed advantages to the CR design are more native joint kinematics, improved proprioception, less bone resection, and better femoral rollback. Victor et al., performed a randomized control trial of PCL-retaining versus PCL-sacrificing TKA assessing functional outcomes and kinematics and found that PCL-retaining implants demonstrated improved femoral rollback with greater posterior displacement of the medial and lateral femoral condyles [48]. It is important to understand that despite overall clinical outcomes remaining similar between CR-TKA and more constrained implants, differences do exist with respect to the kinematics with retaining and sacrificing the PCL. However, the data remains inconsistent as several aforementioned studies suggest that PS-TKA demonstrates modest evidence of improved flexion despite kinematic studies suggesting more native mechanics [42–44].

One benefit of the CR-TKA design is the preservation of bone in the intercondylar notch, since there is no need to accommodate the cam-post design. Studies comparing overall bony resection between CR-TKA and PS-TKA demonstrate decreased bone loss with CR designs [49]. Additional concerns with the cam-post mechanism include increased stress on the polyethylene and the possibility of aseptic loosening. Though the data has not been consistent, few studies have demonstrated increased rates of aseptic loosening in PS-TKA compared to CR-TKA, which may explain some studies citing increased longevity with CR designs [6, 47]. Ultimately, the data has not been consistent in demonstrating superiority over PCL-sacrificing and

PCL-retaining implants, and each implant provides viable options for appropriate patient and surgeon preference.

As implant design continues to evolve to restore native biomechanics and to circumvent some concerns with the cam-post mechanism, designs such as medial-pivot (MP) and ultra-congruent (UC) TKA were introduced as intermediaries. In contrast to the normal mechanics of femoral rollback during knee flexion, biomechanical assessments of CR and PS-TKA have demonstrated concerns for paradoxical motion with initial anterior translation of the femur on the tibia and opposite rotational patterns [50–52]. This can lead to mid-flexion instability and poor patient-reported outcomes. MP designs are aimed to provide increased conformity on the medial tibia with a high anterior wall to promote normal axial rotation along the flatter lateral condyle and facilitate deep knee flexion without anterior subluxation. Similarly, UC designs aim to provide stability by using a deep-dish polyethylene with high anterior and posterior wall with increased congruency of the medial and lateral femoral condyle with the tibia. A recent meta-analysis by Wenzel et al. (2023) demonstrated no clinical differences comparing CR, PS, and UC designs at short-term follow-up [53]. As UC designs become more popular in the United States, kinematic studies as well as long-term studies to assess survivorship will be needed.

Conclusions

Whether to retain or sacrifice the PCL remains an ongoing debate among adult joint reconstruction surgeons. The use of CR versus PS implants in routine primary TKA is often surgeon, institution, or region specific. The United States continues to hold a strong preference for PS-TKA designs, while globally, CR-TKA dominates the landscape. To date, there is no robust and consistent data to suggest one implant design and surgical technique improves patient-reported or functional outcomes. Most surgeons would agree that an incompetent PCL may be a contraindication for using a CR implant, and most surgeons would use more constrained designs. Future research on proper PCL tensioning in TKA may be beneficial for patient outcomes, especially with the use of technology and the possibility of measuring ligamentous tension improves in the future.

References

1. Kurtz S, Ong K, Lau E, et al. Projections of primary and revision hip and knee arthroplasty in the United States from 2005 to 2030. J Bone Joint Surg Am. 2007;89:780–5. https://doi.org/10.2106/jbjs.f.00222.
2. Logterman SL, Wydra FB, Frank RM. Posterior cruciate ligament: anatomy and biomechanics. Curr Rev Musculoskelet Med. 2018;11:510–4. https://doi.org/10.1007/s12178-018-9492-1.

3. Movassaghi K, Patel A, Ghulam-Jelani Z, Levine BR. Modern total knee arthroplasty bearing designs and the role of the posterior cruciate ligament. Arthroplast Today. 2023;21:101130. https://doi.org/10.1016/j.artd.2023.101130.
4. Cho K-Y, Kim K-I, Song S-J, Bae D-K. Does cruciate-retaining total knee arthroplasty show better quadriceps recovery than posterior-stabilized total knee arthroplasty?—objective measurement with a dynamometer in 102 knees. Clin Orthop Surg. 2016;8:379. https://doi.org/10.4055/cios.2016.8.4.379.
5. Purudappa PP, Ramanan SP, Tripathy SK, et al. Intra-operative fractures in primary total knee arthroplasty—A systematic review. Knee Surg Relat Res. 2020;32:40. https://doi.org/10.1186/s43019-020-00054-3.
6. Vertullo CJ, Lewis PL, Lorimer M, Graves SE. The effect on long-term survivorship of surgeon preference for posterior-stabilized or minimally stabilized total knee replacement. J Bone Joint Surg Am. 2017;99:1129–39. https://doi.org/10.2106/jbjs.16.01083.
7. Yang K, Sohn G, Sambandam S. Cruciate-retaining total knee arthroplasty: current concepts review. Cureus. 2023;15:e43813. https://doi.org/10.7759/cureus.43813.
8. Jiang C, Liu Z, Wang Y, et al. Posterior cruciate ligament retention versus posterior stabilization for total knee arthroplasty: a meta-analysis. PLoS One. 2016;11:e0147865. https://doi.org/10.1371/journal.pone.0147865.
9. Bae DK, Song SJ, Kim KI, et al. Intraoperative factors affecting conversion from cruciate retaining to cruciate substituting in total knee arthroplasty. Knee Surg Sports Traumatol Arthrosc. 2016;24:3247–53. https://doi.org/10.1007/s00167-015-3971-3.
10. Banks S, Bellemans J, Nozaki H, et al. Knee motions during maximum flexion in fixed and mobile-bearing arthroplasties. Clin Orthop Relat Res. 2003;(410):131–138. https://doi.org/10.1097/01.blo.0000063121.39522.19.
11. Girgis FG, Marshall JL, Monajem A. The cruciate ligaments of the knee joint. Clin Orthop Relat Res. 1975;(106):216–231. https://doi.org/10.1097/00003086-197501000-00033.
12. Pinskerova V, Johal P, Nakagawa S, et al. Does the femur roll-back with flexion? J Bone Joint Surg Br. 2004;86-B:925–31. https://doi.org/10.1302/0301-620x.86b6.14589.
13. Kim H, Pelker RR, Gibson DH, et al. Rollback in posterior cruciate ligament—retaining total knee arthroplasty. J Arthroplasty. 1997;12:553–61. https://doi.org/10.1016/s0883-5403(97)90179-0.
14. Calvisi V, Paglia A, Ciprietti N, Goderecci R. Cruciate-retaining total knee arthroplasty. In: Primary total knee arthroplasty. 2018. https://doi.org/10.5772/intechopen.74024.
15. Williams A, Logan M. Understanding tibio-femoral motion. Knee. 2004;11:81–8. https://doi.org/10.1016/j.knee.2003.12.004.
16. Browne C, Hermida JC, Bergula A, et al. Patellofemoral forces after total knee arthroplasty: effect of extensor moment arm. Knee. 2005;12:81–8. https://doi.org/10.1016/j.knee.2004.05.006.
17. Sharma A, Leszko F, Komistek RD, et al. In vivo patellofemoral forces in high flexion total knee arthroplasty. J Biomech. 2008;41:642–8. https://doi.org/10.1016/j.jbiomech.2007.09.027.
18. Sass J-O, Johnson K, Darques J-B, et al. Influence of posterior cruciate ligament tension on tibiofemoral and patellofemoral joint contact mechanics in cruciate-retaining total knee replacement: a combined musculoskeletal multibody and finite-element simulation. Comput Methods Biomech Biomed Engin. 2024:1–13. https://doi.org/10.1080/10255842.2024.2329946.
19. Watanabe M, Kuriyama S, Nishitani K, et al. What is the optimal posterior cruciate ligament tension to achieve patient satisfaction in cruciate-retaining total knee arthroplasty? J Arthroplasty. 2023;38:S183. https://doi.org/10.1016/j.arth.2023.01.050.
20. Cromie MJ, Siston RA, Giori NJ, Delp SL. Posterior cruciate ligament removal contributes to abnormal knee motion during posterior stabilized total knee arthroplasty. J Orthop Res. 2008;26:1494–9. https://doi.org/10.1002/jor.20664.
21. Kayani B, Konan S, Horriat S, et al. Posterior cruciate ligament resection in total knee arthroplasty. Bone Joint J. 2019;101-B:1230–7. https://doi.org/10.1302/0301-620x.101b10.bjj-2018-1428.r2.

22. Zhao R, Liu Y, Tian H. Effect of posterior cruciate ligament on knee pressure and gap measured by an electronic sensor during total knee arthroplasty. J Orthop Surg Res. 2023;18:173. https://doi.org/10.1186/s13018-023-03643-6.
23. Heckmann N, Ihn H, Stefl M, et al. Early results from the American Joint Replacement Registry: a comparison with other national registries. J Arthroplasty. 2019;34:S125. https://doi.org/10.1016/j.arth.2018.12.027.
24. Parcells BW, Tria AJ Jr. The cruciate ligaments in total knee arthroplasty. Am J Orthop (Belle Mead NJ). 2016;45(4):E153–60.
25. Emodi GJ, Callaghan JJ, Pedersen DR, Brown TD. Posterior cruciate ligament function following total knee arthroplasty: the effect of joint line elevation. Iowa Orthop J. 1999;19:82–92.
26. Draganich LF, Andriacchi TP, Andersson GB. Interaction between intrinsic knee mechanics and the knee extensor mechanism. J Orthop Res. 1987;5:539–47. https://doi.org/10.1002/jor.1100050409.
27. Laskin RS, O'Flynn HM. Total knee replacement with posterior cruciate ligament retention in rheumatoid arthritis. Clin Orthop Relat Res. 1997;(345):24–28. https://doi.org/10.1097/00003086-199712000-00005.
28. Su EP. Fixed flexion deformity and total knee arthroplasty. J Bone Joint Surg Br. 2012;94-B:112–5. https://doi.org/10.1302/0301-620x.94b11.30512.
29. Archibeck MJ, Berger RA, Barden RM, et al. Posterior cruciate ligament-retaining total knee arthroplasty in patients with rheumatoid arthritis. J Bone Joint Surg Am. 2001;83:1231–6. https://doi.org/10.2106/00004623-200108000-00013.
30. Gill GS, Joshi AB. Long-term results of retention of the posterior cruciate ligament in total knee replacement in rheumatoid arthritis. J Bone Joint Surg. 2001;83:510–2. https://doi.org/10.1302/0301-620x.83b4.11398.
31. Ünkar EA, Öztürkmen Y, Şükür E, et al. Posterior cruciate-retaining versus posterior-stabilized total knee arthroplasty for osteoarthritis with severe varus deformity. Acta Orthop Traumatol Turc. 2017;51:95–9. https://doi.org/10.1016/j.aott.2016.12.008.
32. McAuley JP, Collier MB, Hamilton WG, et al. Posterior cruciate-retaining total knee arthroplasty for valgus osteoarthritis. Clin Orthop Relat Res. 2008;466:2644–9. https://doi.org/10.1007/s11999-008-0436-8.
33. Kubiak P, Archibeck MJ, White RE. Cruciate-retaining total knee arthroplasty in patients with at least fifteen degrees of coronal plane deformity. J Arthroplasty. 2008;23:366–70. https://doi.org/10.1016/j.arth.2007.01.004.
34. Sierra RJ, Berry DJ. Surgical technique differences between posterior-substituting and cruciate-retaining total knee arthroplasty. J Arthroplasty. 2008;23:20–3. https://doi.org/10.1016/j.arth.2008.06.004.
35. Song SJ, Park CH, Bae DK. What to know for selecting cruciate-retaining or posterior-stabilized total knee arthroplasty. Clin Orthop Surg. 2019;11:142. https://doi.org/10.4055/cios.2019.11.2.142.
36. Ritter MA, Faris PM, Keating EM. Posterior cruciate ligament balancing during total knee arthroplasty. J Arthroplasty. 1988;3:323–6. https://doi.org/10.1016/s0883-5403(88)80032-9.
37. Kolisek FR, McGrath MS, Marker DR, et al. Posterior-stabilized versus posterior cruciate ligament-retaining total knee arthroplasty. Iowa Orthop J. 2009;29:23–7.
38. Tanzer M, Smith K, Burnett S. Posterior-stabilized versus cruciate-retaining total knee arthroplasty. J Arthroplasty. 2002;17:813–9. https://doi.org/10.1054/arth.2002.34814.
39. Scott DF. Prospective randomized comparison of posterior-stabilized versus condylar-stabilized total knee arthroplasty: final report of a five-year study. J Arthroplasty. 2018;33:1384–8. https://doi.org/10.1016/j.arth.2017.11.037.
40. Scott DF, Smith RR. A prospective, randomized comparison of posterior stabilized versus cruciate-substituting total knee arthroplasty: a preliminary report with minimum 2-year results. J Arthroplasty. 2014;29:179–81. https://doi.org/10.1016/j.arth.2014.03.050.
41. Bercik MJ, Joshi A, Parvizi J. Posterior cruciate-retaining versus posterior-stabilized total knee arthroplasty. J Arthroplasty. 2013;28:439–44. https://doi.org/10.1016/j.arth.2012.08.008.

42. Tille E, Beyer F, Lützner C, et al. Better flexion but unaffected satisfaction after treatment with posterior stabilized versus cruciate retaining total knee arthroplasty—2-year results of a prospective, randomized trial. J Arthroplasty. 2024;39:368–73. https://doi.org/10.1016/j.arth.2023.08.044.
43. Yoshiya S, Matsui N, Komistek RD, et al. In vivo kinematic comparison of posterior cruciate-retaining and posterior stabilized total knee arthroplasties under passive and weight-bearing conditions. J Arthroplasty. 2005;20:777–83. https://doi.org/10.1016/j.arth.2004.11.012.
44. Li C, Dong M, Yang D, et al. Comparison of posterior cruciate retention and substitution in total knee arthroplasty during gait: a systematic review and meta-analysis. J Orthop Surg Res. 2022;17:152. https://doi.org/10.1186/s13018-022-03047-y.
45. Ben-Shlomo Y, Blom A, Boulton C, Brittain R, Clark E, Dawson-Bowling S, et al. The National Joint Registry 18th annual report 2021. National Joint Registry. 2021.
46. Australian Orthopaedic Association National Joint Replacement Registry (AOANJRR). Hip, knee & shoulder arthroplasty: 2022 annual report, Adelaide: AOA; 2022. p. 1–487.
47. Kanna R, Murali SM, Ramanathan AT, et al. Cruciate retaining total knee arthroplasty has a better 10 year survival than posterior stabilized total knee arthroplasty: a systematic review and meta-analysis. J Exp Orthop. 2023;10:19. https://doi.org/10.1186/s40634-023-00583-2.
48. Victor J, Banks S, Bellemans J. Kinematics of posterior cruciate ligament-retaining and -substituting total knee arthroplasty. J Bone Joint Surg Br. 2005;87-B:646–55. https://doi.org/10.1302/0301-620x.87b5.15602.
49. Wragg R, Khan RJZ, Damasena ITW, Wimhurst J. A comparison of bone loss at total knee replacement: posterior stabilized versus cruciate retaining. J Orthop. 2012;9(1):e1.
50. Dennis DA, Komistek RD, Mahfouz MR, et al. Conventry award paper: multicenter determination of in vivo kinematics after total knee arthroplasty. Clin Orthop Relat Res. 2003;(416):37–57. https://doi.org/10.1097/01.blo.0000092986.12414.b5.
51. Dennis DA, Komistek RD, Mahfouz MR. In vivo fluoroscopic analysis of fixed-bearing total knee replacements. Clin Orthop Relat Res. 2003;(410):114–130. https://doi.org/10.1097/01.blo.0000062385.79828.72.
52. Sabatini L, Risitano S, Parisi G, et al. Medial pivot in total knee arthroplasty: literature review and our first experience. Clin Med Insights Arthritis Musculoskelet Disord. 2018;11:117954411775143. https://doi.org/10.1177/1179544117751431.
53. Wenzel AN, Hasan SA, Chaudhry YP, et al. Ultracongruent designs compared to posterior-stabilized and cruciate-retaining tibial inserts—what does the evidence tell us? A systematic review and meta-analysis. J Arthroplasty. 2023;38:2739. https://doi.org/10.1016/j.arth.2023.05.064.

Chapter 5
Medial Pivot Total Knee Arthroplasty

Seper Ekhtiari, Emilio D. Hernandez, Jesse I. Wolfstadt, and David Backstein

Introduction

Over the decades, total knee arthroplasty (TKA) has been proven to be a safe and effective procedure. Numerous implant designs for primary TKA prostheses have evolved over the years, and several dominant design philosophies have emerged including cruciate retaining (CR), posterior cruciate stabilized (PS), and ultra-congruent (UC). Most designs sacrifice the anterior cruciate ligament while CR designs preserve the PCL. PS designs sacrifice both the ACL and PCL, providing stability and mechanism for femoral rollback using a cam and post. Ultra-congruent devices sacrifice both ligaments and provide stability via the high degree of congruency between the femur and polyethylene insert on both the medial and lateral sides of the joint.

Despite generally excellent results in terms of pain relief, restoration of function, and durability, a sizeable minority of patients (10–15%) remain less than fully satisfied following recovery from TKA surgery [1]. It is also well documented that many modern TKA designs suffer from "paradoxical motion" or the abnormal anterior translation of the femur on the tibia, particularly with activities such as ascent and

S. Ekhtiari (✉)
Granovsky Gluskin Division of Orthopaedics, Sinai Health, Department of Surgery, University of Toronto, Toronto, ON, Canada

Division of Orthopaedic Surgery, Department of Surgery, McMaster University, Hamilton, ON, Canada

E. D. Hernandez · J. I. Wolfstadt
Granovsky Gluskin Division of Orthopaedics, Sinai Health, Department of Surgery, University of Toronto, Toronto, ON, Canada
e-mail: jesse.wolfstadt@sinaihealth.ca

D. Backstein
Hospital for Special Surgery at NCH, Naples, FL, USA

A. J. Tria Jr., G. R. Scuderi (eds.), *The Cruciate Ligaments in Total Knee Arthroplasty*, https://doi.org/10.1007/978-3-031-75992-5_5

descent of stairs. It has been proposed that an implant design which better replicates the stability and kinematics of the normal human knee may improve patient outcomes both in terms of patient satisfaction and objective studies of kinematics [2, 3].

Following the work of investigators such as Pinskirova and Freeman [4], medial pivot TKA design was introduced in 1994 [5]. Using modern imaging and modeling techniques such as dual orthogonal fluoroscopy and three-dimensional magnetic resonance imaging, it has become apparent that normal knee kinematics is highly asymmetrical. On the medial side, the circular femoral condyle spins in place in the concave tibial articulation as the knee moves from extension into flexion. In contrast, in the lateral compartment, the circular femoral condyle rolls over the convex tibial surface. Medial pivot TKA attempts to replicate the normal knee's more congruent and stable medial compartment while allowing for a more mobile lateral compartment [6].

This chapter will provide a detailed review of the current understanding of TKA kinematics and stability while providing an overview of how medial pivot TKA attempts to replicate native knee kinematics more closely. Surgical technical guidance and outcomes following medial pivot TKA will be provided.

Relevant Anatomy

The knee is a complex, composite joint made up of the tibiofemoral and patellofemoral articulations. The tibiofemoral joint is divided into the medial and lateral compartments [7].

Theories of Knee Kinematics

To gain insight into the philosophy behind medial pivot TKA design, it is important to understand the anatomy and kinematics of the native knee joint. Historically, knee joint kinematics was thought of in terms of the "four-bar link" theory, which posits that the knee is made up of a rigid four-bar system, consisting of the ACL, PCL, the distal femur, and the proximal tibia. In this system, as the knee flexes, both femoral condyles translate posteriorly; when the knee is extended, the femoral condyles move anteriorly on the tibia (Fig. 5.1) [9].

As early as 1941, Brantigan and Voshell identified that contrary to the four-bar link theory, the medial femoral condyle acts as the axis of rotation of the knee in the axial plane, allowing for anteroposterior translation of the lateral femoral condyle around a stable and fixed medial compartment [10]. Despite publication in the *Journal of Bone & Joint Surgery*, this theory did not take hold in anatomy or orthopedic teachings. In the 1990s, a highly cited biomechanical study confirmed the same finding to be true during human walking, defining the medial compartment as a "*ball-and-socket*" joint [11]. This nuanced understanding of knee kinematics

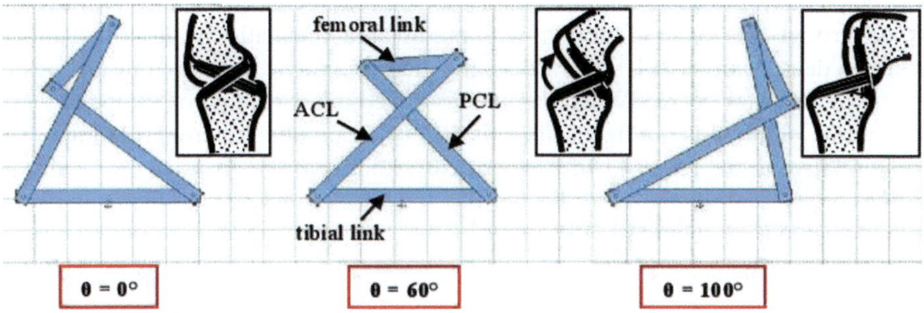

Fig. 5.1 The "four-bar link" theory of knee kinematics [8]

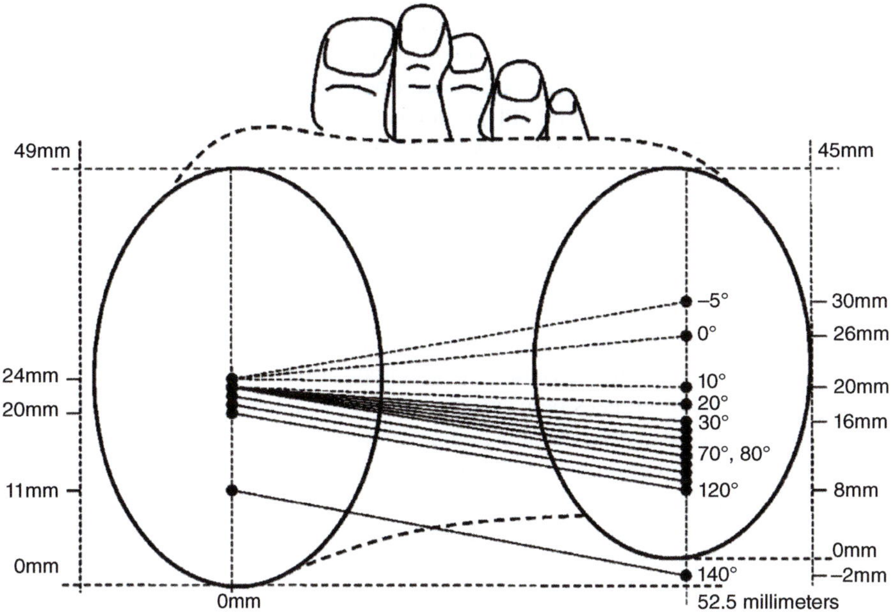

Fig. 5.2 Movement of the medial and lateral femoral condyles on the tibia during flexion and extension while weightbearing [12]

reveals that the medial femoral condyle remains relatively stable in the anteroposterior plane during flexion/extension, while the lateral condyle rolls back posteriorly as the knee moves from extension to flexion (Fig. 5.2).

Knee kinematics differs not only between the medial and lateral compartments, but also changes throughout the arc of motion and depending on whether the foot is fixed or not (i.e., closed vs. open kinetic chain). In terminal extension, particularly when the foot is planted, the femur rotates internally on the tibia (pivoting around the medial compartment), to lock the knee in what is referred to as the "screw-home mechanism" [13–15]. From approximately 20–120°, known as the "fundamental" or “active arc,” the quadriceps and hamstrings work in concert to actively move the knee through this range of motion, with predictable kinematics as described above. Only in deep flexion (>110–120°) does the medial condyle begin to translate posteriorly to a greater degree. When the knee is flexed in the context of an open kinetic chain (i.e., the foot is not fixed), there is also corresponding internal rotation of the tibia relative to the femur [13]. Beyond 120°, known as the “passive arc,” external forces are typically required to further flex the knee, with kneeling being an example of such a movement [13–15].

Role of the Cruciates in Knee Kinematics

The ACL is an intra-articular ligament originating from the medial aspect of the lateral femoral condyle and inserting into the center of the tibia, close to the anterior horn of the lateral meniscus. The ACL is composed of two bundles: the anteromedial (AM) and the posterolateral (PL) bundles. The PL bundle provides anteroposterior and rotational stability with the knee in less than 30° of flexion, while the AM primarily provides stability when the knee is flexed beyond 30° [16]. The PCL has its origin on the medial femoral condyle and its insertion on the posterior aspect of the tibia. The PCL is also composed of two bundles, the anterolateral (AL) and posteromedial (PM) bundles [17]. The AL band is most engaged when the knee is in flexion, while the PM is tightest when the knee is in extension. The main function of the PCL is preventing the excessive posterior translation of the tibia relative to the femur and acts as a secondary rotational stabilizer of the knee [18].

The kinematic differences between the medial and lateral compartments are not surprising when considering the substantial anatomical differences between the two compartments. The medial femoral condyle is larger, with a more spherical radius of curvature, and the medial tibial plateau is concave, in contrast to the convex lateral tibial plateau [19]. As well, the dynamic stabilizers of the medial compartment, including the ligaments, capsule, and meniscus, form a much more complex and stable structure compared to the more mobile and relatively simpler lateral ligamentocapsular complex [20].

History and Rationale of the Medial Pivot TKA

The modern TKA design can be traced back to the 1950s and 1960s, with the Walldius hinged knee design starting to be routinely used as a knee prosthesis [21]. This design did not attempt to recreate the anatomy of the distal femur in any meaningful way, simply replacing the entirety of the knee joint with a relatively simple and symmetrical hinge design, not unlike that of a door hinge [22]. In the late 1970s, Insall et al. introduced the total condylar knee, representing the foundational design from which most modern primary TKA designs have evolved. Insall identified a number of issues with the rigid hinge designs, including excessive levels of constraint and deviation from the natural anatomy of the knee joint [23–25]. Since then, continued improvements have been made on the total condylar prosthesis, with efforts to fine tune various aspects of the joint, including patellofemoral kinematics and optimizing joint stability. However, until recently the TKA has essentially been designed to move through flexion and extension as a relatively simple hinge joint and to ensure reproducibility with relatively rudimentary manual instrumentation. The majority of TKA implants used toward the end of the twentieth century and the early twenty-first century followed the rigid four-bar link theory of knee kinematics. In contrast, the medial pivot TKA prosthesis attempts to reproduce the natural kinematics of the knee as discussed above, aiming to replicate the highly congruent ball-and-socket anatomy of the medial compartment while allowing for a more mobile and less congruent lateral compartment to pivot around it.

Implant Design

To better understand the medial pivot TKA design philosophy, it is useful to compare it to the other commonly used alternative designs. Traditional TKA designs (single- or multi-radius) include PCL sparing or sacrificing designs, which have been complemented with more recent UC and medial congruent designs. Most recently, a "gradually reducing" radius of curvature has also been introduced [26].

The majority of conventional TKA designs adhere to a multi-radius, or "J-curve" design, in which there are multiple different radii of curvature—when looking at the implant in the sagittal plane, there is a larger radius of curvature anteriorly compared to distally, which in turn is larger than the posterior radius of curvature (Fig. 5.3) [27]. These designs did represent an improvement upon historic designs, including allowing deeper flexion and femoral rollback. However, these designs

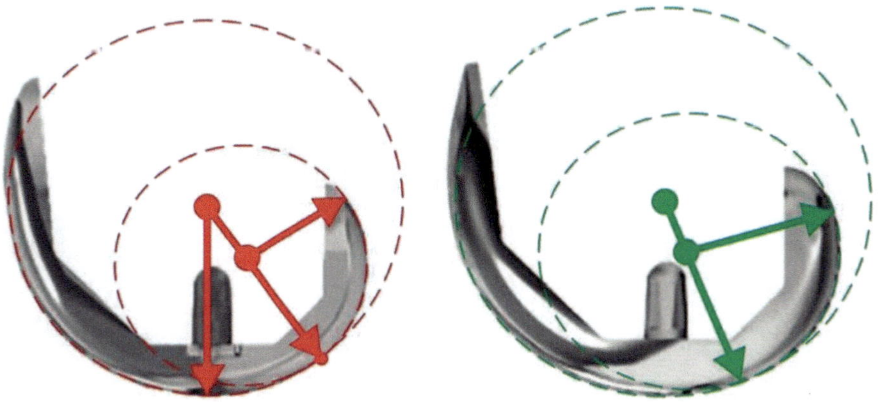

Fig. 5.3 Visual depiction of multiple (left) and single (right) radius TKA designs [26]

have certain limitations, including issues with mid-flexion instability, placing the quadriceps at a mechanical disadvantage, and not accurately reproducing the native femoral rollback, which only happens in the lateral compartment [26].

Another issue encountered by these designs, in particular multi-radius CR knees, is that of "paradoxical anterior motion." This refers to the sudden anterior movement of the femur on the tibia when the knee moves from its larger distal radius curvature to its smaller posterior curvature [28]. This characteristic is often associated with CR designs because the femoral condyles both translate posteriorly on the tibia during flexion, until a sudden change in the radius of curvature engages the PCL, causing a sudden, uncomfortable, and unnatural anterior movement of the femur relative to the tibia [29].

The goal of the medial pivot knee implant is to achieve kinematics more similar to the native knee than those achieved by traditional TKA designs [30]. Crucial to achieving this goal is a highly congruent medial compartment. Thus, rather than a tibial insert which is symmetrical from medial to lateral, the medial portion of the tibial insert is a much deeper dish (simulating the concave medial plateau), with a correspondingly more prominent, larger, and more circular medial femoral condyle on the femoral component [31]. Thus, a highly congruent ball-and-socket joint is reproduced on the medial aspect, as opposed to the traditional hinge joint design. Conversely, the lateral part of the tibial liner is much flatter (simulating the concavity of the lateral plateau), with a smaller and less prominent lateral femoral condyle, thus simulating the native anatomy (Fig. 5.4) [31]. This contrast in design between the compartments allows for the lateral compartment to translate anterior to posterior, pivoting around a stable medial compartment [30, 31]. Critical to the medial pivot concept is the minimal reliance on the medial and lateral collateral ligaments (MCL and LCL) to achieve stability. Instead, the shape of the medial and lateral tibiofemoral articulations provides a system of low compliance on the medial side and higher compliance on the lateral side. In other words, more energy must be imparted to the knee to cause motion between the medial articulation than on the

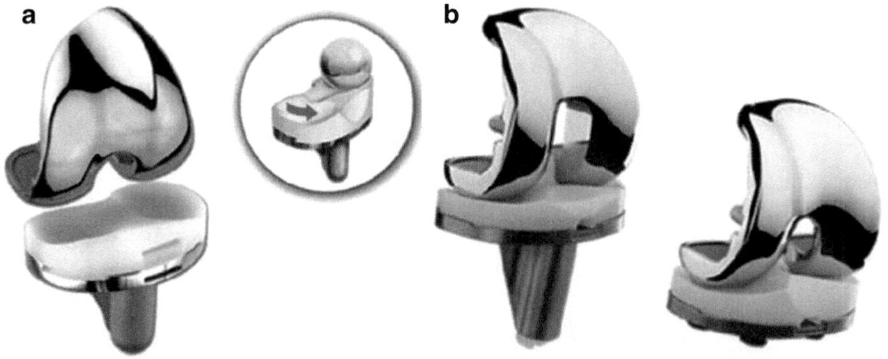

Fig. 5.4 (**a**) medial pivot prosthesis, with the highly congruent ball-and-socket medial compartment, and the more mobile lateral compartment, compared to (**b**) posterior stabilized design with post and cam [32]

lateral side. This results in a TKA which has inherent stability yet remains highly mobile, without requiring equal balance of the collateral ligaments.

The first generation of medial pivot TKAs were introduced in the mid-1990s, with the Medial Rotation Knee (*MRK™, MatOrtho, Surrey, UK*) and the Advance® Medial-Pivot Knee (*Wright Medical, Memphis, TN, USA*). Since then, a range of "second generation" medial pivot designs have been introduced, including the Evolution MP (MicroPort, Shanghai, China), the GMK Sphere (Medacta, Castel San Pietro, Switzerland), among others [33]. All of these designs adhere to the above principles, with newer implants benefiting from improvements in materials technology, surgical technique, and more careful consideration of patellofemoral kinematics.

A number of implant designs have aimed to mimic or approximate the medial pivot philosophy, although they cannot be considered true medial pivot knees. Importantly, a true medial pivot design knee has a single radius around which the medial femoral condyle rotates in both the axial and sagittal planes, while these alternate designs simply increase the congruence of the medial (+/− lateral) compartment(s) to better approximate the bony anatomy of the knee [31]. Thus, if the base implant design is a multi-radius (or J-curve) design, a medial congruent insert cannot fully replicate native knee kinematics [26]. Even with a single sagittal radius design that has a congruent insert option, the axial plane rotation does not adhere to a true ball-and-socket medial pivot philosophy.

Most commonly, these alternate designs include changes in the polyethylene insert of an existing conventional TKA design, whereby a standard TKA implant is "retrofitted" to provide greater congruence between the femoral and tibial components. Among these designs are UC and medial congruent (or "medial stabilized") TKA inserts [31]. Ultra-congruent designs increase congruence in both the medial and lateral compartments and have both an anterior and posterior lip, to compensate for the lack of the cruciate ligaments and avoid femoral sliding in mid-flexion [34]. However, the lack of physiological femoral rollback, axial rotation, and the potential for increased shear stress on the tibial bone surface remain concerning with UC designs [35].

Medial congruent designs aim to address some of these concerns, by providing sagittal plane stability regardless of PCL sparing or sacrificing technique, while theoretically allowing more anteroposterior translation of the lateral compartment [35]. However, in vivo dynamic radiostereometric analysis has demonstrated no difference in terms of actual medial pivoting behavior between UC and medial congruent designs of the same TKA system [35].

Surgical Technique

The overall surgical technique for a medial pivot TKA is similar to a standard TKA, with a few important technical pearls to ensure a successful outcome which respects and leverages the design of the implant. Here we describe the senior authors' preferred surgical technique for a medial pivot TKA.

All patients are evaluated pre-operatively with routine history, physical examination, and a full set of radiographs including anteroposterior, lateral, and skyline views of the affected knee, and full-length standing views of both legs to assess overall alignment. Any patient eligible for a standard primary TKA is typically eligible for a medial pivot implant.

A medial parapatellar approach is used for all cases, including cutting the anterior horn of the medial meniscus and the ACL. A conservative medial exposure is performed off the tibia, sparing the MCL and typically extending no more than halfway from the arthrotomy site to the anterior third of the medial tibial plateau. Avoidance of any iatrogenic damage to the MCL is crucial to maintaining normal kinematics and avoidance of post-operative pain. Release of the MCL to compensate for a loose lateral side in varus knees is not required using this technique. Bone cuts of the femur and tibia are made in a traditional manner; however, the authors' preferred technique includes a distal femoral cut angle of 3° of valgus [36]. It is preferable that the TKA be placed in slightly tighter soft tissue tension in extension than in flexion and slightly tighter medially than laterally.

Outcomes of Medial Pivot TKA

A number of studies have compared medial pivot TKA to other TKA designs, thus the focus in this section will be on studies evaluating knee kinematics and the highest quality clinical studies.

A biomechanical study comparing medial pivot and UC TKA in a full lower body model through a range of daily and physical activity movements demonstrated that medial pivot knees were significantly more likely to replicate the natural motion of the native knee with regard to a stable medial compartment and anteroposterior translation of the lateral compartment during flexion/extension [37]. Interestingly, a study comparing kinematically aligned TKA to mechanically aligned TKA using the same medial pivot implant found that kinematically aligned TKAs replicated the natural medial pivot motion of the knee more closely [38].

A meta-analysis of 15 randomized controlled trials (RCTs) demonstrated no significant difference between medial pivot and PS designs at up to 4 years follow-up in terms of range of motion, mean walking speed, length of stay, radiographic alignment, or complications [39]. Another meta-analysis of 8 RCTs, which included all conventional TKA designs as comparators, also found no significant differences between medial pivot and PS designs at any timepoint up to 2 years for any measured outcome (functional scores, range of motion, complications). They determined that designs other than PS did not have sufficient studies to draw definitive conclusions [40]. Interestingly, an RCT comparing medial pivot TKA to PS and CR TKA simultaneously found that at 6 months, all designs had similar clinical and functional outcomes, but patients with medial pivot TKA had greater satisfaction. At first year, patients in the medial pivot group had significantly better pain scores, function, and quality of life outcomes [41]. Similarly, a retrospective comparison of medial pivot and PS TKAs found that patients in the medial pivot had significantly better forgotten joint score [42, 43].

Considering these findings, it important to keep in mind that the improvements in kinematics which is provided by medial pivot design may not be consciously perceptible by patients, yet they may improve some of the performance of more subtle aspects of daily function.

Technological Advances and Future Directions

The advent of robotic TKA and advanced technologies may help surgeons to achieve their surgical targets more precisely. While the clinical benefits of robotic TKA remain unclear, most high-quality studies evaluating radiographic outcomes have demonstrated that robotic TKA outperforms conventional TKA when it comes to achieving alignment targets and minimizing coronal plane outliers [44]. Thus, at least in theory, the use of advanced technology may help to achieve a medial pivot knee more reliably, by allowing pre- and post-resection measurement of the in situ flexion and extension gaps. However, this has not yet been tested in high quality studies specific to medial pivot kinematics. Gap balancing sensors have also been previously studied in the context of achieving well-balanced knees (though, again, not specifically in relation to medial pivot TKA). A recent meta-analysis found that the use of gap sensors may result in more soft tissue procedures, without a significant difference in outcomes [45]. Some medial pivot TKA systems also include caliper instruments for performing a manual kinematically aligned medial pivot TKA, which may restore a more natural joint line based on the patient's pre-arthritic joint line. While additional information from advanced technologies likely can play a role in improving precision and the ability to achieve a truly medial pivoting knee, that potential has not yet been fully realized. Technologies that are purpose-built for medial pivot implants will be important in helping to achieve this goal, possibly including adjuncts that can track the axial plane kinematics of the knee with flexion and extension during the intra-operative trial.

Conclusions

The design of TKA implants has evolved over time, along with the understanding of the knee joint itself. Originally thought of as a hinge joint with a rigid four-bar link design, the knee is now understood as a much more complex joint, with important differences between the medial and lateral compartments. Medial pivot TKA aims to replicate natural knee kinematics, including the ball-and-socket medial compartment, with a more mobile lateral compartment which rotates around the medial compartment during flexion/extension. Surgical technique is generally similar to a conventional TKA, with a few key differences, including maintaining a more limited release of the medial soft tissues and aiming for a tighter extension gap than flexion and tighter medial than lateral compartment. While biomechanical studies have confirmed that medial pivot designs replicate the native knee kinematics most closely (even compared to "medial stabilized" or "medial congruent" designs), there remains no clear difference in clinical outcomes between medial pivot and PS knees.

References

1. Kahlenberg CA, Nwachukwu BU, McLawhorn AS, Cross MB, Cornell CN, Padgett DE. Patient satisfaction after total knee replacement: a systematic review. HSS J. 2018;14:192–201.
2. Yagishita K, Muneta T, Ju YJ, Morito T, Yamazaki J, Sekiya I. High-flex posterior cruciate-retaining vs posterior cruciate-substituting designs in simultaneous bilateral total knee arthroplasty: a prospective, randomized study. J Arthroplasty. 2012;27(3):368–74.
3. Abdel MP, Morrey ME, Jensen MR, Morrey BF. Increased long-term survival of posterior cruciate-retaining versus posterior cruciate-stabilizing total knee replacements. J Bone Joint Surg Am. 2011;93(22):2072.
4. Iwaki H, Pinskerova V, Freeman MAR. Tibiofemoral movement 1: the shape and relative movements of the femur and tibia in the unloaded cadaver knee. J Bone Joint Surg Br. 2000;82(8):1189.
5. Cacciola G, Mancino F, De Meo F, Di Matteo V, Sculco PK, Cavaliere P, et al. Mid-term survivorship and clinical outcomes of the medial stabilized systems in primary total knee arthroplasty: a systematic review. J Orthop. 2021;24:157.
6. Hodgeson SM, Soeno T, Mears SC, Stambough JB, Barnes CL, Stronach BM. The medial pivot design in total knee arthroplasty. Orthop Clin North Am. 2024;55:49.
7. Chang A, Hubbard JB. Anatomy, bony pelvis and lower limb, femur. StatPearls; 2018.
8. Etoundi AC, Vaidyanathan R, Burgess SC. A bio-inspired condylar knee joint for leg amputees and for knee implants. WIT Trans Ecol Environ. 2012;160:23–34.
9. Pinskerova V, Vavrik P. Knee anatomy and biomechanics and its relevance to knee replacement. In: Personalized hip and knee joint replacement; 2020.
10. Brantigan OC, Voshell AF. The mechanics of the ligaments and menisci of the knee joint. J Bone Joint Surg Am. 1941;23(1):44–66.
11. Lafortune MA, Cavanagh PR, Sommer HJ, Kalenak A. Three-dimensional kinematics of the human knee during walking. J Biomech. 1992;25(4):347.
12. Johal P, Williams A, Wragg P, Hunt D, Gedroyc W. Tibio-femoral movement in the living knee. A study of weight bearing and non-weight bearing knee kinematics using "interventional" MRI. J Biomech. 2005;38(2):269.
13. Vaienti E, Scita G, Ceccarelli F, Pogliacomi F. Understanding the human knee and its relationship to total knee replacement. Acta Biomed. 2017;88:6–16.
14. Nakazoe Y, Yonekura A, Takita H, Miyaji T, Okazaki N, Chiba K, et al. Differences in the flexion and extension phases during kneeling investigated by kinematic and contact point analyses: a cross-sectional study. J Orthop Surg Res. 2022;17(1):192.

15. Freeman MAR, Pinskerova V. The movement of the normal tibio-femoral joint. J Biomech. 2005;38(2):197.
16. Domnick C, Raschke MJ, Herbort M. Biomechanics of the anterior cruciate ligament: physiology, rupture and reconstruction techniques. World J Orthop. 2016;7:82–93.
17. Girgis FG, Marshall JL, Monajem A. The cruciate ligaments of the knee joint. Clin Orthop Relat Res. 1975;106:216.
18. Gollehon DL, Torzilli PA, Warren RF. The role of the posterolateral and cruciate ligaments in the stability of the human knee. A biomechanical study. J Bone Joint Surg Am. 1987;69(2):233.
19. Chaurasia A, Tyagi A, Santoshi JA, Chaware P, Rathinam BA. Morphologic features of the distal femur and proximal tibia: a cross-sectional study. Cureus. 2021;13:e12907.
20. LaPrade RF, Engebretsen AH, Ly TV, Johansen S, Wentorf FA, Engebretsen L. The anatomy of the medial part of the knee. J Bone Joint Surg Am. 2007;89(9):2000.
21. Walldius B. Arthroplasty of the knee using an endoprosthesis. Acta Rheumatol Scand Suppl. 1957;24:1.
22. Merryweather R, Jones GB. Total knee replacement: the Walldius arthroplasty. Orthop Clin North Am. 1973;4(2):585–96.
23. Scuderi GR, Scott WN, Tchejeyan GH. The Insall legacy in total knee arthroplasty. Clin Orthop Relat Res. 2001;392:3.
24. Bargren JH, Freeman MAR, Swanson SAV, Todd RC. ICLH (Freeman/Swanson) arthroplasty in the treatment of arthritic knee: a 2 to 4 year review. Clin Orthop Relat Res. 1976;(120):65–75.
25. Insall J, Scott WN, Ranawat CS. The total condylar knee prosthesis. A report of two hundred and twenty cases. J Bone Joint Surg Am. 1979;61(2):173.
26. Ng JWG, Bloch BV, James PJ. Sagittal radius of curvature, trochlea design and ultracongruent insert in total knee arthroplasty. EFORT Open Rev. 2019;4(8):519.
27. Dall'Oca C, Ricci M, Vecchini E, Giannini N, Lamberti D, Tromponi C, et al. Evolution of TKA design. Acta Biomed. 2017;88:17–31.
28. Komistek RD, Dennis DA, Mahfouz M. In vivo fluoroscopic analysis of the normal human knee. Clin Orthop Relat Res. 2003;410:69.
29. Mirulla AI, Bragonzoni L, Zaffagnini S, Ingrassia T, Zinno R, Innocenti B. Assessment of paradoxical anterior translation in a CR total knee prosthesis coupling dynamic RSA and FE techniques. J Exp Orthop. 2021;8(1):50.
30. Sabatini L, Risitano S, Parisi G, Tosto F, Indelli PF, Atzori F, et al. Medial pivot in total knee arthroplasty: literature review and our first experience. Clin Med Insights Arthritis Musculoskelet Disord. 2018;11:1179544117751431.
31. Movassaghi K, Patel A, Ghulam-Jelani Z, Levine BR. Modern total knee arthroplasty bearing designs and the role of the posterior cruciate ligament. Arthroplast Today. 2023;21:101130.
32. Kulshrestha V, Sood M, Kanade S, Kumar S, Datta B, Mittal G. Early outcomes of medial pivot total knee arthroplasty compared to posterior-stabilized design: a randomized controlled trial. Clin Orthop Surg. 2020;12(2):178.
33. Nisar S, Ahmad K, Palan J, Pandit H, van Duren B. Medial stabilised total knee arthroplasty achieves comparable clinical outcomes when compared to other TKA designs: a systematic review and meta-analysis of the current literature. Knee Surg Sports Traumatol Arthrosc. 2022;30:638.
34. Kim TW, Lee SM, Seong SC, Lee S, Jang J, Lee MC. Different intraoperative kinematics with comparable clinical outcomes of ultracongruent and posterior stabilized mobile-bearing total knee arthroplasty. Knee Surg Sports Traumatol Arthrosc. 2016;24(9):3036.
35. Alesi D, Di Paolo S, Bragonzoni L, Pizza N, Zaffagnini S, Zinno R, et al. No kinematical difference between ultra-congruent and medial-congruent total knee arthroplasty when implanted with mechanical alignment: an in vivo dynamic RSA study. Knee Surg Sports Traumatol Arthrosc. 2022;30(9):2975.
36. Tanifuji O, Blaha JD, Kai S. The vector of quadriceps pull is directed from the patella to the femoral neck knee. Clin Orthop Relat Res. 2013;471(3):1014.

37. Putame G, Terzini M, Rivera F, Kebbach M, Bader R, Bignardi C. Kinematics and kinetics comparison of ultra-congruent versus medial-pivot designs for total knee arthroplasty by multibody analysis. Sci Rep. 2022;12(1):3052.
38. Kaneda K, Niki Y, Kuroyanagi Y, Kobayashi S, Harato K, Iwama Y, et al. Kinematically aligned total knee arthroplasty using medial pivot knee prosthesis enhances medial pivot motion: a comparative kinematic study with mechanically aligned total knee arthroplasty. Arthroplast Today. 2022;13:24.
39. Kakoulidis P, Panagiotidou S, Profitiliotis G, Papavasiliou K, Tsiridis E, Topalis C. Medial pivot design does not yield superior results compared to posterior-stabilised total knee arthroplasty: a systematic review and meta-analysis of randomised control trials. Knee Surg Sports Traumatol Arthrosc. 2023;31(9):3684.
40. Hoskins W, Smith G, Spelman T, Vince KG. Medial pivot designs versus conventional bearing types in primary total knee arthroplasty: a systematic review and meta-analysis of randomized controlled trials. J Am Acad Orthop Surg Glob Res Rev. 2022;6(12):e22.00170.
41. Dowsey MM, Gould DJ, Spelman T, Pandy MG, Choong PF. A randomized controlled trial comparing a medial stabilized total knee prosthesis to a cruciate retaining and posterior stabilized design: a report of the clinical and functional outcomes following total knee replacement. J Arthroplasty. 2020;35(6):1583.
42. Samy DA, Wolfstadt JI, Vaidee I, Backstein DJ. A retrospective comparison of a medial pivot and posterior-stabilized total knee arthroplasty with respect to patient-reported and radiographic outcomes. J Arthroplasty. 2018;33(5):1379.
43. Cassar-Gheiti AJ, Jamieson PS, Radi M, Wolfstadt JI, Backstein DJ. Evaluation of the medial stabilized knee design using data from National Joint Registries and current literature. J Arthroplasty. 2020;35(7):1950.
44. Riantho A, Butarbutar JCP, Fidiasrianto K, Elson E, Irvan I, Haryono H, et al. Radiographic outcomes of robot-assisted versus conventional total knee arthroplasty: a systematic review and meta-analysis of randomized clinical trials. JB JS Open Access. 2023;8(2):e23.00010.
45. Sun C, Zhao Z, Lee WG, Ma Q, Zhang X, Zhu J, et al. Sensor-guided gap balance versus manual gap balance in primary total knee arthroplasty: a meta-analysis. J Orthop Surg Res. 2022;17(1):243.

Chapter 6
PCL Substituting Total Knee Arthroplasty

Zuhdi E. Abdo, Giles R. Scuderi, and Alfred J. Tria Jr

Introduction

The posterior stabilized total knee arthroplasty (PS knee) is one of the two major knee designs which has stood the test of time for the past 40 years. The question for designers has been to preserve the posterior cruciate ligament (PCL) as in the cruciate retaining total knee (CR knee) or to substitute for it as in the PS knee. The PS knee designs utilize a post on the tibial polyethylene that acts as the PCL. Studies have shown that the PS designs tend to have greater range of motion (ROM), more normal kinematics, and more universal application to all degrees of deformity than the CR knees [1]. However, CR knee proponents report a more natural feeling knee for the patient and question the long-term survival of the PS knee post [2, 3]. While recent publications have indicated a decreased usage of the PS knees in the United States, the design remains as one of the major total knee arthroplasties (TKAs) in the world [4].

Z. E. Abdo
Lenox Hill Hospital/Northwell Health, New Hyde Park, NY, USA

G. R. Scuderi
Zucker School of Medicine at Hofstra/Northwell, Hempstead, NY, USA

A. J. Tria Jr (✉)
Rutgers-Robert Wood Johnson Medical School, New Brunswick, NJ, USA

A. J. Tria Jr., G. R. Scuderi (eds.), *The Cruciate Ligaments in Total Knee Arthroplasty*, https://doi.org/10.1007/978-3-031-75992-5_6

History

Early TKA designs were fraught with problems of loosening, wear, and material failures. The Total Condylar Prosthesis (TCP) was one of the earliest knees that showed significant success using dished, congruent tibio-femoral surfaces to address stability and ROM [5, 6]. The TCP II added a prominent tibial post to increase stability of the construct. Because of significant tibial loosening, the post design was modified leading to the Insall-Burstein Knee (IB Knee) that incorporated a cam-post articulation. The modification led to greater ROM and better kinematics [7]. In the late 1980s, the IB-II included a minor modification to the height and position of the tibial post along with multiple femoral, tibial, and polyethylene sizes [8]. The implant was a very successful and reliable implant over the next 10 years, and it was followed by the NexGen Legacy PS (Fig. 6.1) (Zimmer, Warsaw, Indiana). This knee introduced right and left femoral components with a lengthened trochlear groove to address patellar tracking [9]. The NexGen line of implants was the foundation for the NexGen High Flexion Legacy prosthesis (Fig. 6.2) (Zimmer, Warsaw, Indiana) which was designed to accommodate patients with active lifestyles and those with cultural and/or religious practices that require high knee flexion. In order to achieve knee flexion past 140–150°, the geometry of the posterior femoral condyles was altered to improve the contact with the tibial polyethylene articular surface at high flexion, and the anterior lip of the polyethylene was reduced to avoid

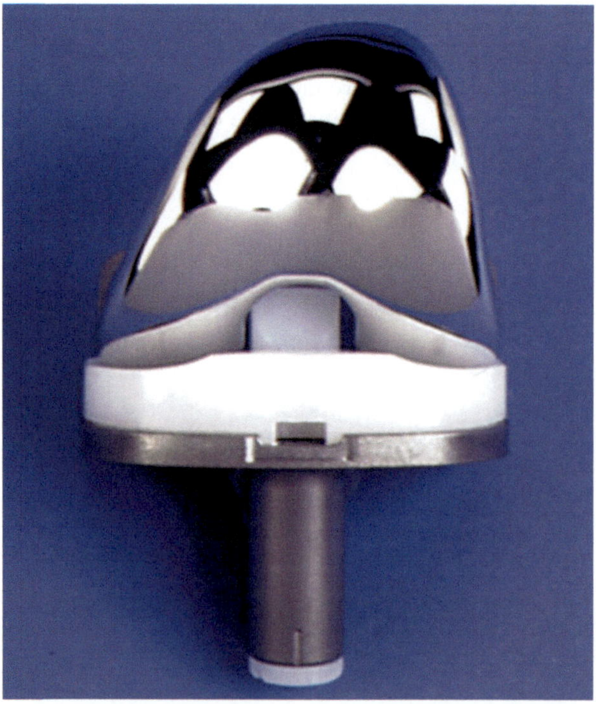

Fig. 6.1 Legacy posterior stabilized prosthesis (LPS)

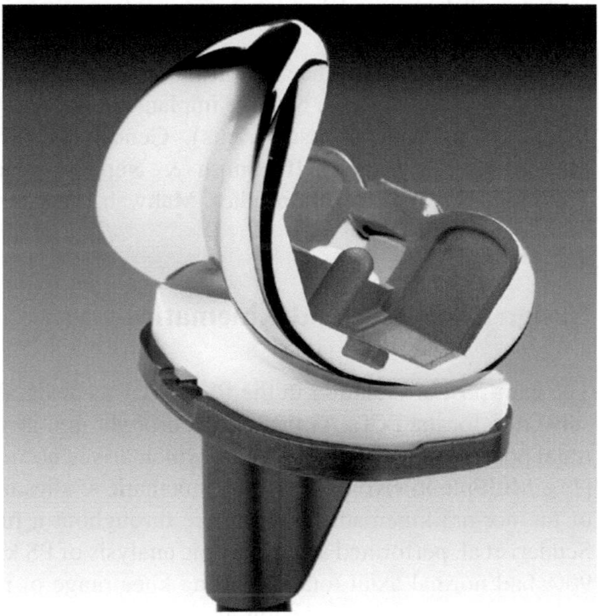

Fig. 6.2 Legacy posterior stabilized high flexion prosthesis (LPS Flex)

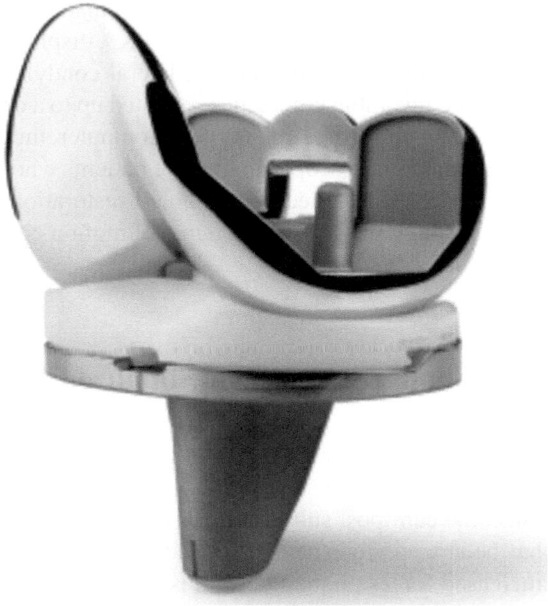

Fig. 6.3 Persona posterior stabilized prosthesis

impingement with the extensor mechanism at high flexion. The Persona PS (Fig. 6.3) (Zimmer, Warsaw, Indiana) is the latest in this PS design and was introduced in 2013 [10]. Notable design changes include an anatomic tibial tray to better fit the anatomy of the proximal tibial surface and a greater inventory of femoral component shapes and sizes.

The Insall-Burstein Knee established the PS knee philosophy and carried over to other modern PS designs. Notable implants in use today include the Attune (DePuy Synthes, Raynham, Massachusetts), Genesis II (Smith & Nephew, Andover, Massachusetts), Journey II (Smith & Nephew, Andover, Massachusetts), and Triathlon PS (Stryker Orthopaedics, Mahwah, New Jersey).

Design Principles and Kinematics

The cam-post articulation in the PS TKA was designed for the IB-II prosthesis to substitute for the PCL. As the knee is brought into flexion between 60 and 90°, the tibial post engages the femoral cam which drives normal posterior femoral rollback [11]. Multiple in vivo fluoroscopic kinematic studies of PS knees found restoration of the normal kinematics of the knee throughout a full range of motion [12–15]. Scuderi et al. performed a fluoroscopic analysis of PS knees in vivo and noted nearly 90% had normal axial rotation during knee range of motion and excellent passive and weightbearing knee flexion angles surpassing 120° [14]. Broberg et al. compared the kinematics and functional outcomes of PS and CR knees and found that the PS knees recreated more normal kinematics and had a faster timed get up and go test than the CR knees [13]. The PS TKA displayed less paradoxical anterior femoral translation on the medial and lateral condyles and greater lateral femoral rollback. The favorable kinematics persisted up to a decade after the procedure. Yoshiya et al. [15] performed an in vivo computer model fitting technique with three-dimensional fluoroscopic analysis of patients who underwent bilateral TKA (one PS knee and one CR knee). They noted restoration of normal kinematics in the PS knees through weightbearing range of motion compared to abnormal kinematics in the CR knees.

Indications for Posterior Stabilized TKA

The PS TKA is a versatile design that can be used for almost all deformities. In the cases where the PCL is insufficient or requires resection to completely balance the knee, the cam-post substitutes for the PCL and controls the knee roll back. If there has been a previous patellectomy, the PS TKA is the design of choice to avoid the increased forces on the PCL if it is retained leading to late rupture.

Surgical Technique

The goal of any knee replacement is restoration of the mechanical axis, equalization of the extension and flexion gaps, and collateral ligament balance with a full ROM. The procedure is initiated with the distal femoral resection that sets the coronal plane alignment and references the mechanical axis of the knee. The tibial resection is completed with a 90-degree angle in the coronal plane and proper sagittal inclination for the specific PS implant that is being used. The PCL is removed with this resection increasing the size of the flexion gap [16, 17]. The gaps are, then, equalized by adjusting the femoral component size (for the flexion gap). The collaterals must be balanced throughout the range of motion. In the varus knee setting, the medial collateral ligament can be lengthened by proximal epicondylar transfer, distal tibial insertion release, or pie crusting [18]. For the valgus knee, the release can be sequential (lateral collateral ligament, iliotibial band, and popliteus tendon releases) or a posterolateral capsular pie crusting [19–21].

With proper external rotation of the femoral and tibial components, the patellar tracking should be in the midline.

Complications

Early iterations of the PS design were associated with a few specific complications including patellar clunk syndrome, tibial post wear, and dislocation.

The patellar clunk occurred as the knee moved from flexion to full extension catching a fibrous nodule at the superior pole of the patella in the femoral box [22]. This was initially treated with quadriceps exercises or arthroscopic excision. Subsequent designs modified the trochlear grove and eliminated this problem [23].

Tibial post wear is uncommon with the present-day designs. It was associated with three surgical errors: knee hyperextension, increased tibial sagittal angle cuts, and flexion instability [24]. The three items all led to excess pressure and wear on the tibial post. Furman reported specific design differences in the PS prostheses that led to post wear without any relationship to age of the implanted device [25].

Dislocation of the early designs of the PS knee (IB-I and IB-II) occurred with high flexion angles that allowed the femoral cam to "jump" over the tibial post [26]. This was subsequently corrected with modification to the post position (moved 2 mm anterior) and increased height of the post (2 mm superior). With the modern-day PS knees, this is no longer a problem.

Outcomes

Long et al. [27] reported long-term follow up on the original cohort of IB-I and IB-II patients. The 30-year survivorship free of any revision was 70.1%. For those patients available for radiographic and clinical follow-up, there was no radiographic evidence of loosening, the average knee flexion was 110°, and they noted significant improvement in preoperative to postoperative Hospital for Special Surgery (HSS) and Knee Society Scores (KSS). Their analysis highlighted a significant difference in survivorship free of aseptic revisions for the monobloc IB-I prosthesis and modular IB-II (68.3% vs 92.3%, respectively). Most TKA systems in use today utilize a modular design that allows for trialing and selection of the desired tibial polyethylene insert.

A 2013 Cochrane Review [1] found a statistically significant difference in knee ROM and Knee Society functional scores favoring the PS over the CR knees. There was no difference in other patient reported outcome categories such as the Western Ontario and McMaster Universities (WOMAC) and Visual Analogue Scale (VAS) pain scores. There was also no difference in the rate of radiolucent lines, implant survival, and complication rates between the groups. A more recent meta-analysis from 2018 evaluated 5407 TKAs across 37 studies comparing the PS and CR designs. The analyses found improvements in knee flexion, knee extension, and Knee Society functional scores favoring the PS knee. There were no significant difference between the PS and CR postoperative complications [28].

Conclusion

The PS knee has remained a tried-and-proven design since its initial inception in the 1970s as the total condylar knee and Insall-Burstein prostheses. Specific complications of the original implants prompted design changes that all but eradicated them in the modern-day implants. Debate continues as to the superior TKA design with systematic reviews demonstrating statistically significant increased postoperative knee flexion and Knee Society functional scores compared to the CR design. The PS knee design can be used for all presenting knee deformities and allows for ease of ligament balancing during the surgical procedure.

References

1. Verra WC, van den Boom LG, Jacobs W, Clement DJ, Wymenga AA, Nelissen RG. Retention versus sacrifice of the posterior cruciate ligament in total knee arthroplasty for treating osteoarthritis. Cochrane Database Syst Rev. 2013;2013(10):CD004803. Published 2013 Oct 11. https://doi.org/10.1002/14651858.CD004803.pub3.

2. Archibeck MJ, Berger RA, Barden RM, et al. Posterior cruciate ligament-retaining total knee arthroplasty in patients with rheumatoid arthritis. J Bone Joint Surg Am. 2001;83:1231–6.
3. Laskin RS, O'Flynn HM. The Insall Award. Total knee replacement with posterior cruciate ligament retention in rheumatoid arthritis. Problems and complications. Clin Orthop Relat Res. 1997;(345):24–28.
4. American Joint Replacement Registry (AJRR): 2022 annual report. Rosemont: American Academy of Orthopaedic Surgeons (AAOS); 2022.
5. Insall J, Scott WN, Ranawat CS. The total condylar knee prosthesis. A report of two hundred and twenty cases. J Bone Joint Surg Am. 1979;61:173.
6. Insall JN, Lachiewicz PF, Burstein AH. The posterior stabilized condylar prosthesis: a modification of the total condylar design. Two to four-year clinical experience. J Bone Joint Surg Am. 1982;64:1317.
7. Agllietti P, Buzzi R, De Felice R, Giron F. The Insall-Burstein total knee replacement in osteoarthritis: a 10-year minimum follow-up. J Arthroplasty. 1999;14(5):560–5.
8. Hossain S, Ayeko C, Anwar M, Elsworth CF, McGee H. Dislocation of Insall-Burstein II modified total knee arthroplasty. J Arthroplasty. 2001;16(2):233–5.
9. Kavolus CH, Hummel MT, Barnett KP, Jennings JE. Comparison of the Insall-Burstein II and the NexGen legacy total knee arthroplasty systems with respect to patella complications. J Arthroplasty. 2008;23(6):822–5.
10. Mathijssen NMC, Verburg H, London NJ, Landsiedl M, Dominkus M. Patient reported outcomes and implant survivorship after total knee arthroplasty with the persona knee implant system: two year follow-up. BMC Musculoskelet Disord. 2019;20:97.
11. Argenson JNA, Scuderi GR, Komistek RD, Scott WN, Kelly MA, Aubaniac JM. In vivo kinematic evaluation and design considerations related to high flexion in total knee arthroplasty. J Biomech. 2005;38(2):277–84.
12. Stiehl JB, Komistek RD, Dennis DA, Paxson RD, Hoff WA. Fluoroscopic analysis of kinematics after posterior-cruciate-retaining knee arthroplasty. J Bone Joint Surg Br. 1995;77(6):884–9.
13. Broberg JS, Ndoja S, MacDonald SJ, Lanting BA, Teeter MG. Comparison of contact kinematics in posterior-stabilized and cruciate-retaining total knee arthroplasty at long-term follow-up. J Arthroplasty. 2020;35(1):272–7. https://doi.org/10.1016/j.arth.2019.07.046.
14. Scuderi GR, Komistek RD, Dennis DA, Insall JN. The impact of femoral component rotational alignment on condylar lift-off. Clin Orthop Relat Res. 2003;(410):148–154. https://doi.org/10.1097/01.blo.0000063603.67412.ca.
15. Yoshiya S, Matsui N, Komistek RD, Dennis DA, Mahfouz M, Kurosaka M. In vivo kinematic comparison of posterior cruciate-retaining and posterior stabilized total knee arthroplasties under passive and weight-bearing conditions. J Arthroplasty. 2005;20(6):777–83.
16. Kayani B, Konan S, Horriat S, Ibrahim MS, Haddad FS. Posterior cruciate ligament resection in total knee arthroplasty: the effect on flexion-extension gaps, mediolateral laxity, and fixed flexion deformity. Bone Joint J. 2019;101(10):1230–7.
17. Warth LC, Deckard ER, Meneghini RM. Posterior cruciate ligament resection does not consistently increase the flexion space in contemporary total knee arthroplasty. J Arthroplasty. 2021;36(3):963–9.
18. Yasgur DJ, Scuderi GR, Insall JN. Medial release for fixed-varus deformity. In: Knee arthroplasty handbook: techniques in total knee and revision arthroplasty. New York: Springer New York; 2006. p. 25–40.
19. Laurencin CT, Scott RD, Volatile TB, Gebhardt EM. Total knee replacement in severe valgus deformity. Am J Knee Surg. 1992;5(3):135–9.
20. Griffin FM, Scuderi GR, Insall JN. Lateral release for fixed-valgus deformity. In: Knee arthroplasty handbook: techniques in total knee and revision arthroplasty. New York: Springer New York; 2006. p. 41–56.
21. Conjeski JM, Scuderi GR. Lateral femoral epicondylar osteotomy for correction of fixed valgus deformity in total knee arthroplasty: a technical note. J Arthroplasty. 2018;33(2):386–90.

22. Maloney W, Schmidt R, Sculco T. Femoral component design and patellar clunk syndrome. Clin Orthop. 2003;410:199–202.
23. Clarke HD, Fuchs R, Scuderi GR, et al. The influence of femoral component design in the elimination of patellar clunk in posterior-stabilized total knee arthroplasty. J Arthroplasty. 2006;21:167.
24. Callaghan JJ, O'Rourke MR, Goetz DD, et al. Tibial post impingement in posterior-stabilized total knee arthroplasty. Clin Orthop. 2002;404:83.
25. Furman BD, Lipman J, Kligman M, Wright TM, Haas SB. Tibial post wear in posterior-stabilized knee replacements is design-dependent. Clin Orthop Relat Res. 2008;466(11):2650–5. https://doi.org/10.1007/s11999-008-0422-1.
26. Lombardi AV Jr, Mallory TH, Vaughn BK, Krugel R, Honkala TK, Sorscher M, Kolczun M. Dislocation following primary posterior-stabilized total knee arthroplasty. J Arthroplasty. 1993;8(6):633–9. https://doi.org/10.1016/0883-5403(93)90012-s.
27. Long WJ, Bryce CD, Hollenbeak CS, Benner RW, Scott WN. Total knee replacement in young, active patients: long-term follow-up and functional outcome: a concise follow-up of a previous report. J Bone Joint Surg Am. 2014;96(18):e159. https://doi.org/10.2106/JBJS.M.01259.
28. Longo UG, Ciuffreda M, Mannering N, D'Andrea V, Locher J, Salvatore G, Denaro V. Outcomes of posterior-stabilized compared with cruciate-retaining total knee arthroplasty. J Knee Surg. 2018;31(4):321–40. https://doi.org/10.1055/s-0037-1603902.

Chapter 7
Bicruciate Substituting Total Knee Arthroplasty

Peter P. Hsiue, Ryan Cheng, Jeffrey A. O'Donnell, and Steven B. Haas

Introduction

Total knee arthroplasty (TKA) continues to be an effective treatment for end-stage arthritis of the knee. However, 15–20% of patients report dissatisfaction after TKA [1–4]. Interestingly, when stratified by age groups, 15% of younger patients (<55 years old) were dissatisfied with 25% of this younger cohort reporting only moderate improvement or less [5, 6]. Given that the projected number of TKA procedures is expected to reach 1.2 million by the year 2040, there has been a persistent effort to improve perioperative factors to improve clinical outcomes [7]. One area of focus has been the implant design in TKA. Since the development of the first modern condylar TKA implant in the early 1970s, surgeons have continued to develop and refine implant designs to restore native knee kinematics and ultimately improve clinical outcomes [8]. This chapter will discuss a new type of implant design: the bicruciate substituting total knee arthroplasty (BCS TKA).

Native Knee Kinematics

In order to appreciate the unique design features that distinguish the BCS TKA, it is critical to understand the kinematics of the native knee. The knee is not a simple hinge joint. Instead, knee motion occurs via flexion-extension, rotation, pivot, and gliding movements. The kinematics that enables this complex interaction involves the three compartments of the knee: the lateral tibiofemoral compartment, the medial tibiofemoral compartment, and the patellofemoral compartment. Specifically,

P. P. Hsiue · R. Cheng · J. A. O'Donnell · S. B. Haas (✉)
Hospital for Special Surgery, New York, NY, USA
e-mail: hsiuep@hss.edu; chengr@hss.edu; odonnellj@hss.edu; haass@hss.edu

A. J. Tria Jr., G. R. Scuderi (eds.), *The Cruciate Ligaments in Total Knee Arthroplasty*, https://doi.org/10.1007/978-3-031-75992-5_7

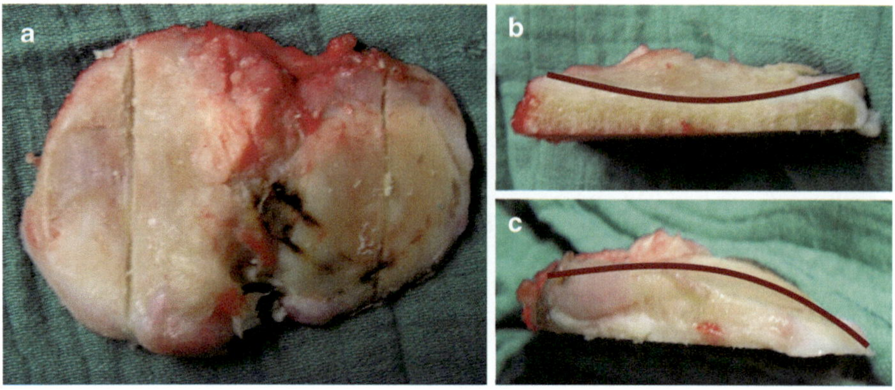

Fig. 7.1 (**a**) The articular surface of the tibia is asymmetric. (**b**) The medial tibial plateau is concave. (**c**) The lateral tibial plateau is convex

as the knee moves from extension to flexion, the medial femoral condyle remains relatively stationary and pivots on the medial tibial plateau, whereas the lateral femoral condyle travels posteriorly on the lateral tibial plateau. This lateral posterior rollback of the femur on the tibia causes the femur to externally rotate as the knee is flexed and is critical for the patella to engage the femoral trochlea and track appropriately. Furthermore, posterior rollback is critical for terminal knee flexion. As the knee continues to flex, the back of the femoral diaphysis will impinge on the tibia around 90°. However, posterior translation of the femur on the tibia increases the amount of flexion allowed prior to impingement [9].

The bony anatomy of the femur and tibia mediate the unique motion of the knee. The radii of curvature of the lateral distal and posterior femoral condyles are smaller than their medial counterparts and facilitate lateral posterior rollback. In contrast, the radii of curvature of the medial distal and posterior femoral condyles are larger which keeps the condyle in place during knee flexion. Elements of tibial plateau anatomy are also crucial for the movements of the knee. The medial tibial plateau is concave and enables the pivoting motion previously described. The lateral tibial plateau is flat, if not somewhat convex, and mediates posterior rollback of the lateral femoral condyle (Fig. 7.1) [10].

Finally, the soft tissues within the knee joint also play a critical role during knee motion. The BCS TKA attempts to substitute for both the anterior cruciate ligament (ACL) and posterior cruciate ligament (PCL). The ACL primarily functions to prevent anterior subluxation of the tibia. In addition, as the knee transitions from full extension to flexion (approximately from 15 to 30°), the ACL is active in mediating lateral femoral condyle rollback. At mid-flexion, the tension on the ACL gradually decreases and the tension at the PCL increases. This transfer of tension from the ACL to the PCL in mid-flexion prevents posterior subluxation of the tibia which enables proper posterior rollback of the femur [11].

BCS TKA Design Features

Traditional TKA implant designs, including cruciate retaining (CR) and posterior stabilized (PS) designs, do not restore native knee kinematics [12]. The CR TKA implant design retains the native PCL to prevent anterior translation of the femur during knee flexion. However, studies investigating CR TKA designs have demonstrated a paradoxical anterior femoral translation during deep knee flexion as well as a lateral pivot as the knee moves from extension to flexion [13–15]. On the other hand, PS TKA designs sacrifice the PCL during surgery and utilize a cam on the femur and a post on the tibia to engage during deep flexion (40–90°). The interaction of the cam and post pushes the femur posteriorly and mimics native posterior rollback. Studies comparing PS TKA kinematics to native knee kinematics have shown that PS TKA do exhibit posterior rollback of the femur on the tibia although the magnitude of rollback was less than that of the native knee [14, 16]. More importantly, PS TKA implants do not confer any additional constraint during early knee flexion prior to cam and post engagement. Instead, the surface geometries of the tibial liner and femoral implant are what dictate knee kinematics during this early range of motion [12]. Therefore, an improved TKA implant would have to account for the aforementioned shortcomings of previous TKA designs.

The BCS TKA implant aims to better recreate native knee kinematics via new design features such as an asymmetric bearing geometry with high sagittal conformity medially and substitutions for both the ACL and PCL. The first iteration of the BCS TKA (JOURNEY I; Smith and Nephew; Memphis, TN, USA) featured a dual cam-post design which substituted for the ACL and PCL. These features were intended to promote normal knee kinematics and increase coronal stability throughout the range of motion. The design was successful in recreating lateral rotation and posterior translation patterns of the native knee [17, 18]. The femoral component and tibial liner are asymmetric and provide a medial concave surface and a lateral convex surface which promotes a medial pivot and lateral posterior rollback, respectively (Fig. 7.2) [19]. Furthermore, the implant resting position was designed to be midline in the sagittal plane, thereby restoring the knee's normal position, optimizing musculature efficiency during range of motion, and promoting more natural patella tracking. Zambianchi et al. in their 2018 study evaluated the knee kinematics in 16 second-generation BCS TKA (JOURNEY II; Smith and Nephew; Memphis, TN, USA) using video fluoroscopy and compared the results to historical first-generation BCS TKA data. They demonstrated that the design adjustments of the second-generation BCS TKA adequately limited the excessive posterior translation of the femoral condyles while maintaining kinematics similar to those of the native knee [20].

One additional noteworthy design feature of the BCS TKA is the asymmetry of the implants in the coronal plane. Specifically, the tibial insert has a built-in 3 degrees of varus and the femoral component has a built-in 3 degrees of valgus. To understand the rationale behind these features, it is important to briefly review the new system for describing knee phenotypes, the Coronal Plane Alignment of the

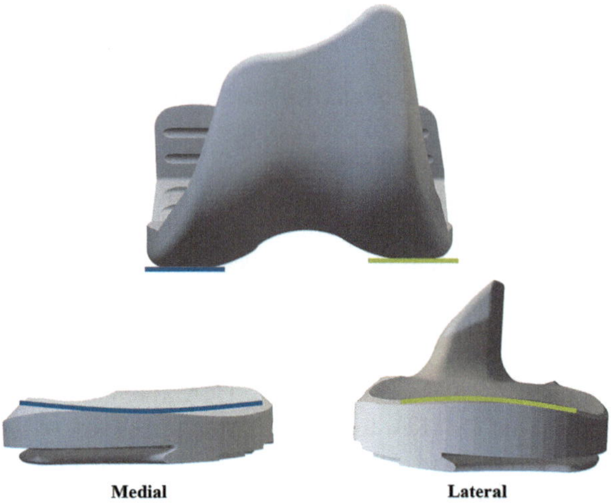

Fig. 7.2 Femoral component and tibial liner are asymmetric. The tibial liner provides a medical concave surface and lateral convex surface to facilitate medial pivot and lateral posterior rollback, respectively

Knee (CPAK), which was described in the 2021 study by MacDessi et al. [21] Their study found that >75% of patients fell within cohorts in which there was a valgus femur and a varus tibia, regardless of whether or not their overall alignment was varus, valgus, or neutral [21]. Utilization of traditional symmetric implant with bone resections that vary 3° from 90-degree cuts would recreate anatomy that only represents approximately 24% of the population based on CPAK. However, use of the BCS TKA asymmetric implant designs with the same bone resections would recreate anatomy that represents approximately 90% of the population on CPAK.

Clinical Results

Multiple studies have demonstrated that the BCS TKA exhibits overall kinematic patterns that are more similar to the native knee [11, 19, 20, 22, 23]. Victor et al. in their 2010 study evaluated the in vivo kinematics of 86 BCS TKA implanted by three different surgeons (JOURNEY I; Smith and Nephew; Memphis, TN, USA) using fluoroscopy during a weightbearing deep bend of the knee. They found that overall axial rotation patterns were similar to the native knee. Interestingly, their study showed differences in kinematic measurements between surgeons which suggests that surgical technique, specifically soft tissue management, impacts the ultimate outcome with the BCS TKA [19]. A similar study was performed using the second-generation BCS TKA. Grieco et al. in their 2018 study compared the in vivo kinematics of 40 knees which had undergone TKA with a second-generation BCS TKA implant (JOURNEY II BCS; Smith and Nephew; Memphis, TN, USA) to 10 normal asymptotic knees. Using fluoroscopy, their group was able to analyze knee kinematics throughout a range of motion. They found similar femoral rollback and axial rotation patterns from 0 to 30° and 60 to 90° and beyond. However, there was negligible anterior-posterior motion during mid-flexion (30–60°) which was attributed to the discrete nature of the dual cam-post mechanism [11]. Interestingly, LaCour et al. in their 2024 study compared the in vivo kinematics of 20 unconstrained BCS TKA versus 20 constrained BCS TKA during deep knee flexion using fluoroscopic surveillance and three-dimensional modeling. They found that both the constrained and unconstrained BCS TKA designs achieved similar, albeit slightly decreased in magnitude, amounts of lateral femoral rollback compared to the native knee. Thus, their conclusion was that the utilization of a constrained insert in a BCS TKA did not result in a kinematic conflict [24].

When compared to traditional TKA implant designs, such as PS TKA and CR TKA, the BCS TKA has demonstrated in vivo knee kinematics that were more similar to that of the native knee. Ishibashi et al. in their 2021 retrospective observational study compared in vivo knee kinematics of 17 BCS TKA (JOURNEY II BCS; Smith and Nephew; Memphis, TN, USA) to 12 PS TKA (LEGION; Smith and Nephew; Memphis, TN, USA) using fluoroscopy. Their study showed increased overall femoral external rotation of the BCS TKA compared to the PS TKA. However, despite these kinematic differences postoperative 2011 Knee Society Scores were not significantly different. They attributed the kinematic differences to the different surface geometries of the BCS TKA and PS TKA implants [25]. Ishibashi et al. performed a similar study in 2022 which compared 17 BCS TKA (JOURNEY II BCS; Smith and Nephew; Memphis, TN, USA) to 18 CR TKA (JOURNEY II CR; Smith and Nephew; Memphis, TN, USA); of note, both the BCS TKA and CR TKA implants in this study had similar surface geometries. Their study demonstrated increased posterior femoral bicondylar rollback and greater maximum flexion angle in BCS TKA versus CR TKA. The CR TKA demonstrated paradoxical anterior motion. Despite these differences in knee kinematics, there were no significant differences in postoperative 2011 Knee Society Scores [25].

The high sagittal medial conforming articular geometry that is utilized in the BCS TKA can be broadly categorized as a medial pivot (MP) TKA. Again, the conforming medial compartment attempts to limit anterior-posterior movement while allowing for more lateral compartment movement [26]. Of note, while most MP TKA designs can be cruciate retaining, cruciate sacrificing, medial pivot designs can incorporate cruciate ligament substitution as well [27]. There is limited data directly comparing the in vivo kinematics or clinical outcomes between the different types of MP TKA designs. However, kinematic studies have shown that retention of the PCL in MP TKA can improve lateral femoral rollback, but does not alter clinical outcomes [28, 29]. However, when comparing MP TKA to traditional PS or CR designs, studies have demonstrated improved in vivo kinematics and patient-reported outcomes. Specifically, Pritchett et al. in their 2011 randomized-controlled trial evaluated 440 patients who underwent staged bilateral TKA with different TKA designs. Their results showed that patients preferred a MP TKA design 76.2% of the time when compared to a standard PS TKA design and 76.0% of the time when compared to a standard CR TKA design [30]. As the popularity of MP TKA increases, it will be important to compare both in vivo kinematics between different MP TKA designs as well as evaluate corresponding clinical outcomes.

With respect to clinical outcomes, multiple studies have demonstrated that the BCS TKA is a safe and effective implant design for TKA [31]. Numerous in vivo kinematic studies have shown consistent rotation and lateral rollback that is similar to the natural knee. Clinical studies have also reported high satisfaction as well as significant improvements in pain and function. Harris et al. in their 2018 study reviewed 209 BCS TKA and evaluated radiographic, clinical, and patient-reported outcomes. They found an increase in both Knee Society Scores and patient-reported satisfaction and functional activity scores. The cumulative incidence of reoperation at 2-years was 1.48% [31]. Kosse et al. in their 2020 prospective study evaluated postoperative maximum knee flexion and patient-reported outcome scores in 62 patients who underwent TKA with a BCS TKA (JOURNEY II BCS; Smith and Nephew; Memphis, TN, USA). Their findings demonstrated postoperative maximum flexion comparable to preoperative ranges as well as improved clinical and functional outcomes in patients with increased flexion [32]. Of note, the first-generation BCS TKA implants were associated with an increased risk of iliotibial band pain as well as increased risk of tibiofemoral dislocation. Christen et al. in their 2018 retrospective study compared the complication and revision rates of the first-generation BCS TKA (JOURNEY I BCS; Smith and Nephew; Memphis, TN, USA) to the second-generation BCS TKA (JOURNEY II BCS; Smith and Nephew; Memphis, TN, USA). Their findings demonstrated decreased risk of reoperation and revision surgery in the second-generation BCS TKA patients which they attributed to the improved design of the implant [33].

Conclusion

In an effort to improve patient satisfaction after TKA, the BCS TKA implant was designed to recreate native knee kinematics. Recent studies of the new second-generation BCS TKA implant have demonstrated consistently improved knee kinematics and patient-reported outcomes. Future studies are warranted to not only evaluate the long-term outcomes of the second-generation BCS TKA, but also compare them to other popular TKA designs including CR TKA and PS TKA.

References

1. Scott CE, Howie CR, MacDonald D, Biant LC. Predicting dissatisfaction following total knee replacement: a prospective study of 1217 patients. J Bone Joint Surg Br. 2010;92(9):1253–8. https://doi.org/10.1302/0301-620X.92B9.24394.
2. Bourne RB, Chesworth BM, Davis AM, Mahomed NN, Charron KD. Patient satisfaction after total knee arthroplasty: who is satisfied and who is not? Clin Orthop Relat Res. 2010;468(1):57–63. https://doi.org/10.1007/s11999-009-1119-9.

3. Noble PC, Gordon MJ, Weiss JM, Reddix RN, Conditt MA, Mathis KB. Does total knee replacement restore normal knee function? Clin Orthop Relat Res. 2005;(431):157–165. https://doi.org/10.1097/01.blo.0000150130.03519.fb.
4. Noble PC, Conditt MA, Cook KF, Mathis KB. The John Insall Award: patient expectations affect satisfaction with total knee arthroplasty. Clin Orthop Relat Res. 2006;452:35–43. https://doi.org/10.1097/01.blo.0000238825.63648.1e.
5. Lange JK, Lee YY, Spiro SK, Haas SB. Satisfaction rates and quality of life changes following total knee arthroplasty in age-differentiated cohorts. J Arthroplasty. 2018;33(5):1373–8. https://doi.org/10.1016/j.arth.2017.12.031.
6. Weiss JM, Noble PC, Conditt MA, Kohl HW, Roberts S, Cook KF, Gordon MJ, Mathis KB. What functional activities are important to patients with knee replacements? Clin Orthop Relat Res. 2002;(404):172–188. https://doi.org/10.1097/00003086-200211000-00030.
7. Shichman I, Roof M, Askew N, Nherera L, Rozell JC, Seyler TM, Schwarzkopf R. Projections and epidemiology of primary hip and knee arthroplasty in Medicare patients to 2040-2060. JB JS Open Access. 2023;8(1):e22.00112. https://doi.org/10.2106/JBJS.OA.22.00112.
8. Ranawat CS. History of total knee replacement. J South Orthop Assoc. 2002;11(4):218–26. https://www.ncbi.nlm.nih.gov/pubmed/12597066.
9. Angerame MR, Holst DC, Jennings JM, Komistek RD, Dennis DA. Total knee arthroplasty kinematics. J Arthroplasty. 2019;34(10):2502–10. https://doi.org/10.1016/j.arth.2019.05.037.
10. Pinskerova V, Vavrik P. Chapter 14. Knee anatomy and biomechanics and its relevance to knee replacement. In: Rivière C, Vendittoli PA, editors. Personalized hip and knee joint replacement [Internet]. Cham: Springer; 2020. https://www.ncbi.nlm.nih.gov/books/NBK565765/. https://doi.org/10.1007/978-3-030-24243-5_14.
11. Grieco TF, Sharma A, Dessinger GM, Cates HE, Komistek RD. In vivo kinematic comparison of a bicruciate stabilized total knee arthroplasty and the Normal knee using fluoroscopy. J Arthroplasty. 2018;33(2):565–71. https://doi.org/10.1016/j.arth.2017.09.035.
12. Zingde SM, Slamin J. Biomechanics of the knee joint, as they relate to arthroplasty. Orthop Trauma. 2017;31(1):1–7, issn:1877–1327. https://doi.org/10.1016/j.mporth.2016.10.001.
13. Dennis DA, Komistek RD, Mahfouz MR, Walker SA, Tucker A. A multicenter analysis of axial femorotibial rotation after total knee arthroplasty. Clin Orthop Relat Res. 2004;(428):180–189. https://doi.org/10.1097/01.blo.0000148777.98244.84.
14. Dennis DA, Komistek RD, Mahfouz MR, Haas BD, Stiehl JB. Multicenter determination of in vivo kinematics after total knee arthroplasty. Clin Orthop Relat Res. 2003;(416):37–57. https://doi.org/10.1097/01.blo.0000092986.12414.b5.
15. Haas BD, Komistek RD, Stiehl JB, Anderson DT, Northcut EJ. Kinematic comparison of posterior cruciate sacrifice versus substitution in a mobile bearing total knee arthroplasty. J Arthroplasty. 2002;17(6):685–92. https://doi.org/10.1054/arth.2002.33550.
16. Mueller J, Komistek RD, Dennis DA. Kinematics of the implanted and non-implanted knee. In: Insall & Scott surgery of the knee. 5th ed. Philadelphia: Churchill Livingstone; 2012.
17. Kuroyanagi Y, Mu S, Hamai S, Robb WJ, Banks SA. In vivo knee kinematics during stair and deep flexion activities in patients with bicruciate substituting total knee arthroplasty. J Arthroplasty. 2012;27(1):122–8. https://doi.org/10.1016/j.arth.2011.03.005.
18. van Duren BH, Pandit H, Price M, Tilley S, Gill HS, Murray DW, Thomas NP. Bicruciate substituting total knee replacement: how effective are the added kinematic constraints in vivo? Knee Surg Sports Traumatol Arthrosc. 2012;20(10):2002–10. https://doi.org/10.1007/s00167-011-1796-2.
19. Victor J, Mueller JK, Komistek RD, Sharma A, Nadaud MC, Bellemans J. In vivo kinematics after a cruciate-substituting TKA. Clin Orthop Relat Res. 2010;468(3):807–14. https://doi.org/10.1007/s11999-009-1072-7.
20. Zambianchi F, Fiacchi F, Lombari V, Venturelli L, Marcovigi A, Giorgini A, Catani F. Changes in total knee arthroplasty design affect in-vivo kinematics in a redesigned total knee system: a fluoroscopy study. Clin Biomech (Bristol, Avon). 2018;54:92–102. https://doi.org/10.1016/j.clinbiomech.2018.03.014.

21. MacDessi SJ, Griffiths-Jones W, Harris IA, Bellemans J, Chen DB. Coronal plane alignment of the knee (CPAK) classification. Bone Joint J. 2021;103-B(2):329–37. https://doi.org/10.1302/0301-620X.103B2.BJJ-2020-1050.R1.
22. Catani F, Innocenti B, Belvedere C, Labey L, Ensini A, Leardini A. The Mark Coventry Award: articular contact estimation in TKA using in vivo kinematics and finite element analysis. Clin Orthop Relat Res. 2010;468(1):19–28. https://doi.org/10.1007/s11999-009-0941-4.
23. Morra EA, Rosca M, Greenwald JF, Greenwald AS. The influence of contemporary knee design on high flexion: a kinematic comparison with the normal knee. J Bone Joint Surg Am. 2008;90 Suppl 4:195–201. https://doi.org/10.2106/JBJS.H.00817.
24. LaCour MT, Dessinger GM, Haas SB, Komistek RD. In vivo weight-bearing kinematics for constrained versus traditional bicruciate stabilized total knee arthroplasty cohorts compared to the normal knee. J Arthroplasty. 2024;39(6):1589–94. https://doi.org/10.1016/j.arth.2023.11.033.
25. Ishibashi T, Tomita T, Yamazaki T, Tsuji S, Yoshikawa H, Sugamoto K. Kinematics of bicruciate and posterior stabilized total knee arthroplasty during deep knee flexion and stair climbing. J Orthop Res. 2021;39(6):1262–70. https://doi.org/10.1002/jor.24773.
26. Hamilton LD, Shelburne KB, Rullkoetter PJ, Barnes CL, Mannen EM. Kinematic performance of medial pivot total knee arthroplasty. J Arthroplasty. 2024;39(6):1595–1601.e1597. https://doi.org/10.1016/j.arth.2023.11.038.
27. Hodgeson SM, Soeno T, Mears SC, Stambough JB, Barnes CL, Stronach BM. The medial pivot design in total knee arthroplasty. Orthop Clin North Am. 2024;55(1):49–59. https://doi.org/10.1016/j.ocl.2023.06.007.
28. Miyazaki Y, Nakamura T, Kogame K, Saito M, Yamamoto K, Suguro T. Analysis of the kinematics of total knee prostheses with a medial pivot design. J Arthroplasty. 2011;26(7):1038–44. https://doi.org/10.1016/j.arth.2010.08.015.
29. Budhiparama NC, Lumban-Gaol I, Novito K, Hidayat H, De Meo F, Cacciola G, Cavaliere P. PCL retained is safe in medial pivot TKA—a prospective randomized trial. Knee Surg Sports Traumatol Arthrosc. 2023;31(12):5856–63. https://doi.org/10.1007/s00167-023-07634-2.
30. Pritchett JW. Patients prefer a bicruciate-retaining or the medial pivot total knee prosthesis. J Arthroplasty. 2011;26(2):224–8. https://doi.org/10.1016/j.arth.2010.02.012.
31. Harris AI, Luo TD, Lang JE, Kopjar B. Short-term safety and effectiveness of a second-generation motion-guided total knee system. Arthroplast Today. 2018;4(2):240–3. https://doi.org/10.1016/j.artd.2017.11.007.
32. Kosse NM, Heesterbeek PJC, Defoort KC, Wymenga AB, van Hellemondt GG. Maximal flexion and patient outcomes after TKA, using a bicruciate-stabilizing design. Arch Orthop Trauma Surg. 2020;140(10):1495–501. https://doi.org/10.1007/s00402-020-03491-7.
33. Christen B, Kopjar B. Second-generation bi-cruciate stabilized total knee system has a lower reoperation and revision rate than its predecessor. Arch Orthop Trauma Surg. 2018;138(11):1591–9. https://doi.org/10.1007/s00402-018-3019-5.

Chapter 8 Bicruciate Retaining Total Knee Arthroplasty

Alfred J. Tria Jr and Giles R. Scuderi

Introduction

Bicruciate retaining total knee arthroplasty (BCR TKA) is not a new concept and was the original intention of designers in the early 1970s [1–3]. These total knee arthroplasties (TKA) attempted to resurface the knee and retain as much of the presenting anatomy as possible. The unicondylar knee prostheses (UKA) preserved both cruciate ligaments and have continued this approach up to the present day [4–6]. The TKA is a much more difficult design to develop. The cruciate ligaments coordinate the knee range of motion (ROM) with the surface anatomy of the femur and tibia. TKA does not duplicate the exact surface anatomy of the knee and, thus, the retained cruciates are asked to function with a changed anatomical picture. If the surface anatomy of the TKA is too constrained, there can be a kinematic conflict with the retained cruciates leading to early loosening (as seen with the designs in the 1970s) [1, 2]. Unconstrained surfaces can lead to instability despite the retention of the cruciates [7]. Thus, there is a fine line of balance between cruciate ligament retention and prosthetic surface anatomy.

A. J. Tria Jr (✉)
Rutgers-Robert Wood Johnson Medical School, New Brunswick, NJ, USA

G. R. Scuderi
Zucker School of Medicine at Hofstra/Northwell, Hempstead, NY, USA

A. J. Tria Jr., G. R. Scuderi (eds.), *The Cruciate Ligaments in Total Knee Arthroplasty*, https://doi.org/10.1007/978-3-031-75992-5_8

Prosthetic Designs

The primary problem for the BCR knee is the tibial surface fixation. Preservation of the cruciates requires the maintenance of a central bone island that precludes the possibility of a stem for intramedullary fixation (Fig. 8.1). In order to improve the fixation, designers have turned to modified keels or screws (Fig. 8.2). These modifications have improved the results but require unique instrumentation with greater emphasis on surgical technique.

The Geomedic knee was designed in 1972 at The Mayo Clinic and was initially well received; however, it presented a kinematic conflict with the cruciates driving ROM and the surfaces forcing constraint [7]. The subsequent tibial loosenings discouraged surgeons and interest in cruciate retention diminished.

During the period of time from the 1980s until the year 2000, some designers maintained interest in the BCR knee and published results that were comparable to the results for the posterior stabilized and PCL retaining knees [8–10]. The surgical techniques were more challenging, and the adoption rate was not that high. However, long-term follow-up studies did report that clinical results were similar to many other designs of the same time period [11, 12].

With the introduction of robotics and computer-controlled replacements, it became evident that the kinematics of the knee replacements was often not similar to that of the native knee [13]. Correlating this with the fact that 15% of patients are dissatisfied with their replacement, some designers sought to return to designs that more closely replicated the original native knee anatomy and kinematics [14, 15].

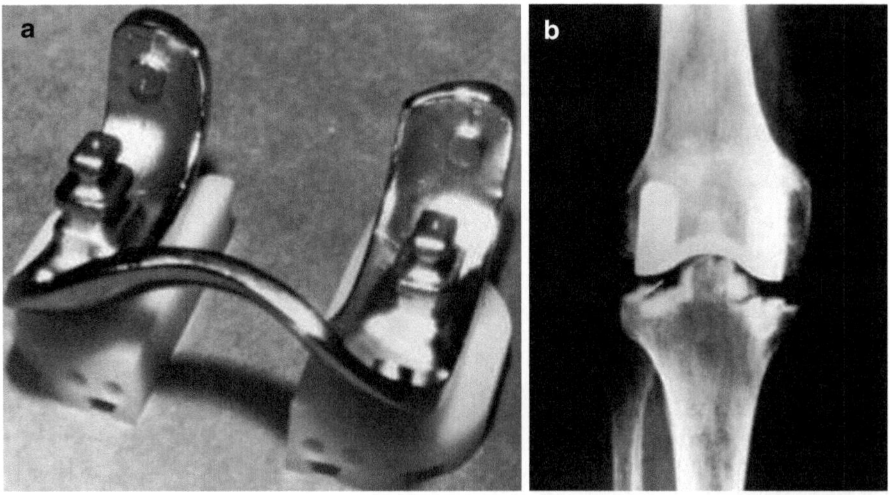

Fig. 8.1 The duocondylar knee prosthesis utilized separate medial and lateral tibial surfaces in order to preserve the cruciates. (Figure 20.5 Page 591, From Surgery of the Knee, edited by John N Insall, Churchill Livingstone, New York, 1984)

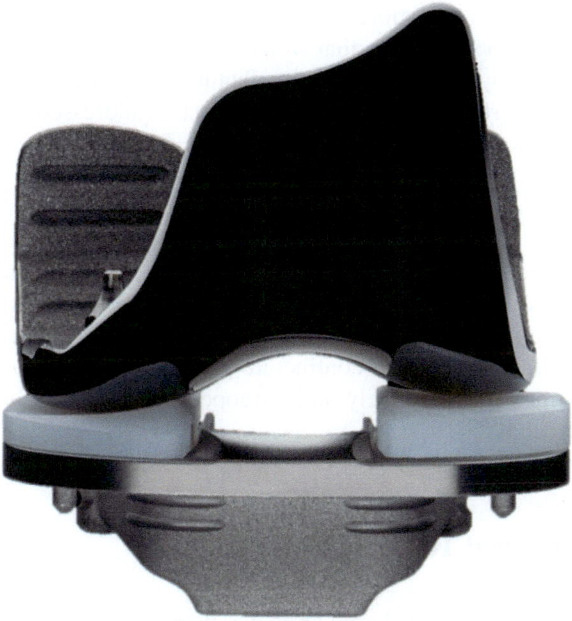

Fig. 8.2 Bicruciate retaining TKA with a tibial keel for fixation (Journey II XR Knee from Smith and Nephew)

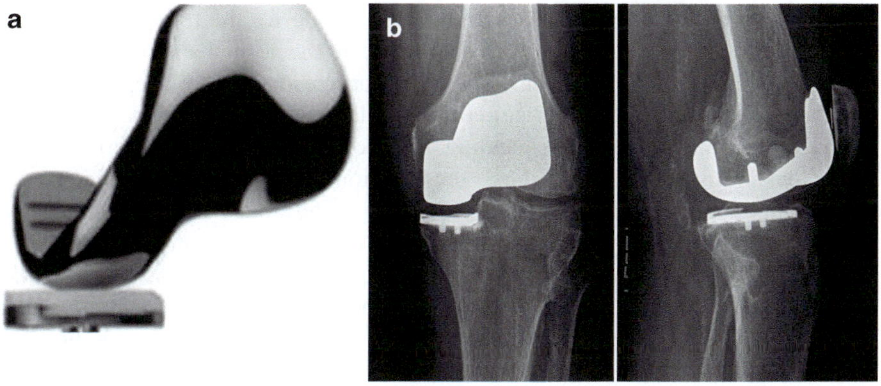

Fig. 8.3 (**a**) The arthroplasty preserved both cruciates and resurfaced the medial and patellofemoral compartments with a single piece femur (Journey Deuce Knee from Smith and Nephew). (**b**) AP and lateral X-ray of a left knee with the Journey-Deuce knee arthroplasty

Newer Designs

Thus, in the early 2000s, there was a gradual increase in interest in the BCR designs. One design group moved from the unicondylar concept to a bicompartmental knee that spared the cruciates and resurfaced the medial and patellofemoral compartments (Journey Deuce Knee Arthroplasty) [16, 17]. This was a monolithic design and had a single piece femoral component (Fig. 8.3a, b). Once again, the surgical procedure was more demanding and it was difficult to coordinate the appropriate sizing for each knee that would accommodate the two compartments. This was followed by a design that manufactured a CT-based prosthesis for each knee (iDuo Knee Arthroplasty from Conformis) that addressed the mismatch between the patellofemoral and medial compartments. The prostheses were difficult to implant and did not always match the underlying anatomy of the actual knee [18].

The attempts to preserve the cruciates led to a rebirth of the BCR knee that resurfaced all of the knee compartments and preserved both cruciates. The selection process has been modified. Patients must be well motivated with a clear understanding of the advanced rehab protocols. The BMI is limited (best <30). The ROM of the knee should be greater than 120° with no varus/valgus fixed deformity greater than 10° and no flexion contracture greater than 5°. Cruciate integrity should be confirmed preoperatively and intraoperatively with clear maintenance throughout the procedure [19].

Surgical Technique

This technique is based upon the instrumentation designed to implant the Journey II XR knee from Smith and Nephew, Memphis, Tennessee.

The surgical procedure begins with the resurfacing for the femoral component, which is anatomically designed to closely replicate the normal anatomy. The resection is carried out to remove only the bone surface that will be replaced by the prosthetic thickness with preservation of the intercondylar notch. The tibial resection is more complicated and demanding. Rotation, depth of resection, cruciate ligament tensioning, and bone island preservation must all be considered. The instruments for the resection are prosthesis specific and unique in their design (Fig. 8.4). The instrument incorporates protective pins that prevent any undercutting of the bone island. If the bone island lifts upward, it is possible to add screw fixation; but this requires thorough evaluation of the resulting cruciate stability. There are also some techniques that utilize robotically assisted instrumentation; however, they have not seen high adoption rates because of the learning curve, expense, and additional operative times. Once the tibial resection is completed, it is critical to confirm that the knee has a full range of motion without a flexion contracture or hyperextension, good medial-lateral balance, and no significant anterior or posterior laxity. With proper femoral and tibial rotation, the patella should track midline without requiring releases. Combining all of these factors can be mentally challenging and surgically demanding.

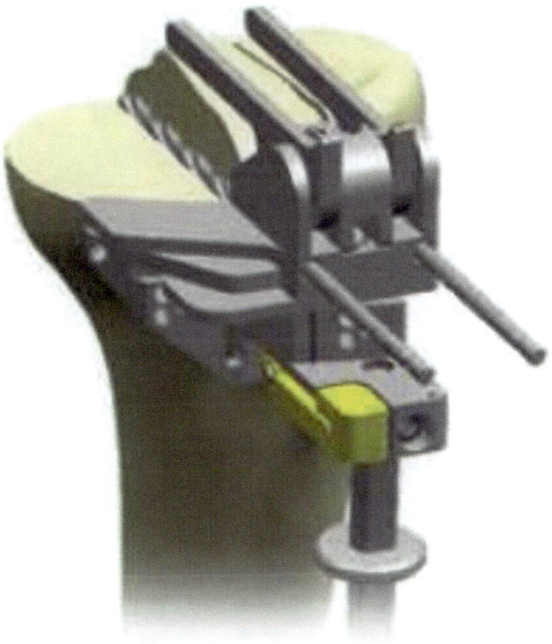

Fig. 8.4 A tibial cutting guide that protects the bone island with parallel pins (From Journey II XR Knee system, Smith and Nephew, Memphis, Tenn)

Results

In the early 2000s, two new BCR prostheses were developed (The Journey II XR Knee from Smith and Nephew, and The XP Total knee from Biomet) (Figs. 8.2 and 8.5). The early results were encouraging but only one design (The Journey II XR Knee) went on to demonstrate acceptable midterm findings (Table 8.1 lists the major BCR results reported in the literature) [23, 24, 30].

Complications

There have been reports of scarring around the cruciate ligaments (cyclops lesion) that can lead to a flexion contracture. Arthroscopic debridement of the lesion along with a manipulation has been somewhat effective in correcting this [31, 32]. There are other reports of a higher frequency of reoperation with an increased incidence of radiolucent lines [24]. Cementing the tibial component is extremely demanding because there is no central intramedullary stem. The designs incorporate either a keel or posts that do not afford the same fixation as the stemmed tibia. Intraoperative avulsion of the tibial spine can sometimes be corrected with the use of screw for

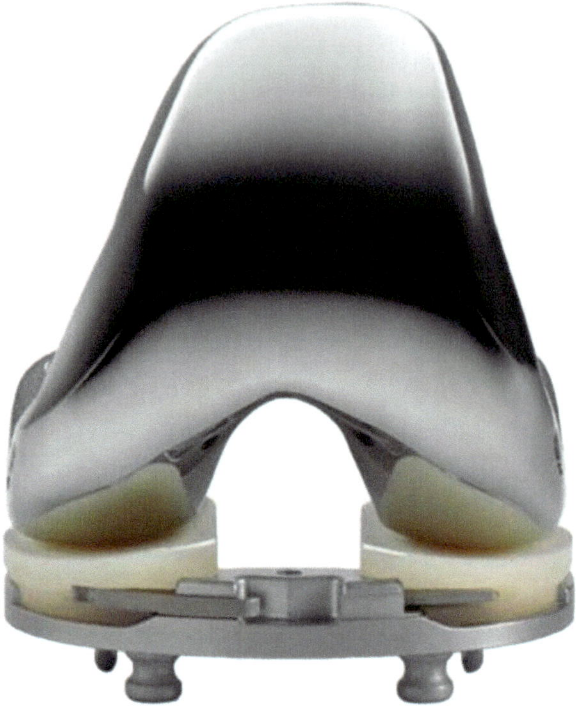

Fig. 8.5 XP cruciate retaining TKA (From Biomet)

fixation; however, if the fixation is tenuous, it is best to abandon the procedure. There is the possibility that the ACL may rupture after surgery leading to instability that can require revision.

Patients do appear to prefer the BCR knee over the PS or CR designs [33]. There is no doubt that this design requires thorough preoperative evaluation of the presenting knee. The operative procedure is different than the other approaches, and the postoperative management requires continued observation to assure good range of motion without compromising the cruciate bone island. With all of this considered, the BCR knee is probably best for a small percentage of patients with the right indications, the right attitude, and the right surgical procedure.

The question remains concerning the long-term results, the patient satisfaction, and the kinematics of the replacements [33–36]. In the future, refinements of the imaging process, kinematic correlations, and more sophisticated intraoperative controls may lead to greater use of this design with improved satisfaction and longevity.

Summary

Advantages of the BCR TKA are as follows:

Table 8.1 Major BCR results reported in the literature

Reference	Prosthesis	# Knees	Follow-up	Results
Sabouret et al. [2]	Hermes 2C (Cloutier)	163	22 years	82% survival, 4.3% aseptic loosening
Goutallier et al. [20]	Hermes (Cloutier)	41	8 years	2 loosenings
Townley [9]	Anatomic knee	532	2–11 years	2% tibial loosening 89% excellent/good
Lavoie et al. [21]	BCR	39	5 years	Equal to PS group, but 5 adverse events in BCR
Pritchett [11]	Anatomic knee	537	23 years	94% survivorship, 5.6% revised (mostly poly wear), 2 late ACL ruptures
Beuchel and Pappas [10]	Low contact stress knee, meniscal bearing	46	12 years	91% survivorship
Stiehl et al. [12]	LCS BCR	324	14 years	79% survivorship
Pelt et al. [22]	BCR	107	3 years	88% survivorship, 19 revisions, 5 tibial loosening
Eggenberger et al. [23]	XP	195	5.2 years	9.7% tibial loosening
Christensen et al. [24]	BCR Zimmer-Biomet	66	2–32 months	5% revision
Alnachoukati et al. [25]	BCR	146	1–33 months	1.4% revision 94% neutral or higher satisfaction
Pritchett [26]	BCRvsPCL	91	2–14 years	BCR vs. PCL 73.6% preferred BCR
Troelsen et al. [27]	XPvsCR	23/22	2 years	No RSA diff.no PROM diff. 1 BCR rev and 3 manipulations
Singh et al. [28]	BCR	133	2–2.87 years	6 reoperations 96.2% survivorship
Baumann et al. [29]	BCRvsUKAvsPS	34/34/34	18 months	FJS for BCR = UKA

1. Improved kinematics
2. Increased ROM
3. More rapid recovery
4. Fewer complaints of clicking or patellar clunk
5. Better patient satisfaction

Disadvantages of the BCR TKA are as follows:

1. Design is only for a limited number of patients (selection is critical)
2. Surgical technique is demanding
3. Tibial loosening and/or tibial tray breakage can be a problem
4. Cruciate ligament degeneration after the BCR may lead to revision
5. Scarring around the ACL (cyclops lesion) can lead to loss of full extension

BCR TKA is not for all knees or all surgeons. The surgical technique is more demanding than standard PCL sparing or PS TKA. If the correct knee is chosen, and the surgical procedure is well monitored, the clinical results at midterm follow-up are similar to other designs. Preservation of the presenting anatomy has always led to excellent results in all orthopedic surgeries.

References

1. Gunston FH. Polycentric knee arthroplasty. Prosthetic simulation of normal knee movement. J Bone Joint Surg Br. 1971;53(2):272–7.
2. Sabouret P, Lavoie F, Cloutier JM. Total knee replacement with retention of both cruciate ligaments: a 22-year follow-up study. Bone Joint J. 2013;95-B(7):917–22.
3. Ranawat CS, Insall J, Shine J. Duo-condylar knee arthroplasty: Hospital for Special Surgery Design. Clin Orthop Relat Res. 1976;(120):76–82.
4. Romanowski MR, Repicci JA. Minimally invasive unicondylar arthroplasty: eight year follow-up. J Knee Surg. 2002;15(1):17–22.
5. Hurst JM, Berend KR. Mobile-bearing unicondylar knee arthroplasty: the Oxford experience. Orthop Clin North Am. 2015;46(1):113–24.
6. Marmor L. Unicompartmental arthroplasty of the knee with a minimum of 10-year follow-up. Clin Orthop Relat Res. 1988;228:171–7.
7. Riley D, Woodyard E. Long-term results of geomedic total knee replacement. J Bone Joint Surg Br. 1985;67(4):548–50.
8. Sabouret P, Lavoie F, Cloutier M. Total knee replacement with retention of both cruciate ligaments: a 22-year follow-up study. Bone Joint J. 2013;95-B(7):917–22.
9. Townley CO. The anatomic total knee resurfacing arthroplasty. Clin Orthop Relat Res. 1985;(192):82–96.
10. Beuchel FF, Pappas MJ. Long-term survivorship analysis of cruciate -sparing versus cruciate sacrificing knee prostheses using meniscal bearings. Clin Orthop Relat Res. 1990;260:162–9.
11. Pritchett JW. Bicruciate-retaining total knee replacement provides satisfactory function and implant survivorship at 23 years. Clin Orthop Relat Res. 2015;473(7):2327–33.
12. Stiehl J, Hamelynck KJ, Voorhorst PE. International multi-centre survivorship analysis of mobile bearing total knee arthroplasty. Int Orthop. 2006;30:190–9.
13. Angerame MR, Holst DC, Jennings JM, Komistek RD, Dennis DA. Total knee arthroplasty kinematics. J Arthroplasty. 2019;34(10):2502–10.
14. Noble PC, Gordon MJ, Weiss JM, Reddix RN, Conditt MA, Mathis KB. Does total knee replacement restore normal knee function? Clin Orthop Relat Res. 2005;431:157–65.
15. Gunaratne R, Pratt DN, Banda J, Fick DP, Khan RJK, Robertson BW. Patient dissatisfaction following total knee arthroplasty: a systematic review of the literature. J Arthroplasty. 2017;32:3854–60.
16. Rolston L, Bresch J, Engh G, Franz A, Kreuzer S, Nadaud M, Puri L, Wood D. Bicompartmental knee arthroplasty: a bone-sparing, ligament-sparing, and minimally invasive alternative for active patients. Orthopedics. 2007;30(8 Suppl):70–3.
17. Rolston L, Siewert K. Assessment of knee alignment after bicompartmental knee arthroplasty. J Arthroplasty. 2009;24:1111–4.
18. Steinert AF, Beckmann J, Holzapfel BM, Rudert M, Arnholdt J. Bicompartmental individualized knee replacement : use of patient-specific implants and instruments (iDuo™). Oper Orthop Traumatol. 2017;29(1):51–8.
19. Tria AJ Jr. A contemporary bicruciate total knee arthroplasty. Semin Arthroplast. 2017;28:65–70.

20. Goutallier D, Manicom O, Van Driessche S. Total knee arthroplasty with bicruciate preservation: comparison versus the same posterostabilized design at eight years follow-up. Rev Chir Orthop Reparatrice Appar Mot. 2008;94(6):585–595.
21. Lavoie F, Denis A, Chergui S, Al-Shakfa F, Sabouret P. Bicruciate-retaining total knee arthroplasty non-inferior to posterior-stabilized prostheses after 5 years: a randomized, controlled trial. Knee Surg Sports Traumatol Arthrosc. 2023;31(3):1034–42.
22. Pelt CE, Sandifer PA, Gililland JM, Anderson MB, Peters CL. Mean three-year survivorship of a new bicruciate retaining total knee arthroplasty: are revisions still higher than expected? J Arthroplasty. 2019;34:1957–62.
23. Eggenberger EE, Hurst JM, Morris MJ, Berend KR, Lombardi AV, Crawford DA. Midterm outcomes of a bicruciate retaining compared with the bicruciate sacrificing knee system. J Arthroplasty. 2022;37:S2145–249.
24. Christensen JC, Brothers J, Stoddard GJ. Higher frequency of reoperation with a new bicruciate-retaining total knee arthroplasty. Clin Orthop Relat Res. 2017;475:62–9.
25. Alnachoukati OK, Emerson RH, Diaz E, Ruchaud E, Ennin KA. Modern day bicruciate-retaining arthroplasty: a short-term review of 146 knees. J Arthroplasty. 2018;33:2485–90.
26. Pritchett JW. Patients prefer a bicruciate-retaining or the medial pivot total knee prosthesis. J Arthroplasty. 2011;26(2):224–8.
27. Troelsen A, Ingelsrud LH, Thomsen MG, Muharemovic O, Otte KS, Husted H. Are there differences in micromotion on radiostereometric analysis between bicruciate and cruciate-retaining designs in TKA? Randomized controlled trial. Clin Orthop Relat Res. 2020;478(9):2045–53.
28. Singh V, Yeroushalmi D, Christensen T, Bieganowski T, Tang A, Schwarzkopf R. Early outcomes of a novel bicruciate-retaining knee system: a 2-year minimum retrospective cohort study. Arch Orthop Trauma Surg. 2023;143(1):503–9.
29. Baumann F, Krutsch W, Worlilcek M, Kerschbaum M, Zeliner J, Schmitz P, Nerlich M, Tibesku C. Reduced joint-awareness in bicruciate-retaining total knee arthroplasty. Arch Orthop Trauma Surg. 2018;138(2):273–9.
30. De Windt TS, Van Laarhoven SN, Van Hellemondt GG. Bicruciate-retaining total knee arthroplasty: state of the art for the younger and active population? A systematic review and future prospective. Appl Sci. 2022;12:10721.
31. Klaassen MA, Aikins JL. The cyclops lesion after bicruciate-retaining total knee replacement. Arthroplast Today. 2017;3(4):242–6.
32. Winston BA, Jones J, Ries MD. Flexion contracture due to cyclops lesion after bicruciate-retaining total knee arthroplasty. Arthroplast Today. 2019;5(4):442–5.
33. Pritchett JW. Patients prefer a bicruciate retaining or medial pivot knee prosthesis. J Arthroplasty. 2011;26(2):224–8.
34. Zhou C, Peng Y, An S, Bedair H, Li G. Does contemporary bicruciate retaining total knee arthroplasty restore the native knee kinematics? A descriptive literature review. Arch Orthop Trauma Surg. 2022;142(9):2313–22.
35. De Faoite D, Ries C, Foster M, Boese CK. Indications for bi-cruciate retaining total knee replacement: an international survey of 346 knee surgeons. PLoS One. 2020;15:e0234616. https://doi.org/10.1371/journal.pone.0234616.
36. Boese CK, Ebohon S, Ries C, De Faoite D. Bi-cruciate retaining total knee arthroplasty: a systematic literature review of clinical outcomes. Arch Orthop Trauma Surg. 2021;141(2):293–304.

Chapter 9
Partial Knee Arthroplasties

Todd E. Bertrand, Patricia R. Melvin, and Adolph V. Lombardi Jr

Historical Perspective

Partial knee arthroplasty, specifically as it relates to the medial side of the knee joint, has gained popularity for the treatment of end-stage anteromedial osteoarthritis (AMOA) with multiple studies showing higher patient satisfaction, quicker overall recovery, and lower risk of major medical complications compared to total knee arthroplasty (TKA) [1, 2]. However, the initial reports at the advent of medial unicompartmental knee arthroplasty (UKA) were not as promising with results inferior to total knee arthroplasty reported by multiple authors [3, 4].

Goodfellow and O'Connor were among the first to report on a large case series of medial unicompartmental knee arthroplasties with a modern prosthetic design. In their study in 1988, they looked at 103 cases of the Oxford mobile bearing medial unicompartmental arthroplasty system (Zimmer Biomet, Warsaw, IN) performed between 1982 and 1985 with 76 medial and 27 lateral compartment replacements with absence of the anterior cruciate ligament (ACL) not considered a contraindication. Absence of the posterior cruciate ligament (PCL) was not encountered. The authors noted a strong association between failure of the arthroplasty and the state of the ACL, whether intact or deficient, particularly in the medial compartment, with 4/5 (80%) of tibial components with aseptic loosening being in ACL-deficient knees. In addition, the only case of meniscal bearing dislocation noted in their series was also in a knee that was noted to be ACL deficient at the time of surgery. Their conclusion was that medial UKA with a mobile bearing prosthesis in the setting of ACL deficiency failed 10 times more frequently (21.4% vs. 2.1%) than in those knees with an intact ACL [5].

T. E. Bertrand · P. R. Melvin · A. V. Lombardi Jr (✉)
JIS Orthopedics, New Albany, OH, USA
e-mail: LombardiAV@jisortho.com

A. J. Tria Jr., G. R. Scuderi (eds.), *The Cruciate Ligaments in Total Knee Arthroplasty*, https://doi.org/10.1007/978-3-031-75992-5_9

The proposed mechanism of increased failure, specifically aseptic loosening of the tibial component, was two-fold. First, the increased force of the hamstrings exerted as a secondary restraint to anterior tibial translation in ACL deficiency is countered by an equal force exerted from the quadriceps to avoid paradoxical flexion of the knee. This increased muscle force is thought to increase contact pressures in the joint and produce overloading, possibly leading to loosening. Secondly, if the anterior tibial translation in ACL deficiency is uncompensated by hamstring action, the femoral component will edge load the tibial component, possibly leading to a rocking-type phenomena and subsequent loosening. Interestingly, in the lateral compartment, there was not an association between ACL deficiency and failure of lateral UKA.

In addition to the ACL status alone, Hernigou et al. in 2004 evaluated the effect of slope of the tibial implant in mobile bearing medial UKA comparing ACL-intact and ACL-deficient knees. In 99 patients undergoing medial UKA, at the time of implantation 50 knees had a normal appearing ACL, 31 knees had a damaged ACL, and 18 knees had complete ACL deficiency. In all, 77 knees had not been revised at final follow-up and mean anteroposterior (AP) tibial translation on weight bearing lateral radiographs was 3.7 mm with average posterior slope of the tibial implant of 4.3°. Five ruptures of the ACL were documented postoperatively after the index procedure and in all of these knees the posterior slope was greater than or equal to 13°. Interestingly, in the 18 knees implanted with known ACL deficiency, 11 were un-revised at final follow-up with average posterior tibial slope of less than 5°. However, in the 7 knees that were revised with known ACL deficiency, the posterior tibial slope was greater than 8°. The conclusion was that posterior tibial slope of greater than 7° should be avoided, particularly in ACL-deficient knees if concomitant cruciate ligament reconstruction is not performed. This work was formative in establishing early guidelines for the posterior slope of the tibial implant in both the ACL-intact and ACL-deficient knee for an optimal outcome [6].

Pathoanatomy

Anteromedial osteoarthritis, as described by Goodfellow and White, is the arthritic pattern seen in an ACL-intact knee involving the anterior and central portions of the medial tibial plateau [7]. Given that the ACL is intact the posterior tibial cartilage remains intact secondary to the tibia not having excessive anterior translation. As the knee goes into flexion, the posterior femoral condyle rolls out of the central defect on the tibia and up onto intact posterior tibial cartilage, thereby maintaining the length of the medial collateral ligament and preventing a fixed varus deformity (Fig. 9.1). However, the natural history of anteromedial osteoarthritis over time if not treated can lead to functional ACL damage, potentially from notch osteophytes that develop, thereby allowing anterior translation of the tibia and subsequent posterior tibial cartilage wear. This results in a more diffuse pattern of wear on the medial tibial plateau and patients often complain of pain as a presenting symptom

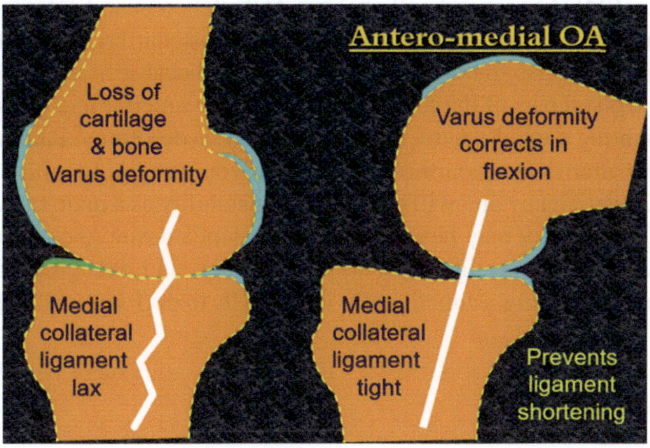

Fig. 9.1 Schematic representation of anteromedial osteoarthritis of the knee showing intact posterior cartilage on the femur and tibia as the knee goes into flexion

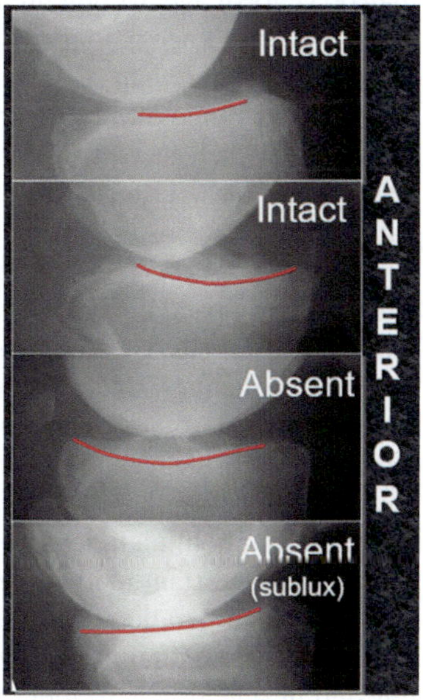

Fig. 9.2 Lateral radiographs of ACL-intact and ACL-absent knees showing translation of the femoral-tibial dwell point posteriorly

rather than instability as the soft tissue contracture along with the development of posterior and notch osteophytes provide a stability to the knee even in the setting of ACL deficiency (Fig. 9.2).

In contrast, patients who otherwise have a normal knee without signs or symptoms of osteoarthritis who develop ACL deficiency, traumatically or otherwise, and do not undergo reconstruction will oftentimes have normal appearing tibial cartilage in the anterior and central third with full thickness posterior wear secondary to anterior tibial translation. This pattern of osteoarthritis, known as posteromedial osteoarthritis (PMOA) is specifically seen in ACL-deficient and patients who do not undergo reconstruction and who had a knee void of osteoarthritis prior to the injury. In PMOA, the MCL also maintains its normal length because as the knee comes into extension, the distal part of the femur rolls onto intact anterior and central cartilage, thereby preventing medial contracture and fixed varus deformity. Patients who present with this pattern of osteoarthritis tend to be younger fitting with the traumatic nature of ACL deficiency and will tend to have instability as a main complaint rather than pain. This possibly may be related to the patient's desire to continue with high impact activities that may involve cutting, pivoting, and changing directions, all such motions that require a functionally intact ACL to perform well [8].

Criteria for UKA

Kozinn and Scott were the first to develop a standardized set of criteria for assessing patients' candidacy for UKA. These criteria involved the exclusion of patients less than 60 years of age, weight greater than 82 kg (180 lbs), absence of a bone-on-bone defect, anterior knee pain as the only presenting symptom, and cumulative angular deformity greater than 15°. Inclusion criteria for UKA were physically active patients with range of motion greater than 90°, a knee flexion contracture less than 5°, minimal pain at rest, non-inflammatory arthropathy, and an intact ACL [9]. Based upon these criteria, it has been estimated that only between 2 and 15% of patients with knee osteoarthritis (OA) would be candidates for UKA [8].

Given the rigid selection criteria of Kozinn and Scott, the criteria set forth by the Nuffield Orthopaedic Care Centre, referred to as the Nuffield criteria, for medial mobile bearing UKA were less strict and felt to be more inclusive of a greater proportion of patients with knee OA. These criteria involved bone-on-bone medial cartilage loss, anteromedial osteoarthritis with preserved posterior cartilage/bone, intact lateral cartilage, and a functionally competent ACL (Fig. 9.3) [10–12]. Despite the more relaxed nature of the Nuffield criteria compared to the original Kozinn and Scott criteria, both include a functionally intact ACL as necessary for UKA, likely owing to the substantial kinematic preservation afforded by an intact ACL.

More recent studies have looked at performing medial UKA in patients with ACL deficiency. Patient selection is key to achieving a good outcome, and an essential step in selection is to identify patients who are considered "copers" and "non-copers" [13, 14]. Patients with a history of traumatic ACL rupture without reconstruction can develop posteromedial wear leading to varus deformity with PMOA, which can be seen as posterior wear on the lateral radiograph. In contrast, patients who develop AMOA with secondary ACL disruption over time secondary to chronic anterior tibial translation and/or the development of notch osteophytes will have both anteromedial and posteromedial OA patterns showing more diffuse wear on lateral radiographs. When pain instead of knee instability is the main

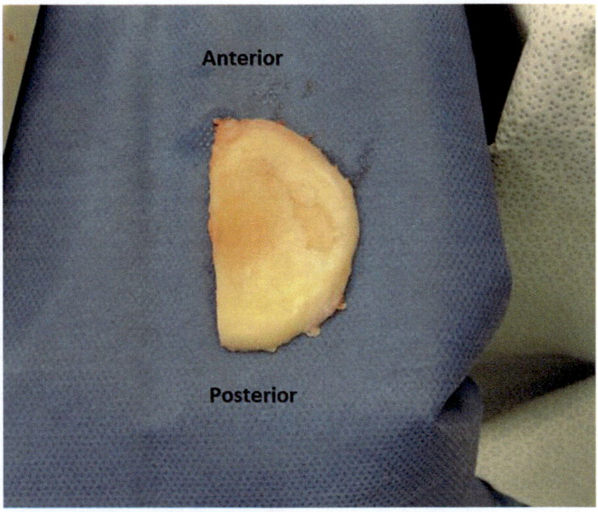

Fig. 9.3 Tibial bone specimen showing anteromedial osteoarthritis with preserved posterior tibial cartilage

symptom and other criteria for medial UKA are satisfied, medial UKA combined with or without ACL reconstruction is indicated. The decision on whether to pursue ACL reconstruction concurrently with medial UKA revolves around patient age and activity levels, with older patients or those with more sedentary lifestyles benefiting from fixed bearing medial UKA without ACL reconstruction [15, 16].

Prosthetic Design

Unicompartmental arthroplasties can be broadly divided into mobile bearing and fixed bearing as it pertains to how the polyethylene component moves (mobile bearing) or locks (fixed bearing) in relation to the tibial baseplate. Given the nature of UKA, the cruciate ligaments located centrally in the intercondylar notch and tibial eminences are not resected as part of the procedure. However, as it relates to the cruciate ligaments, specifically the ACL, preparation and placement of the tibial baseplate are paramount. Whether performing fixed or mobile bearing medial UKA, the tibial baseplate preparation revolves around maximizing medial tibial plateau coverage to distribute implant stresses across a broader area and decrease the risk of medial tibial plateau fracture and subsequent baseplate subsidence. To accomplish this, the vertical cut going anterior to posterior for baseplate preparation will involve the medial aspect of the ACL tibial eminence without causing injury to intact ACL fibers (Fig. 9.4). The design of modern-day tibial baseplates involves a metal lateral wall that will lie flush against the anterior-posterior tibial bone cut and is recessed along the proximal portion of the lateral vertical wall to avoid ACL irritation against the metal implant (Fig. 9.5).

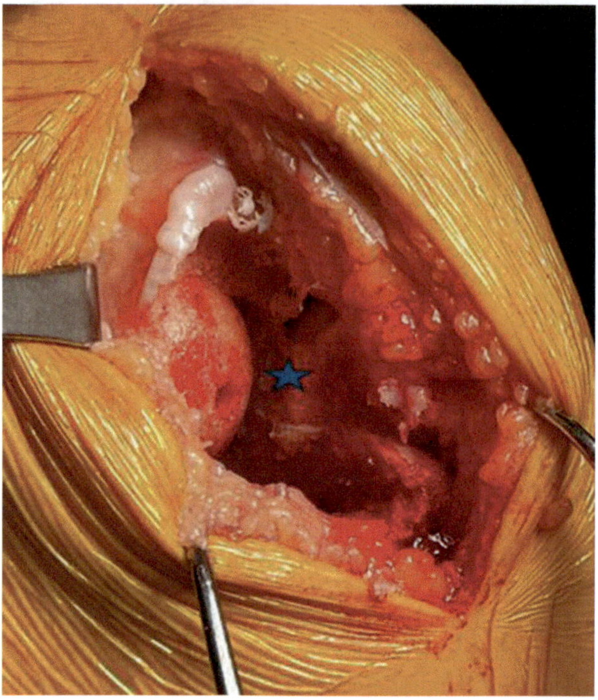

Fig. 9.4 Intraoperative image showing relationship of ACL footprint (☆) to the anterior-posterior cut along the medial tibia for baseplate preparation

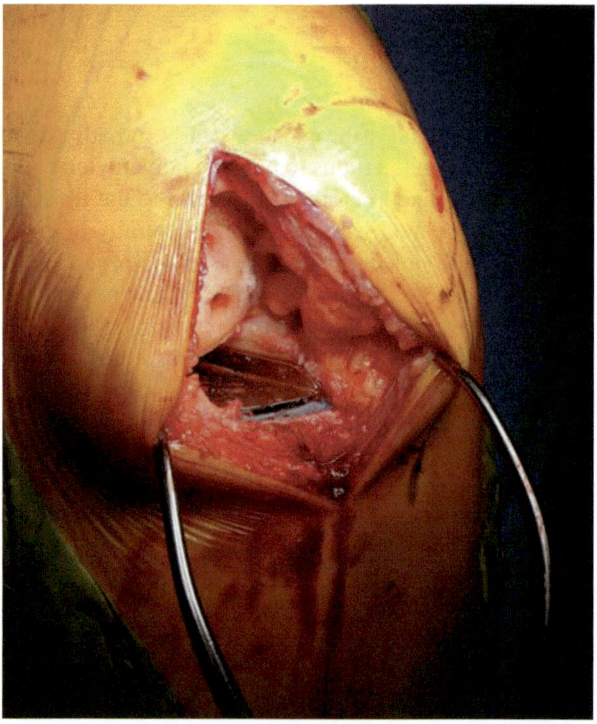

Fig. 9.5 Tibial implant of Oxford medial partial knee (Zimmer Biomet, Warsaw, IN) with the lateral wall of the implant recessed below the proximal portion of the tibia

Surgical Technique

Medial UKA with Intact ACL

The surgical technique for medial UKA will be outlined specifically as it pertains to the Oxford medial UKA (Zimmer Biomet, Warsaw, IN); however, the surgical principles, especially pertaining to tibial baseplate preparation, share similarities across all UKAs.

The patient is placed supine on a regular table either with the leg straight or on a leg-holder with the foot of the bed dropped to be perpendicular to the floor to help to obtain maximal amount of flexion for instrumentation and trialing. In the event the UKA should be aborted in favor of a TKA in the hanging-leg position, the foot of the bed can be raised and new drapes placed beneath to prevent contamination. A thigh high tourniquet should also be used to help achieve a clean, dry bone-cement interface if cementation is the chosen fixation technique. After arthrotomy, the lateral compartment and ACL should be visually inspected to confirm that the UKA is appropriate [17, 18].

Once the decision has been made to proceed with UKA, the medial tibia is exposed with care taken to ensure that no release of the medial collateral ligament is performed to avoid over correction beyond the pre-disease state of the knee. The tibial resection guide is placed and should be set to take as minimal a tibial cut as possible. The Oxford medial UKA (Zimmer Biomet, Warsaw IN) uses spoons that can minimize bone cuts based on relation to the distal posterior femoral condyles. The pins for the tibial guide should be placed away from the medial cortex and care should be taken to not perforate the far cortex with the pin. Taking multiple passes with the pin should be avoided to prevent stress risers and postoperative fracture [19].

The vertical tibial cut should be made with the saw blade perpendicular to the flexion/extension axis of the knee, coplanar with the medial tibial spine to maximize tibial coverage. One should avoid raising the saw as this will lead to a deeper posterior vertical cut which can predispose to tibial plateau fracture [20]. Alignment outside of 6° or more of varus and any degree of valgus has been shown to place increased stress on the tibial baseplate which may lead to early loosening or collapse. For similar reasons, excessive tibial slope should also be avoided [19]. Once tibial preparation is completed, the tibial baseplate should be sized to the maximal fit possible without overhanging. Undersized tibial components may lead to increased poly wear, and oversized tibial components may cause pain [20, 21]. By closely opposing the tibial baseplate to the vertical cut, one may achieve additional rotational stability.

Using an intramedullary alignment rod, the drill guide for the femoral component is connected by a coupler and centered over the femoral condyle. Drill holes are then made through the femoral drill guide both for performing the posterior femoral resection and for the use of spigots and reamers to balance the flexion and extension gaps. Once the posterior resection is completed, the distal femur is then reamed with a cylindrical reamer to convert the femoral condyle into a spherical shape to match the curvature of the femoral component. The flexion and extension gaps are then balanced within less than 1 mm of each other using gap spoons and spigots. After gap balancing is completed, the final tibial preparation is done, and trials are inserted. The femoral component is inset into the femoral condyle using an anterior recess reamer, thereby preventing any possibility of articulation with the patellofemoral joint.

Meticulous attention should be paid to handling of the cement as cement can act as a loose body and be a cause of early revision or failure [21]. Cleaning out cement from the tibia is much simpler in modular metal-backed tibia baseplates as opposed to nonmodular components where the view is obstructed by the polyethylene. Removal of excess cement and osteophytes especially posteriorly minimizes impingement of the polyethylene bearing and, thereby lessens the risks of bearing dislocation.

Medial UKA in ACL Deficiency

In patients undergoing medial UKA with ACL deficiency without plans for reconstruction, the tibial slope is reduced from the standard 7° to minimize anterior tibial translation. Otherwise, the surgery proceeds as stated above for the ACL-intact knee with maximal tibial implant coverage and adequate tension of the medial collateral ligament. An important point to remember if ACL reconstruction is not chosen is that only selective removal of notch osteophytes is warranted, as these may be providing functional stability and removal could render the knee unstable [8].

Surgical technique in patients undergoing concurrent medial UKA and ACL reconstruction differs from the technique for just medial UKA alone. In the combined technique, the anterior-posterior (AP) tibial resection should be several millimeters medial to the ACL footprint to avoid interference of the implant with the tibial tunnel for the ACL graft [22]. In contrast, the AP cut for medial UKA alone should be at the level of the ACL tibial eminence to maximize tibial baseplate coverage. In addition, the slope of the tibial implant is more anatomic and not lessened as in the ACL-deficient knee not undergoing ligament reconstruction. The femoral cuts are performed in the standard fashion [13, 23].

Tibial tunnel placement for the ACL graft is critical, and it is located immediately adjacent to the tibial tuberosity, more laterally located than in ACL reconstruction alone, to minimize risk of medial tibial plateau fracture as well as to help avoid ACL graft impingement on the implant (Fig. 9.6a, b). If a cemented UKA prosthesis is chosen, great care must be taken to avoid cement penetration into the ACL graft tunnel, as the UKA implant is typically fixated prior to ACL graft placement in the tibial tunnel. Oftentimes, a tibial reamer the same size as the graft tunnel is placed into the tunnel prior to cementation to prevent cement intrusion and after cementing

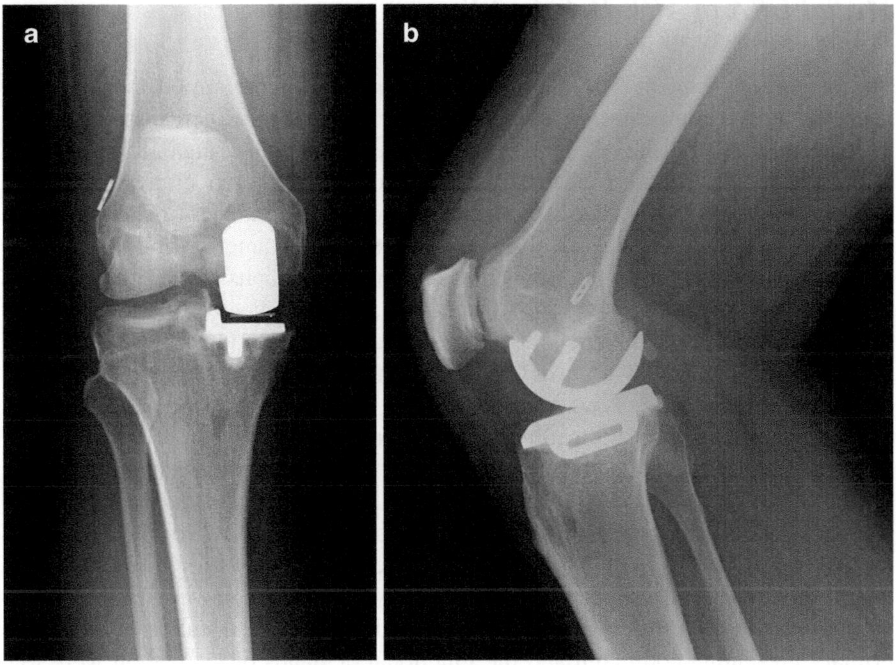

Fig. 9.6 (**a**) AP and (**b**) lateral radiograph of the right knee showing combined medial UKA and ACL reconstruction with suspensory fixation on the femoral side and interference screw fixation on the tibial side. Note the tibial tunnel placement is slightly more lateral and adjacent to the tibial baseplate of the implant

arthroscopic visualization of the tunnel can be performed to facilitate removal of any unintended cement that may be present in the tunnel [24].

Clinical Outcomes

Medial UKA in ACL-Intact Knees

Medial UKA in the setting of an intact ACL has excellent long-term survivorship with multiple registries showing results just slightly inferior to total knee arthroplasty [25, 26]. The reasons for this have been elucidated previously where survivorship may be compromised from early revision for non-pathological indications such as "physiologic" radiolucency around the tibial baseplate [27]. For pathologic indications, early revision of medial UKA predominantly involves aseptic loosening, infection, tibial plateau fracture, and bearing dislocation, in the case of mobile bearing designs [28]. Late revisions of medial UKA tend to be more for progression of OA in other compartments as well as aseptic loosening [20].

Medial UKA in ACL-Deficient Knees

The outcomes of medial UKA in ACL deficiency are more varied than in those knees with ACL competency. Deschamps et al. found that the inclusion of measuring anterior tibial translation on preoperative lateral weight bearing radiographs was important for determining whether patients would have better clinical outcomes following medial UKA. In their study, they found an approximately 25% failure rate among 79 medial UKAs in ACL-deficient knees and that anterior tibial translation of greater than 10 mm on lateral weight bearing radiographs had a higher rate of failure at a minimum follow-up of 60 months, likely indicative of excessive AP instability from ACL deficiency [29]. In a separate study, Goodfellow et al. showed a high failure rate in 28 ACL-deficient patients undergoing medial UKA with a mobile bearing prosthesis, with most failures being related to eccentric or edge loading of the tibial implant leading to aseptic loosening [5].

Mancuso et al. noted a significantly higher failure rate in patients undergoing medial UKA without ACL reconstruction (12.3%) versus those patients who received a combined procedure with ACL reconstruction (3.7%). The most common reasons for failure in the UKA alone group were tibial loosening, progression of lateral OA, pain, and weight bearing instability, with most converted to TKA for definitive management. However, it was concluded that if AP instability was not the primary presenting complaint and the functional demands of the patient were low such as in elderly individuals, then fixed bearing medial UKA can produce good clinical results with low complication rates, but patient selection is paramount [30].

Similarly, in a recent meta-analysis, Du et al., evaluated 8 studies with a mean age of 66 years and mean follow-up of 6.9 years and found that patients in both ACL-deficient and ACL-intact groups improved in clinical scores postoperatively without a significant difference in revision or complication rates. They concluded that ACL-deficient patients undergoing medial UKA without ligament reconstruction can achieve clinical scores and low revision rates similar to ACL-intact patients, especially among middle-aged and elderly individuals [31].

The role of posterior tibial implant slope has been previously evaluated by Suero et al., in a cadaveric model where leveling of the posterior tibial slope close to neutral by a reduction of around 8° correlated with around 5 mm of anterior tibial translation on Lachman testing which was found to be close to physiologic in the ACL-intact knee. Thus, it was recommended to reduce posterior tibial slope in ACL-deficient knees to aid in AP stability [32]. Historically, this was seen by Hernigou and Deschamps with a posterior tibial slope of greater than 7° in a fixed bearing medial UKA showing a substantial increase in rates of aseptic loosening [6]. However, while Plancher et al. did find that posterior tibial slope greater than 7° led to higher postoperative pain, they did not find any effect on revision to TKA [33].

Plancher et al. described pes anserine bursitis as a temporary complication following UKA in ACL-deficient knees without reconstruction. This is secondary to the compensatory pull of the hamstring tendons to help minimize anterior tibial translation and usually occurred within a few weeks of surgery. The time course in most patients was found to be limited with treatment consisting of corticosteroid injections into the pes anserine bursa if needed and most cases resolving by 6 months postoperatively [13].

Medial UKA and Combined ACL Reconstruction

Pandit et al. have proposed an algorithm for treatment of patients with medial UKA and ACL reconstruction in one or two steps depending on their initial presenting complaint. If pain is the main presenting complaint, then medial UKA and ACL reconstruction are performed in the same surgical procedure, whereas if instability in the main complaint, then ACL reconstruction is performed with medial UKA reserved for only those situations in which pain persists or worsens after ACL reconstruction and is attributable to end-stage AMOA [15].

Legnani et al. evaluated 12 patients with end-stage medial compartment OA and ACL deficiency who were felt to be candidates for medial UKA with combined ACL reconstruction and compared clinical outcomes and radiological results to a match set of 26 patients undergoing TKA. At 10-year follow-up, there was no difference in patient-reported outcome measures between groups and no notable differences in radiographic assessment including implant loosening or pathologic radiolucent lines. Given this, the authors concluded that medial UKA with ACL reconstruction is comparable to TKA at long-term follow-up regarding both clinical and radiographic outcomes with no increased risk of complications seen [34].

Similarly, Jaber et al. evaluated 23 knees that underwent combined medial UKA with the Oxford mobile bearing prosthesis (Zimmer Biomet, Warsaw, IN) with an average 10-year follow-up. All clinical outcome scores showed significant improvement over pre-operative values with estimated implant survivorship of 91.4% at 14.5 years with only 2 revisions noted for trauma and progression of lateral knee OA. The authors concluded that medial UKA combined with ACL reconstruction is an effective treatment option for patients with ACL deficiency and medial compartment OA [35].

In terms of fixed bearing vs. mobile bearing design, there is limited data to suggest superiority of one over the other in the setting of medial UKA with ACL reconstruction. Although the majority of the literature for this combined surgery has been done with mobile bearing designs, Kurien et al. evaluated 24 patients undergoing combined ACL reconstruction and fixed bearing medial UKA with the Physica ZUK prosthesis (Lima Corporate, Udine Italy) with a mean follow-up of 5.1 years and showed excellent clinical and radiographic outcomes with no revisions performed during the study period [36]. Similarly in a retrospective study performed by Tecame et al. looking at 2 groups of patients who underwent combined ACL reconstruction and medial UKA, 9 patients with mobile bearing prostheses and 14 patients with fixed bearing designs, there was no difference seen in clinical outcomes of implant loosening at most recent follow-up [37].

Medial UKA in PCL Deficiency

Although less has been published on the role of posterior cruciate ligament (PCL) deficiency and the survivorship of medial UKA, it has been generally believed that an intact PCL is necessary for long-term survivorship of the implant. Prior finite element analysis by Lee et al. has shown that in simulated patient models of PCL-deficient patients undergoing medial UKA, AP translation significantly increased at high-flexion angles and the contact stresses in the patellofemoral joint and articular cartilage increased significantly in the setting of PCL deficiency. Based upon this, it has been proposed that performing UKA in patients with PCL deficiency may increase the risk of prosthesis wear, loosening, and progression of OA in other knee compartments [38]. There has been one case report of a patient undergoing combined PCL reconstruction with medial UKA with good clinical and functional outcomes at early follow-up [39].

However, a retrospective study by Li et al. looked at the outcome of mobile bearing medial UKA performed in 9 patients with PCL deficiency with an average patient age of 51 years and follow-up of 6 years. They found 8 out of 9 patients had good to excellent clinical outcomes based on the Oxford Knee Score with only 1 revision for bearing dislocation performed 9 years after the index procedure. Despite the overall positive outcomes, the number of patients was small and surgical indications were poorly defined; therefore, no firm recommendations could be made. The authors concluded that PCL deficiency should continue to be a relative contraindication to medial UKA; however, more studies are needed with larger numbers to determine whether patients with PCL deficiency can benefit from medial UKA [40].

Summary

Partial knee arthroplasty, specifically medial UKA for treatment of end-stage AMOA, has historically been dependent upon having intact cruciate ligaments secondary to early studies showing an increased rate of aseptic loosening of the tibial baseplate in the setting of cruciate ligament deficiency. Current implant design has allowed for preservation of the ACL as well as minimal impingement to maximize normal kinematic motion of the knee. The surgical technique attempts to maximize tibial baseplate coverage of the medial tibial plateau in ACL-intact knees while attempting to maintain posterior tibial slope of approximately 7°. In patients with ACL-deficient knees who are undergoing medial UKA with combined ACL reconstruction, the tibial baseplate is shifted medially to allow for tibial tunnel placement for the ACL graft, with graft fixation occurring after implant placement, and in patients with knees not undergoing ACL reconstruction, tibial slope is minimized to decrease excessive AP translation.

Early clinical studies of medial UKA in ACLdeficient knees and less so in PCL-deficient knees not undergoing concomitant reconstruction have shown increased rates of failure and need for revision surgery secondary to implant loosening on the tibial side. However, more recent studies have shown that proper patient selection is of paramount importance with less active or elderly patients having acceptable clinical and radiographic outcomes with medial UKA alone without undergoing cruciate ligament reconstruction. Combined medial UKA and ACL reconstruction has been shown to have excellent clinical and radiographic long-term follow-up and comparable to matched patients undergoing TKA.

References

1. Pongcharoen B, Liengwattanakol P, Boontanapibul K. Comparison of functional recovery between unicompartmental and total knee arthroplasty: a randomized controlled trial. J Bone Joint Surg Am. 2023;105(3):191–201. https://doi.org/10.2106/JBJS.21.00950.
2. Suarez JC, Saxena A, Arguelles W, Watson Perez JM, Ramamoorthy V, Hernandez Y, Osondu CU. Unicompartmental knee arthroplasty vs total knee arthroplasty: a risk-adjusted comparison of 30-day outcomes using National Data from 2014 to 2018. Arthroplast Today. 2022;17:114–9. https://doi.org/10.1016/j.artd.2022.06.017.
3. Mallory TH, Danyi J. Unicompartmental total knee arthroplasty. A five- to nine-year follow-up study of 42 procedures. Clin Orthop Relat Res. 1983;(175):135–8.
4. Insall J, Aglietti P. A five to seven-year follow-up of unicondylar arthroplasty. J Bone Joint Surg Am. 1980;62(8):1329–37.
5. Goodfellow JW, Kershaw CJ, Benson MK, O'Connor JJ. The Oxford knee for unicompartmental osteoarthritis. The first 103 cases. J Bone Joint Surg Br. 1988;70(5):692–701. https://doi.org/10.1302/0301-620X.70B5.3192563.
6. Hernigou P, Deschamps G. Posterior slope of the tibial implant and the outcome of unicompartmental knee arthroplasty. J Bone Joint Surg Am. 2004;86(3):506–11. https://doi.org/10.2106/00004623-200403000-00007.
7. White SH, Ludkowski PF, Goodfellow JW. Anteromedial osteoarthritis of the knee. J Bone Joint Surg Br. 1991;73(4):582–6. https://doi.org/10.1302/0301-620X.73B4.2071640.
8. Adravanti P, Budhiparama NC, Berend KR, Thienpont E. ACL-deficient knee and unicompartmental OA: state of the art. J ISAKOS. 2017;2(3):162–70.
9. Kozinn SC, Scott R. Unicondylar knee arthroplasty. J Bone Joint Surg Am. 1989;71(1):145–50.
10. Cartier P, Sanouiller JL, Grelsamer RP. Unicompartmental knee arthroplasty surgery. 10-year minimum follow-up period. J Arthroplasty. 1996;11(7):782–8. https://doi.org/10.1016/s0883-5403(96)80177-x.
11. van der List JP, McDonald LS, Pearle AD. Systematic review of medial versus lateral survivorship in unicompartmental knee arthroplasty. Knee. 2015;22(6):454–60. https://doi.org/10.1016/j.knee.2015.09.011.
12. Yoshida K, Tada M, Yoshida H, Takei S, Fukuoka S, Nakamura H. Oxford phase 3 unicompartmental knee arthroplasty in Japan—clinical results in greater than one thousand cases over ten years. J Arthroplasty. 2013;28(9 Suppl):168–71. https://doi.org/10.1016/j.arth.2013.08.019.
13. Plancher KD, Dunn AS, Petterson SC. The anterior cruciate ligament-deficient knee and unicompartmental arthritis. Clin Sports Med. 2014;33(1):43–55. https://doi.org/10.1016/j.csm.2013.08.006.

14. Daniel DM, Stone ML, Dobson BE, Fithian DC, Rossman DJ, Kaufman KR. Fate of the ACL-injured patient. A prospective outcome study. Am J Sports Med. 1994;22(5):632–44. https://doi.org/10.1177/036354659402200511.
15. Pandit H, Beard DJ, Jenkins C, Kimstra Y, Thomas NP, Dodd CA, Murray DW. Combined anterior cruciate reconstruction and Oxford unicompartmental knee arthroplasty. J Bone Joint Surg Br. 2006;88(7):887–92. https://doi.org/10.1302/0301-620X.88B7.17847.
16. Weston-Simons JS, Pandit H, Jenkins C, Jackson WF, Price AJ, Gill HS, Dodd CA, Murray DW. Outcome of combined unicompartmental knee replacement and combined or sequential anterior cruciate ligament reconstruction: a study of 52 cases with mean follow-up of five years. J Bone Joint Surg Br. 2012;94(9):1216–20. https://doi.org/10.1302/0301-620X.94B9.28881.
17. Hurst JM, Berend KR. Mobile-bearing unicondylar knee arthroplasty: the Oxford experience. Orthop Clin North Am. 2015;46(1):113–24. https://doi.org/10.1016/j.ocl.2014.09.007.
18. Morris MJ, Frye BM, Ekpo TE, Berend KR. Unicompartmental knee replacement with new Oxford instruments. Oper Tech Orthop. 2012;22(4):189–95. https://doi.org/10.1053/j.oto.2012.11.003.
19. Crawford DA, Berend KR, Lombardi AV. Management of the failed medial unicompartmental knee arthroplasty. J Am Acad Orthop Surg. 2018;26(20):e426–33. https://doi.org/10.5435/JAAOS-D-17-00107.
20. van der List JP, Zuiderbaan HA, Pearle AD. Why do medial unicompartmental knee arthroplasties fail today? J Arthroplasty. 2016;31(5):1016–21. https://doi.org/10.1016/j.arth.2015.11.030.
21. Ghosh P, Mohammad HR, Martin B, Campi S, Murray DW, Mellon SJ. Low polyethylene creep and wear following mobile-bearing unicompartmental knee replacement. Knee Surg Sports Traumatol Arthrosc. 2021;29(10):3433–42. https://doi.org/10.1007/s00167-020-06243-7.
22. Krishnan SR, Randle R. ACL reconstruction with unicondylar replacement in knee with functional instability and osteoarthritis. J Orthop Surg Res. 2009;4:43. https://doi.org/10.1186/1749-799X-4-43.
23. Engh GA, Ammeen DJ. Unicondylar arthroplasty in knees with deficient anterior cruciate ligaments. Clin Orthop Relat Res. 2014;472(1):73–7. https://doi.org/10.1007/s11999-013-2982-y.
24. Adravanti P. Unicompartmental knee replacement with ACL reconstruction. In: Insall & Scott surgery of the knee, 6th ed. Elsevier; 2016.
25. Australian. Australian Orthopaedic Association: National Joint Replacement Registry Hip and Knee Arthroplasty annual report 2012; 2012.
26. The National Joint Registry. NJR 11th annual report; 2014.
27. Kennedy JA, Palan J, Mellon SJ, Esler C, Dodd CAF, Pandit HG, Murray DW. Most unicompartmental knee replacement revisions could be avoided: a radiographic evaluation of revised Oxford knees in the National Joint Registry. Knee Surg Sports Traumatol Arthrosc. 2020;28(12):3926–34. https://doi.org/10.1007/s00167-020-05861-5.
28. Vasso M, Antoniadis A, Helmy N. Update on unicompartmental knee arthroplasty: current indications and failure modes. EFORT Open Rev. 2018;3(8):442–8. https://doi.org/10.1302/2058-5241.3.170060.
29. Deschamps G, Lapeyre B. [Rupture of the anterior cruciate ligament: a frequently unrecognized cause of failure of unicompartmental knee prostheses. Apropos of a series of 79 Lotus prostheses with a follow-up of more than 5 years]. Rev Chir Orthop Reparatrice Appar Mot. 1987;73(7):544–551.
30. Mancuso F, Dodd CA, Murray DW, Pandit H. Medial unicompartmental knee arthroplasty in the ACL-deficient knee. J Orthop Traumatol. 2016;17(3):267–75. https://doi.org/10.1007/s10195-016-0402-2.
31. Du G, Qiu H, Zhu J, Wang H, Xiao Q, Zhang Z, Lin X, Zheng G. No difference unicompartmental knee arthroplasty for medial knee osteoarthritis with or without anterior cruciate ligament deficiency: a systematic review and meta-analysis. J Arthroplasty. 2023;38(3):586–593.e1. https://doi.org/10.1016/j.arth.2022.10.018.
32. Suero EM, Citak M, Cross MB, Bosscher MR, Ranawat AS, Pearle AD. Effects of tibial slope changes in the stability of fixed bearing medial unicompartmental arthroplasty in ante-

rior cruciate ligament deficient knees. Knee. 2012;19(4):365–9. https://doi.org/10.1016/j.knee.2011.07.004.

33. Plancher KD, Shanmugam JP, Brite JE, Briggs KK, Petterson SC. Relevance of the tibial slope on functional outcomes in ACL-deficient and ACL intact fixed-bearing medial unicompartmental knee arthroplasty. J Arthroplasty. 2021;36(9):3123–30. https://doi.org/10.1016/j.arth.2021.04.041.
34. Legnani C, Borgo E, Macchi V, Terzaghi C, Ventura A. Unicompartmental knee replacement combined with anterior cruciate ligament reconstruction provides comparable results to total knee replacement with no increased risk of complications. SICOT J. 2024;10:10. https://doi.org/10.1051/sicotj/2024005.
35. Jaber A, Kim CM, Barié A, Streit M, Schmitt H, Clarius M, Merle C, Bangert Y. Combined treatment with medial unicompartmental knee arthroplasty and anterior cruciate ligament reconstruction is effective on long-term follow-up. Knee Surg Sports Traumatol Arthrosc. 2023;31(4):1382–7. https://doi.org/10.1007/s00167-022-07102-3.
36. Kurien T, Stragier B, Senevirathna S, Geutjens G. Excellent outcomes with combined single stage Physica ZUK medial unicompartment knee replacement and anterior cruciate ligament reconstruction results in young, active patients with instability and osteoarthritis with a mean follow up of 5 years. Knee. 2022;36:114–9. https://doi.org/10.1016/j.knee.2022.04.008.
37. Tecame A, Savica R, Rosa MA, Adravanti P. Anterior cruciate ligament reconstruction in association with medial unicompartmental knee replacement: a retrospective study comparing clinical and radiological outcomes of two different implant design. Int Orthop. 2019;43(12):2731–7. https://doi.org/10.1007/s00264-019-04341-x.
38. Lee JA, Koh YG, Kim PS, Kang KW, Kwak YH, Kang KT. Biomechanical effect of tibial slope on the stability of medial unicompartmental knee arthroplasty in posterior cruciate ligament-deficient knees. Bone Joint Res. 2020;9(9):593–600. https://doi.org/10.1302/2046-3758.99.BJR-2020-0128.R1.
39. Zheng T, Du L, Chu Z, Li L, Li B, Zhang B, Li X, Liu P, Lu Q. Unicompartmental knee arthroplasty combined with posterior cruciate ligament reconstruction: a case report. BMC Musculoskelet Disord. 2024;25(1):370. https://doi.org/10.1186/s12891-024-07492-0.
40. Li P, Kennedy J, Mohammad HR, Pang Z, Mellon S, Jackson W, Price A, Dodd C, Murray D. Acceptable outcomes with unicompartmental knee replacement and PCL deficiency are achievable: a case series of nine patients. Knee Surg Sports Traumatol Arthrosc. 2021;29(10):3272–8. https://doi.org/10.1007/s00167-020-06112-3.

Part IV
Surgical Techniques

Chapter 10
Kinematic Approach

Alexander J. Nedopil, Sahil A. Sanghavi, Stephen M. Howell, and Maury L. Hull

Introduction

This book chapter begins by defining kinematically aligned (KA) total knee arthroplasty and briefly outlining its advantages. Next, the chapter describes the salient surgical steps of KA TKA, including an accuracy comparison between manual and robotic instrumentation. The section describing the tibial resection includes a method on how to preserve the tibial PCL insertion. Following the tibial resection, the chapter guides the surgeon through the three balancing steps that kinematically align a TKA, including using the insert goniometer, which helps the surgeon identify the optimal insert thickness. Next, the chapter reviews biomechanical and clinical studies, which conclude that an insert with medial 1:1 ball-in-socket conformity can provide anterior-posterior stability, thus replicating anterior cruciate ligament function. Least, a summary of in vivo evidence shows that the only conditions that restore native external tibial orientation (i.e., screw-home) in extension and internal

A. J. Nedopil (✉)
Department of Orthopaedic Surgery, König-Ludwig-Haus, University of Würzburg, Würzburg, Germany

S. A. Sanghavi
Department of Arthroplasty, Sancheti Institute for Orthopaedics and Rehabilitation, Pune, India

S. M. Howell
Department of Biomedical Engineering, University of California at Davis, Davis, CA, USA

M. L. Hull
Department of Biomedical Engineering, University of California at Davis, Davis, CA, USA

Department of Mechanical Engineering, University of California at Davis, Davis, CA, USA

Department of Orthopaedic Surgery, University of California at Davis, Davis, CA, USA
e-mail: mlhull@ucdavis.edu

A. J. Tria Jr., G. R. Scuderi (eds.), *The Cruciate Ligaments in Total Knee Arthroplasty*, https://doi.org/10.1007/978-3-031-75992-5_10

tibial orientation at 90° flexion are the combination of KA, which resurfaces the patient's pre-arthritic knee without releasing ligaments, and an insert with a medial 1:1 ball-in-socket and a lateral flat articular surface along with PCL retention.

Definition and Advantages of Kinematically Aligned Total Knee Arthroplasty

Kinematically aligned (KA) total knee arthroplasty resurfaces the patient's pre-arthritic knee to restore the articular surfaces, limb alignment, and joint line obliquity. Using components that restore the articular surface geometry and soft tissue constraints of the native knee, these steps align the knee's three kinematic axes with the axes of the femoral and tibial components [1–3]. Resurfacing the pre-arthritic knee retains the native resting lengths of the collateral ligaments and the posterior cruciate ligament (PCL), thus eliminating the need for their release [4].

The high long-term implant survival rates at 7, 13, and 16 years after KA TKA are comparable to or higher than survival rates after mechanically aligned TKA [5–7]. Furthermore, radio-stereometric analysis (RSA) of tibial baseplate migration after unrestricted kinematically aligned TKA with posterior cruciate ligament (PCL) retaining components has shown that the risk of tibial baseplate loosening at 1 and 2 years is low and comparable to or less than mechanically aligned TKA, even up to 9° of varus alignment [8–10]. The high Forgotten Joint Scores (FJS) and Oxford Knee Scores (OKS) and the restoration of native knee medial and lateral tibial compartment forces can encourage surgeons to explore the advantages of resurfacing the patient's pre-arthritic knee, thus avoiding costly and time-consuming physical therapy, and enabling early functional recovery [1, 11–17].

Performing the KA TKA Surgical Technique While Preserving the PCL with Manual Instruments and Caliper Measurements Offers Greater Accuracy than Robotics

Because KA resurfaces the knee by matching the resection thickness of the distal and posterior femoral condyles to the thickness of the femoral component, KA TKA is a surgery based on millimeter measurements and not angular measurements.

Surgical Steps for Resurfacing the Pre-Arthritic Femur with Manual Instruments and Four Caliper Measurements

The surgeon relies on four caliper measurements of the femoral resections to verify that the femoral component resurfaces the patient's pre-arthritic articular surface (Fig. 10.1). After inspection of the distal and posterior femoral condyles, partially worn cartilage is removed to expose subchondral bone. Worn cartilage is compensated with augments that reduce the thickness of the resected condyle by 2 mm [18] (Fig. 10.2). After the caliper measurement of the resected condyle, each femoral resection is corrected so that its thickness equals that of the condyle of the femoral component after compensating 2 mm for cartilage loss and 1 mm for the kerf made by the saw blade to limit deviations from the pre-arthritic distal and posterior femoral articular surfaces to within 0 ± 0.5 mm [19].

Accuracy with Manual Instruments

Two studies that used manual instruments to perform KA TKA reported that the most inaccurate distal and posterior medial femoral resections deviated from 0.9 mm over-resection to a −1.5 mm under-resection [20, 21]. These studies also reported the effect of surgeons' experience and the learning curve of performing KA TKA accurately, which was negligible. Three studies that used robotic instrumentation to perform mechanically aligned TKA reported the most inaccurate distal and posterior medial femoral resections deviated from a 2.3 mm over-resection to a −0.9 mm under-resection [22–24]. These deviations due to inaccuracy can be devastating because 1 mm or more over-resections from the medial pre-arthritic femoral articular surface worsen the FJS (100 best, 0 worst) and OKS (48 best, 0 worst) by a minimum of 31 and 7 points [25].

Surgical Steps for Resurfacing the Pre-Arthritic Tibia with Manual Instruments and Four Caliper Measurements

To set the proximal tibia parallel to the patient's pre-arthritic varus-valgus (V-V) orientation and medial tibial slope, the surgeon first sets the tibial resection guide 8 mm distal to the tibial articular surface and parallel to its V-V orientation after visually compensating for cartilage and bone wear. Next, they set an angle wing, inserted through the tibial guide's medial slot, parallel to the patient's pre-arthritic slope. When stabilizing the tibial resection guide to the bone the surgeon adjusts the I-E orientation of the guide to match the anterior-posterior axis of the oval-shaped lateral tibial plateau. After performing the proximal tibial resection, two caliper measurements verify that the tibial resection sets the tibial component's V-V

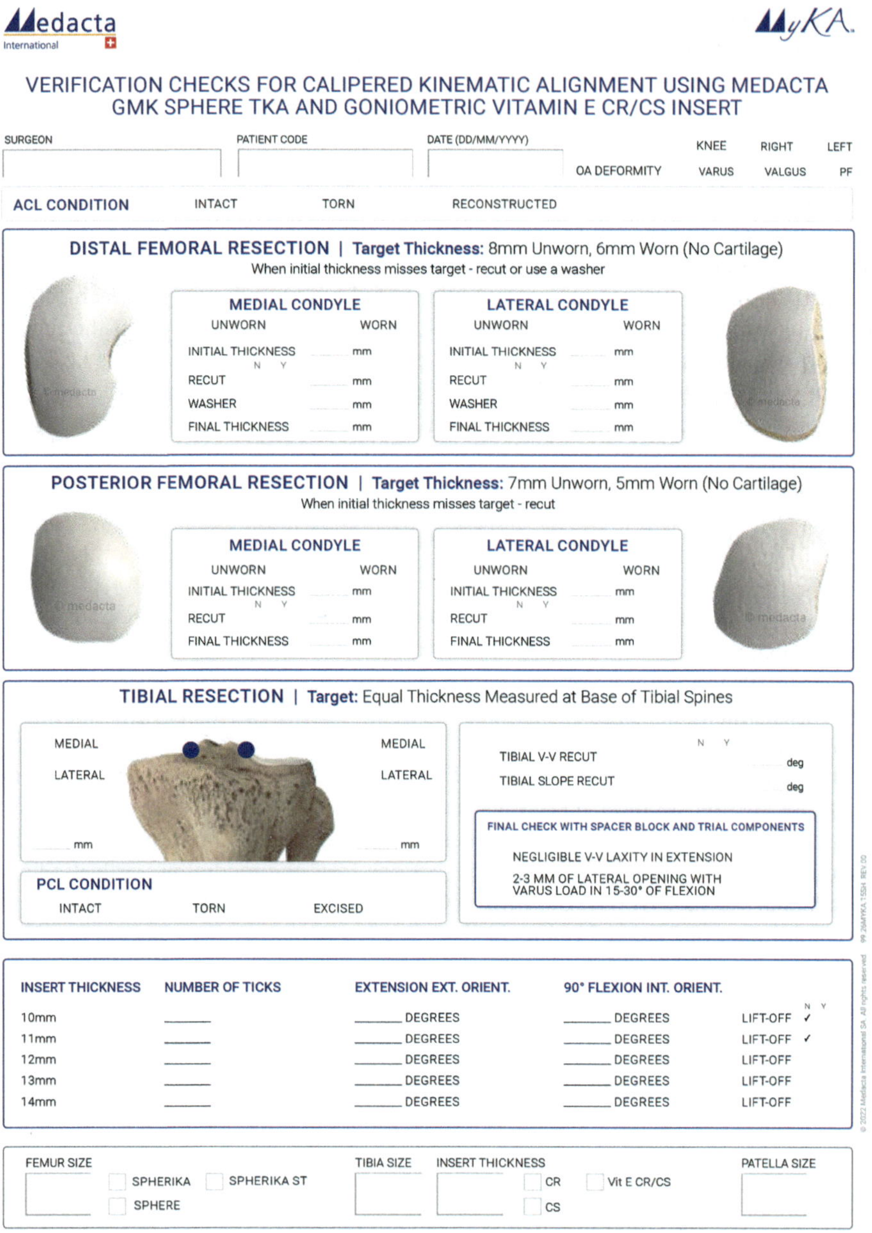
Medacta International

MyKA

VERIFICATION CHECKS FOR CALIPERED KINEMATIC ALIGNMENT USING MEDACTA GMK SPHERE TKA AND GONIOMETRIC VITAMIN E CR/CS INSERT

SURGEON | PATIENT CODE | DATE (DD/MM/YYYY) | KNEE RIGHT LEFT

OA DEFORMITY VARUS VALGUS PF

ACL CONDITION INTACT TORN RECONSTRUCTED

DISTAL FEMORAL RESECTION | Target Thickness: 8mm Unworn, 6mm Worn (No Cartilage)

When initial thickness misses target - recut or use a washer

MEDIAL CONDYLE (UNWORN / WORN)		LATERAL CONDYLE (UNWORN / WORN)	
INITIAL THICKNESS	mm	INITIAL THICKNESS	mm
RECUT (N Y)	mm	RECUT (N Y)	mm
WASHER	mm	WASHER	mm
FINAL THICKNESS	mm	FINAL THICKNESS	mm

POSTERIOR FEMORAL RESECTION | Target Thickness: 7mm Unworn, 5mm Worn (No Cartilage)

When initial thickness misses target - recut

MEDIAL CONDYLE (UNWORN / WORN)		LATERAL CONDYLE (UNWORN / WORN)	
INITIAL THICKNESS	mm	INITIAL THICKNESS	mm
RECUT (N Y)	mm	RECUT (N Y)	mm
FINAL THICKNESS	mm	FINAL THICKNESS	mm

TIBIAL RESECTION | Target: Equal Thickness Measured at Base of Tibial Spines

MEDIAL LATERAL mm — MEDIAL LATERAL mm

TIBIAL V-V RECUT (N Y) deg

TIBIAL SLOPE RECUT deg

FINAL CHECK WITH SPACER BLOCK AND TRIAL COMPONENTS

NEGLIGIBLE V-V LAXITY IN EXTENSION

2-3 MM OF LATERAL OPENING WITH VARUS LOAD IN 15-30° OF FLEXION

PCL CONDITION INTACT TORN EXCISED

INSERT THICKNESS	NUMBER OF TICKS	EXTENSION EXT. ORIENT.	90° FLEXION INT. ORIENT.	(N Y)
10mm	______	______ DEGREES	______ DEGREES	LIFT-OFF ✓
11mm	______	______ DEGREES	______ DEGREES	LIFT-OFF ✓
12mm	______	______ DEGREES	______ DEGREES	LIFT-OFF
13mm	______	______ DEGREES	______ DEGREES	LIFT-OFF
14mm	______	______ DEGREES	______ DEGREES	LIFT-OFF

FEMUR SIZE SPHERIKA SPHERIKA ST SPHERE | TIBIA SIZE | INSERT THICKNESS CR CS Vit E CR/CS | PATELLA SIZE

© 2022 Medacta International SA. All rights reserved 99.26MYKA.15SH REV.00

Fig. 10.1 The image shows the intraoperative verification worksheet the surgeon completes for each kinematically aligned total knee arthroplasty. It includes the patient number, surgeon name, sex, age, BMI, date of surgery, right or left knee, type of primary deformity (varus, valgus, or patellofemoral), condition of ACL and PCL, target thickness of femoral resections, initial and corrected caliper-measured thickness of each femoral and tibial resection, and the implanted component sizes

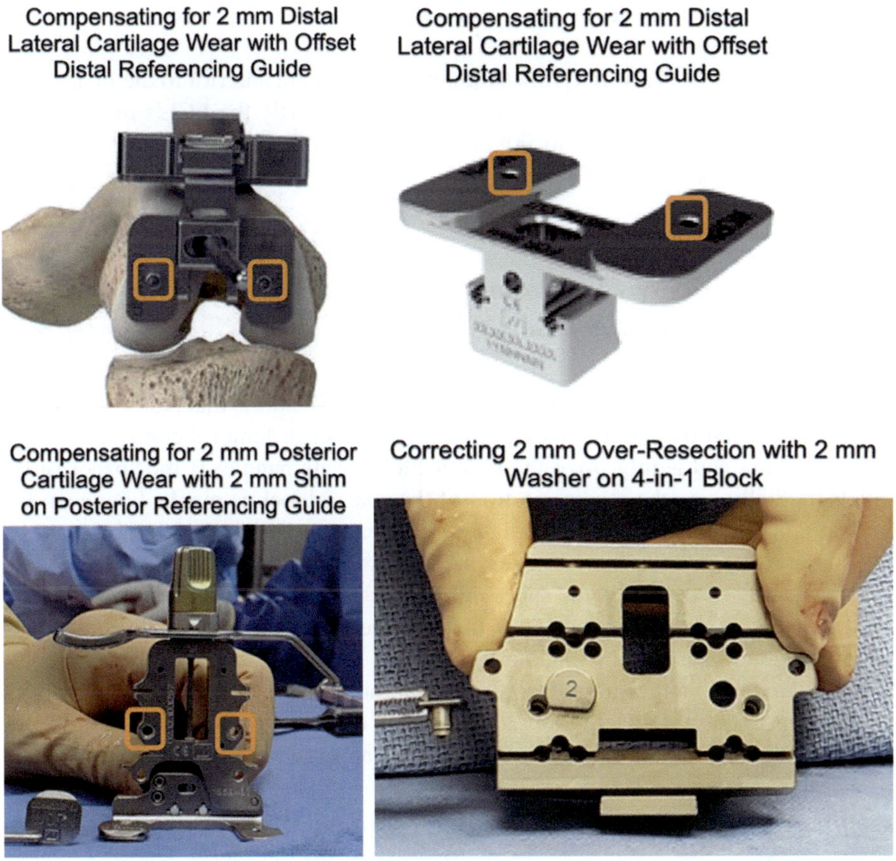

Fig. 10.2 The composite of images shows the manual instruments used to make the distal and posterior femoral resections. The features include an offset distal referencing guide with two holes (orange squares) for compression screws (upper left and right), a posterior referencing guide set at 0° with small, medium, and large width posterior feet with two holes (orange squares) for compression screws and removable shims to compensate for 2 mm of distal and posterior cartilage wear (lower left), and a washer, available in 1 and 2 mm (shown) thicknesses, to correct for an over-resection of wear (lower left), and a washer, available in 1 and 2 mm (shown) thicknesses, to correct for an over-resection of a distal femoral condyle (lower right)

orientation, and the inspection of the medial tibial resection in conjunction with two caliper measurements verifies that the tibial resection matches the patient's pre-arthritic slope. When necessary, differences between the medial and lateral thicknesses of the tibial resection are fine-tuned by recutting the tibia to correct the difference. Equalization of these two thicknesses is the initial verification that the V-V orientation of the tibial resection is correct. When necessary, differences between the medial anterior and posterior thicknesses are fine-tuned by recutting the tibia to correct the difference, which sets the posterior slope [26].

Protecting the PCL by Inserting a Pin Anterior to the PCL Fossa

To maintain the PCL's integrity, the surgeon can drill a pin anterior to the PCL fossa, which blocks the saw from posterior translation. To verify the PCL's integrity, the surgeon should flex the knee to 90°, inspect, and palpate the PCL to confirm its maintained tension (Fig. 10.3).

Three Surgical Steps for Balancing the KA TKA that Use a Spacer Block and the Insert Goniometer

At 90° flexion, the surgeon chooses the spacer block thickness that restores a medial pivot. They insert the spacer block between the posterior femoral condyles and the proximal tibia and gently pivot the spacer block at its handle. If the spacer block pivots medially, i.e., the medial portion of the spacer block is pinched between the medial condyle and tibia while its lateral portion translates anteriorly posteriorly, the surgeon extends the knee to examine the extension space. If the spacer block pivots laterally or centrally, the surgeon increases the thickness of the spacer block until a medial pivot is restored. They then proceed to examine the extension space using the same spacer block thickness.

At full extension, the surgeon confirms that the spacer block thickness restores a rectangular extension space. They apply a V-V moment to the knee and look for lift-off of the medial and lateral femoral and tibial resection from the spacer block.

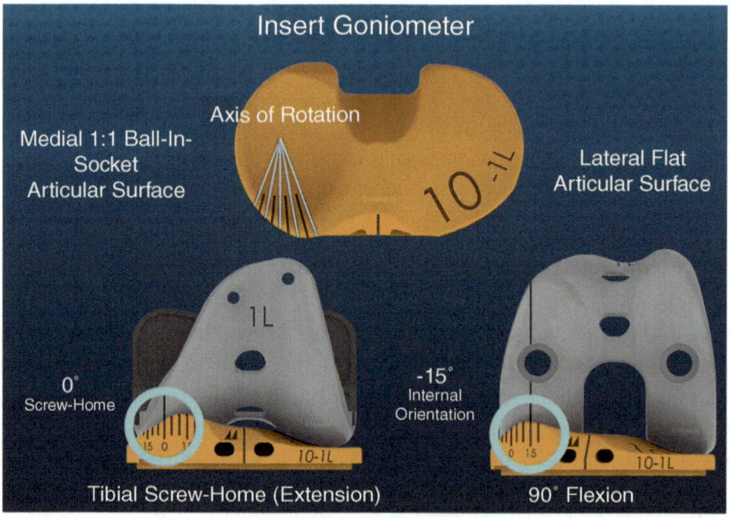

Fig. 10.3 The composite of a right knee with valgus deformity demonstrates an additional technique to preserve the PCL's insertion when resecting the proximal tibia (left) and the confirmatory step to ensure its integrity (right)

The tibial resection is fine-tuned by removing additional tibia until the extension space becomes rectangular [27]. The surgeon refrains from releasing collateral ligaments and the PCL. Hence, when a KA TKA appears too tight, the surgeon readjusts the tibial resection so that the tibial component's orientation resurfaces the knee's pre-arthritic articulation.

The final step of balancing the KA TKA occurs with trial components at full extension and 90° flexion. The surgeon uses the insert goniometer to determine the optimal insert thickness after matching an anatomically shaped tibial baseplate to the tibial resection surface [28, 29]. The design of the insert goniometer consists of markings in front of the medial compartment that are calibrated to the axis of rotation and define the orientation of the insert in relation to the femoral component. The insert goniometer measures tibial orientation relative to a reference line, laser etched vertically on the center of the trial femoral component's medial condyle. Combining an angular scale on the medial insert and a vertical line on the medial femoral condyle enables the surgeon to measure tibial orientation in extension and at 90° flexion intraoperatively during passive knee positioning (Fig. 10.4).

The surgeon selects the ideal insert thickness by observing changes between different insert thicknesses in the external orientation of the tibia in extension and internal tibial orientation in 90° flexion as measured by an insert goniometer. The surgeon records the extension and flexion tibial orientations for each insert

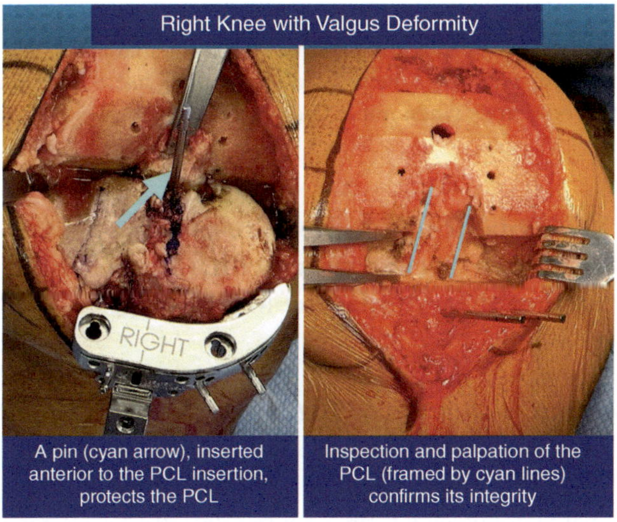

Fig. 10.4 The composite shows left trial components, which measure the tibial internal-external orientations relative to the femur in extension and at 90° flexion. The markings in the front of the insert's medial compartment are calibrated to the axis of rotation within the medial socket (top). The intersection of the vertical line along the femoral component's medial condyle with the insert's markings defines the tibial orientation, which measured 0° in extension (bottom left) and −15° internal at 90° flexion (bottom right)

thickness. The optimal thickness is the insert that provides the greatest orientations in extension and/or 90° flexion [28].

Restoring ACL Stability Requires a Medial 1:1 Ball-in-Socket Insert Conformity to Restore a Medial Pivot

The kinematics of the knee in the axial plane during extension largely depend on the intact anterior cruciate ligament (ACL) and the geometry of the articular surfaces [30, 31]. During knee flexion-extension, the medial femoral condyle is a sphere (=ball) that rotates on the medial tibial plateau and the medial meniscus (=socket) to produce a combination of flexion-extension and I-E rotation [31]. Because the medial condyle hardly translates from anterior to posterior during a flexion motion, the medial compartment of the knee is analogous to a constrained ball-in-socket joint. The ACL aids in the medial condyle's anterior-posterior (A-P) stability. The stable position of the medial condyle contributes to the isometry of the medial collateral ligament (MCL) during range of motion [32]. A medial 1:1 ball-in-socket insert conformity restores the stable position of the femoral component's medial condyle during gait, downhill walking, and stair descent in contrast to low-conforming PCL retaining or posterior stabilized insert conformities [33, 34]. In vivo fluoroscopic evaluation of KA TKA with PCL retention and a 1:1 ball-in-socket insert conformity reported restoration of close to native tibiofemoral kinematics. In contrast, a low-conforming PCL retaining insert exhibits a loss of a medial pivot indicative of abnormal tibiofemoral kinematics [1, 35]. Restoring a native medial pivot with a 1:1 medial ball-in-socket insert conformity improves patient-reported outcomes when implanted with KA principles [12, 36].

Restoring I-E Tibial Rotation Requires an Intact PCL, a Medial 1:1 Ball-In-Socket Insert with a Lateral Flat Articular Surface that Mimics the Morphology of the Native Knee

Tibial External Orientation in Extension Tightens the Lateral Collateral Ligament

While the medial femoral condyle does not translate, the lateral condyle flexes but also translates from anterior to posterior during a flexion motion. The convex shape of the lateral tibial plateau and the mobile lateral meniscus permit this coupled motion of the lateral condyle. The coupling of a stable medial condyle with a lateral condyle that translates from anterior to posterior during flexion translates into internal tibial rotation during flexion. The anterior position of the lateral condyle (i.e., external tibial orientation) during knee extension increases the distance between the lateral collateral ligament's femoral origin and its insertion on the fibula head, thus tightening the lateral collateral ligament (LCL) [32]. Hence, the external tibial rotation during terminal knee extension (=screw-home) is essential to tension the LCL and to restore a rectangular extension space.

Tibial Internal Orientation at 90° Flexion Reduces the Q-Angle

As the native knee flexes, the PCL tension drives the tibia's internal rotation. This, in turn, reduces the Q-angle and optimizes the tension in the retinacular ligaments, which enables optimal patellofemoral tracking during knee flexion [37–39]. Ideally, a TKA should restore this native tibial internal orientation at 90° flexion, promoting patellofemoral tracking. As the native knee moves from extension to 90° flexion, the tibia internally rotates by an average of 17°–18° [37, 40–42].

PCL Retention Promotes Internal Tibial Rotation During Flexion

A well-known consequence of PCL excision is an increased flexion space laxity, which is inconsistent and unpredictable between knees [43–45]. In addition, PCL excision causes a loss of about half of the internal tibial rotation from extension to 90° flexion [39]. Trying to compensate for the loss of internal tibial rotation by reducing the posterior slope does not solve the problem [46]. In a cadaveric study, four surgeons performed a KA TKA with a medial ball-in-socket and lateral flat tibial articular design. Before and after PCL excision, they compared the internal-external orientation of the tibia in extension and at 90° flexion. With retention of the PCL, the mean internal tibial orientation was 15°, whereas with excision of the PCL, the mean internal tibial orientation decreased to 7°. This implies that retention of the PCL helped the prosthetic knee achieve mean internal tibial orientation (15°) that was comparable to the native knee (18°) (Fig. 10.5). The loss of PCL-driven internal tibial rotation can, in turn, predispose the knee to patella maltracking and anterior knee pain.

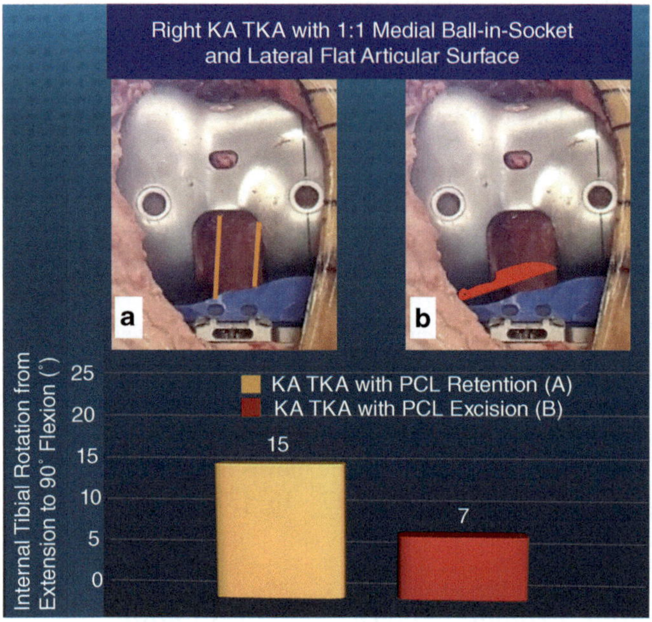

Fig. 10.5 The bar chart illustrates the difference in internal tibial rotation during cadaveric KA TKA, which occurs from a flexion motion from 0° to 90°, before (**a**) and after PCL excision (**b**), which caused a loss of about half of the internal tibial rotation

An Insert with Medial 1:1 Ball-In-Socket Conformity and a Lateral Flat Articular Surface Restores I-E Tibial Rotation

The sagittal plane conformity of the insert on the medial side determines passive knee kinematics. Medial Stabilized (MS) inserts from different manufacturers have varying levels of spherical conformity in the medial compartment. A study of 21 patients undergoing caliper-verified KA TKA with PCL retention compared the degree of internal tibial rotation between inserts with a 1:1 medial ball-in-socket or spherical conformity and one with a less than spherical medial ball-in-socket conformity. Both inserts had an identical lateral flat articular surface [47]. The mean tibial orientation for both insert conformities was similar in extension. In 90° and 120° flexion, the 1:1 ball-in-socket conformity demonstrated 2° and 3° more internal tibial orientation, respectively (Fig. 10.6). Inserts with less than spherical conformity allow the tibia to move anteriorly, thereby reducing the tension in the PCL. PCL tension is required for optimal internal tibial rotation. However, whether this minor increase in internal tibial rotation is clinically relevant remains to be seen.

An equally important condition for restoring native knee kinematics, in addition to a medial 1:1 ball-in-socket conformity, is the sagittal plane geometry of the lateral compartment of the insert. Posterior stabilized (PS), cruciate retaining (CR),

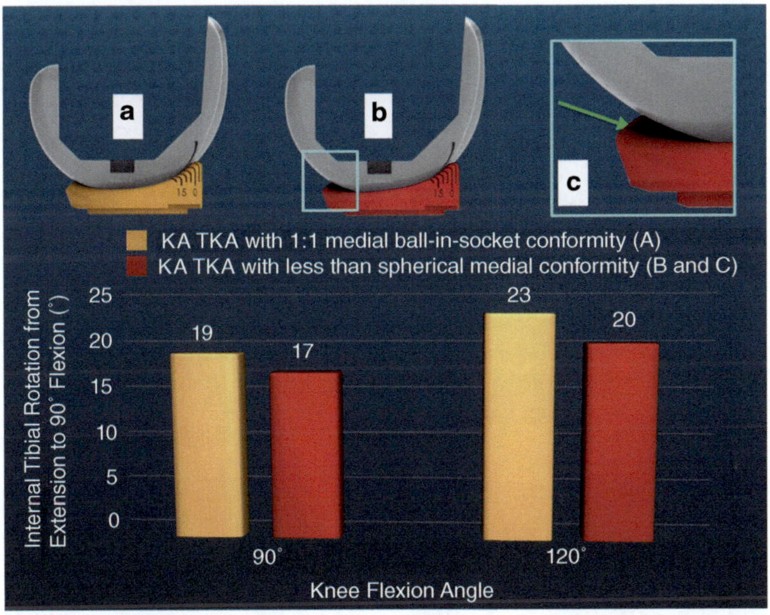

Fig. 10.6 The bar chart illustrates the difference in PCL-driven internal tibial rotation during KA TKA, which occurs during a flexion motion from 0° to 90° and 120°, between an insert with a lateral flat articular surface and a 1:1 medial ball-in-socket conformity (**a**) and a less than spherical medial conformity (**b** and **c**). The insert with less than spherical medial conformity reduces internal tibial rotation by 2° to 3°

and ultra-congruent (UC) insert geometries that have an anterolateral and posterolateral rim cause a mechanical stop of the tibial screw-home during knee extension and block internal tibial rotation during knee flexion. A study quantitated the reduction in tibial rotation caused by an anterolateral and posterolateral rim. Two surgeons treated 23 patients undergoing KA with PCL retention [48]. They determined the difference in tibial rotation between inserts with a lateral flat articulation surface (F), low-congruent (LC), and ultra-congruent (UC) inserts. Compared to the lateral flat surface, the LC and UC surfaces decreased the magnitude of tibial rotation by reducing the external tibial orientation in extension and internal tibial orientation at 90° flexion (Fig. 10.7). Thus, a medial ball-in-socket insert with a lateral flat articular surface allows the PCL to drive tibial rotation during knee extension and flexion. This axial plane motion is less likely with other insert geometries with lateral concavities, where the posterolateral rim functions as a "chock-block" [39].

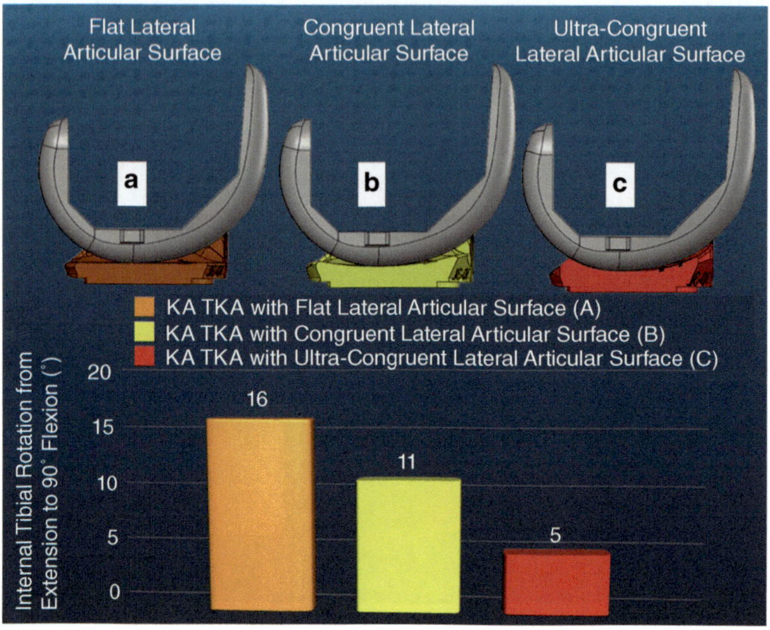

Fig. 10.7 The bar chart illustrates the difference in PCL-driven internal tibial rotation during KA TKA, which occurs during a flexion motion from 0° to 90°, between a 1:1 medial ball-in-socket conformity with a flat (**a**), congruent (**b**), and ultra-congruent lateral articular surface (**c**). The congruent and ultra-congruent lateral articular surfaces reduced internal tibial rotation by 5° and 11°, respectively

Conclusions

In summary, KA TKA resurfaces the patient's pre-arthritic knee and refrains from releasing collateral ligaments and the PCL, which promotes long-term survivorship and high patient function. The surgeon must verify each femoral resection's thickness with a caliper and fine-tune the tibial resection to restore a rectangular extension space. The insert goniometer, which measures external tibial orientation in extension and internal tibial orientation at 90° flexion, can help the surgeon identify the optimal insert thickness. The conformity of the insert ideally mimics the native knee to restore anterior-posterior stability with a medial 1:1 ball-in-socket conformity, replicating ACL function and in combination with a lateral flat articular surface providing a medial pivot. To restore the native knee's V-V laxity and optimize patellofemoral tracking, a TKA needs native external tibial orientation (i.e., screw-home) in extension, internal tibial orientation at 90° flexion, and an intact PCL.

References

1. Elorza SP, O'Donnell E, Nedopil AJ, Howell SM, Hull ML. A new tibial insert design with ball-in-socket medial conformity and posterior cruciate ligament retention closely restores native knee tibial rotation after unrestricted kinematic alignment. J Exp Orthop. 2023;10(1):115.
2. Nicolet-Petersen S, Saiz A, Shelton T, Howell S, Hull ML. Kinematically aligned TKA restores physiological patellofemoral biomechanics in the sagittal plane during a deep knee bend. Knee Surg Sports Traumatol Arthrosc. 2020;28(5):1497–507.
3. Riviere C, Iranpour F, Harris S, et al. The kinematic alignment technique for TKA reliably aligns the femoral component with the cylindrical axis. Orthop Traumatol Surg Res. 2017;103(7):1069–73.
4. Howell SM, Papadopoulos S, Kuznik KT, Hull ML. Accurate alignment and high function after kinematically aligned TKA performed with generic instruments. Knee Surg Sports Traumatol Arthrosc. 2013;21(10):2271–80.
5. Dossett HG, Arthur JR, Makovicka JL, et al. A randomized controlled trial of kinematically and mechanically aligned total knee arthroplasties: long-term follow-up. J Arthroplast. 2023;38(6S):S209–14.
6. Howell SM, Akhtar M, Nedopil AJ, Hull ML. Reoperation, implant survival, and clinical outcome after kinematically aligned total knee arthroplasty: a concise clinical follow-up at 16 years. J Arthroplast. 2024;39(3):695–700.
7. Klasan A, de Steiger R, Holland S, Hatton A, Vertullo CJ, Young SW. Similar risk of revision after kinematically aligned, patient-specific instrumented total knee arthroplasty, and all other total knee arthroplasty: combined results from the Australian and New Zealand Joint Replacement Registries. J Arthroplast. 2020;35(10):2872–7.
8. Laende EK, Richardson CG, Dunbar MJ. A randomized controlled trial of tibial component migration with kinematic alignment using patient-specific instrumentation versus mechanical alignment using computer-assisted surgery in total knee arthroplasty. Bone Joint J. 2019;101-B(8):929–40.
9. Niesen AE, Tirumalai PA, Howell SM, Hull ML. Risk of tibial baseplate loosening is low in patients following unrestricted kinematic alignment total knee arthroplasty using a cruciate-retaining medial conforming insert: a study using radiostereometric analysis (RSA) at 2 years. Knee Surg Sports Traumatol Arthrosc. 2024;32(3):693–703.
10. Niesen AE, Garverick AL, Howell SM, Hull ML. Low tibial baseplate migration 1 year after unrestricted kinematically aligned total knee arthroplasty using a medial conforming implant design. Knee Surg Sports Traumatol Arthrosc. 2023;31(4):1433–42.
11. Elbuluk AM, Jerabek SA, Suhardi VJ, Sculco PK, Ast MP, Vigdorchik JM. Head-to-head comparison of kinematic alignment versus mechanical alignment for total knee arthroplasty. J Arthroplast. 2022;37(8S):S849–S51.
12. French SR, Munir S, Brighton R. A single surgeon series comparing the outcomes of a cruciate retaining and medially stabilized total knee arthroplasty using kinematic alignment principles. J Arthroplast. 2020;35(2):422–8.
13. Scott DF, Gray CG. Outcomes are better with a medial-stabilized vs a posterior-stabilized total knee implanted with kinematic alignment. J Arthroplast. 2022;37(8S):S852–S8.
14. Yaron BZ, Ilan S, Tomer K, Eran B, Gabriel A, Noam S. Patients undergoing staged bilateral knee arthroplasty are less aware of their kinematic aligned knee compared to their mechanical knee. J Orthop. 2021;23:155–9.
15. Shelton TJ, Nedopil AJ, Howell SM, Hull ML. Do varus or valgus outliers have higher forces in the medial or lateral compartments than those which are in-range after a kinematically aligned total knee arthroplasty? Limb and joint line alignment after kinematically aligned total knee arthroplasty. Bone Joint J. 2017;99-B(10):1319–28.
16. Pacheco Elorza S, O'Donnell E, Delman C, Howell SM, Hull ML. Posterior cruciate ligament retention with medial ball-in-socket conformity promotes internal tibial rotation and knee flexion while providing high clinical outcome scores. Knee. 2023;43:153–62.

17. Akhtar M, Howell SM, Nedopil AJ, Hull ML. Similar recovery rate for patients aged between 50 and 89 years that go home on the surgery day and self-administer their rehabilitation after kinematically aligned total knee arthroplasty. J Pers Med. 2024;14(5):504.
18. Nam D, Lin KM, Howell SM, Hull ML. Femoral bone and cartilage wear is predictable at 0 degrees and 90 degrees in the osteoarthritic knee treated with total knee arthroplasty. Knee Surg Sports Traumatol Arthrosc. 2014;22(12):2975–81.
19. Nedopil AJ, Howell SM, Hull ML. Deviations in femoral joint lines using calipered kinematically aligned TKA from virtually planned joint lines are small and do not affect clinical outcomes. Knee Surg Sports Traumatol Arthrosc. 2020;28(10):3118–27.
20. Howell SM, Nedopil AJ, Hull ML. Negligible effect of surgeon experience on the accuracy and time to perform unrestricted caliper verified kinematically aligned TKA with manual instruments. Knee Surg Sports Traumatol Arthrosc. 2022;30(9):2966–74.
21. Nedopil AJ, Dhaliwal A, Howell SM, Hull ML. A surgeon that switched to unrestricted kinematic alignment with manual instruments has a short learning curve and comparable resection accuracy and outcomes to those of an experienced surgeon. J Pers Med. 2022;12(7):1152.
22. Li C, Zhang Z, Wang G, et al. Accuracies of bone resection, implant position, and limb alignment in robotic-arm-assisted total knee arthroplasty: a prospective single-centre study. J Orthop Surg Res. 2022;17(1):61.
23. Seidenstein A, Birmingham M, Foran J, Ogden S. Better accuracy and reproducibility of a new robotically-assisted system for total knee arthroplasty compared to conventional instrumentation: a cadaveric study. Knee Surg Sports Traumatol Arthrosc. 2021;29(3):859–66.
24. Rossi SMP, Sangaletti R, Perticarini L, Terragnoli F, Benazzo F. High accuracy of a new robotically assisted technique for total knee arthroplasty: an in vivo study. Knee Surg Sports Traumatol Arthrosc. 2023;31(3):1153–61.
25. Rak D, Rugamer T, Klann L, Nedopil AJ, Rudert M. Setting the distal and posterior condyle of the femoral component to restore the medial pre-arthritic femoral articular surface results in better outcomes after total knee arthroplasty. Knee Surg Sports Traumatol Arthrosc. 2023;31:5319–31.
26. Johnson JM, Mahfouz MR, Midillioglu MR, Nedopil AJ, Howell SM. Three-dimensional analysis of the tibial resection plane relative to the arthritic tibial plateau in total knee arthroplasty. J Exp Orthop. 2017;4(1):27.
27. Nedopil AJ, Singh AK, Howell SM, Hull ML. Does calipered kinematically aligned TKA restore native left to right symmetry of the lower limb and improve function? J Arthroplast. 2018;33(2):398–406.
28. Nedopil AJ, Howell SM, Hull ML. Measurement of tibial orientation helps select the optimal insert thickness to personalize PCL tension in a medial ball-in-socket TKA. J Pers Med. 2022;12(9):1427.
29. Nedopil AJ, Zamora T, Shelton T, Howell SM, Hull M. A best-fit of an anatomic tibial baseplate closely parallels the flexion-extension plane and covers a high percentage of the proximal tibia. J Knee Surg. 2021;34(13):1486–94.
30. Hamada D, Wada K, Takasago T, et al. Native rotational knee kinematics are lost in bicruciate-retaining total knee arthroplasty when the tibial component is replaced. Knee Surg Sports Traumatol Arthrosc. 2018;26(11):3249–56.
31. Martelli S, Pinskerova V. The shapes of the tibial and femoral articular surfaces in relation to tibiofemoral movement. J Bone Joint Surg Br. 2002;84(4):607–13.
32. Rivière C, Vendittoli P-A. Personalized hip and knee joint replacement. Cham (CH): Springer; 2020.
33. Gray HA, Guan S, Young TJ, Dowsey MM, Choong PF, Pandy MG. Comparison of posterior-stabilized, cruciate-retaining, and medial-stabilized knee implant motion during gait. J Orthop Res. 2020;38(8):1753–68.
34. Schutz P, Taylor WR, Postolka B, et al. Kinematic evaluation of the GMK sphere implant during gait activities: a dynamic videofluoroscopy study. J Orthop Res. 2019;37(11):2337–47.

35. Delman CM, Ridenour D, Howell SM, Hull ML. The posterolateral upslope of a low-conforming insert blocks the medial pivot during a deep knee bend in TKA: a comparative analysis of two implants with different insert conformities. Knee Surg Sports Traumatol Arthrosc. 2021;31:3627–36.
36. Scott DF, Gray CG. Outcomes are better with a medial-stabilized vs a posterior-stabilized total knee implanted with kinematic alignment. J Arthroplast. 2022;37(8S):S852–8.
37. Freeman MA, Pinskerova V. The movement of the knee studied by magnetic resonance imaging. Clin Orthop Relat Res. 2003;410:35–43.
38. Li G, Gill TJ, DeFrate LE, Zayontz S, Glatt V, Zarins B. Biomechanical consequences of PCL deficiency in the knee under simulated muscle loads--an in vitro experimental study. J Orthop Res. 2002;20(4):887–92.
39. Nedopil AJ, Howell SM, Hull ML. More passive internal tibial rotation with posterior cruciate ligament retention than with excision in a medial pivot TKA implanted with unrestricted caliper verified kinematic alignment. Knee Surg Sports Traumatol Arthrosc. 2023;31(3):852–60.
40. Freeman MA, Pinskerova V. The movement of the normal tibio-femoral joint. J Biomech. 2005;38(2):197–208.
41. Hill PF, Vedi V, Williams A, Iwaki H, Pinskerova V, Freeman MA. Tibiofemoral movement 2: the loaded and unloaded living knee studied by MRI. J Bone Joint Surg Br. 2000;82(8):1196–8.
42. Komistek RD, Dennis DA, Mahfouz M. In vivo fluoroscopic analysis of the normal human knee. Clin Orthop Relat Res. 2003;(410):69–81.
43. Hino K, Ishimaru M, Iseki Y, Watanabe S, Onishi Y, Miura H. Mid-flexion laxity is greater after posterior-stabilised total knee replacement than with cruciate-retaining procedures: a computer navigation study. Bone Joint J. 2013;95-B(4):493–7.
44. Kayani B, Konan S, Horriat S, Ibrahim MS, Haddad FS. Posterior cruciate ligament resection in total knee arthroplasty: the effect on flexion-extension gaps, mediolateral laxity, and fixed flexion deformity. Bone Joint J. 2019;101-B(10):1230–7.
45. Warth LC, Deckard ER, Meneghini RM. Posterior cruciate ligament resection does not consistently increase the flexion space in contemporary total knee arthroplasty. J Arthroplast. 2021;36(3):963–9.
46. Nedopil AJ, Thadani PJ, McCoy TH, Howell SM, Hull ML. Adjusting insert thickness and tibial slope do not correct internal tibial rotation loss caused by PCL resection: in vitro study of a medial constraint TKA implanted with unrestricted calipered kinematic alignment. J Knee Surg. 2023;36(5):507–14.
47. Nedopil AJ, Shekhar A, Howell SM, Hull ML. An insert with less than spherical medial conformity causes a loss of passive internal rotation after calipered kinematically aligned TKA. Arch Orthop Trauma Surg. 2021;141(12):2287–94.
48. Nedopil AJ, Howell SM, Hull ML. A TKA insert with a lateral flat articular surface maximizes external and internal tibial orientations without anterior lift-off relative to low-and ultracongruent surfaces. J Pers Med. 2022;12(8):1274.

Chapter 11
Ligament Gap Balancing Approach

Martin Roche, Tsun Law, Gabrielle Dituri, and Ebony James

Introduction

Total Knee Arthroplasty (TKA) has long been recognized as one of the most successful interventions for end-stage osteoarthritis, significantly improving patient mobility and quality of life. However, despite its widespread success, the growing incidence of revision TKA (rTKA) reflects the persistent challenges faced by surgeons, particularly in achieving optimal postoperative outcomes. Recent data indicate that between 10 and 30% of patients report dissatisfaction post-TKA, with instability, persistent pain, infection, and aseptic loosening being the primary culprits [1]. Instability remains a significant contributor to rTKA, with registry data from the USA and Australia highlighting its role in approximately 13% of cases (Fig. 11.1a, b). The need for revision rTKA is increasing annually causing a financial burden on the US healthcare system [2]. This issue is not reserved to the USA. In a study conducted using data from the Australian Orthopaedic Association National Joint Replacement Registry (AOANJRR), instability as a cause for a patient's first rTKA procedures reached 13% in 2010 [3].

Ultimate knee function requires precise implant positioning and alignment. Furthermore, soft tissue balancing in the coronal, rotational, and sagittal planes is critical for successful TKA function. The debate has been on how to technically achieve these targets that are thought to improve post-op knee satisfaction and survivorship.

Instability can be due to excessive laxity in one or more planes leading to pain, swelling, and decreased post-op function (Fig. 11.2) [1]. Over tensioning in one or

---

The original version of the chapter has been revised. A correction to this chapter can be found at https://doi.org/10.1007/978-3-031-75992-5_17

M. Roche · T. Law (✉) · G. Dituri · E. James
Hospital for Special Surgery Florida, West Palm Beach, FL, USA
e-mail: Rochem@hss.edu; lawt@hss.edu

A. J. Tria Jr., G. R. Scuderi (eds.), *The Cruciate Ligaments in Total Knee Arthroplasty*, https://doi.org/10.1007/978-3-031-75992-5_11

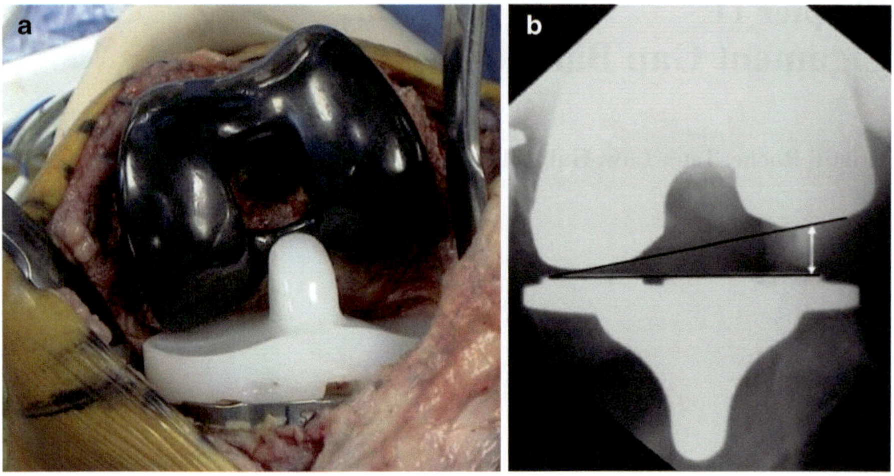

Fig. 11.1 (**a**) Intraoperative picture of flexion gap asymmetry and instability. (**b**) shows a post-op X-ray stress view revealing excessive asymmetric opening in flexion laterally

multiple planes can lead to pain and stiffness post-op, leading to decreased function as well [4].

Insall [5] taught us that a TKR is a soft tissue procedure and described flexion and extension gap balancing in total knee arthroplasty (TKA) over 30 years ago but up to recently we have not had the adequate tools to define appropriate soft tissue tension. Now that we do have objective inputs from advancing technology, we now need to define the appropriate targets.

The focus on equal "gaps" in flexion and extension came from the teaching of obtaining balance by replacing the required space from bone resections (Fig. 11.3). The approach to obtaining equal gaps has been largely divide into a measured resection technique in an attempt to recreate the boney cuts based on anatomic landmarks and then balance the knee by soft tissue releases or implant constraint; vs a traditional gap balance technique utilizing a planar tibial cut with a distraction force to enable the soft tissue constraints that define femoral rotation and position to achieve equal gaps [6].

The extension gap is measured at full extension (0° of flexion) and the flexion gap at 90° of flexion. Utilizing sensor-based technology, the soft tissue tension was seen to decrease from 0° to 30° as the weight of the leg and screw home mechanism unlocks and the posterior capsule relaxes [7, 8]. The extension and flexion gaps are further divided into medial and lateral compartments. The medial compartment is more isometric due to the medial collateral (MCL) positioning and the subjective distraction of 1–2 mm throughout the range of motion is commonly defined as an acceptable gap. The lateral compartment has more inherent laxity due to the lateral collateral ligament (LCL) positioning and dynamic expansion of the posterior lateral compartment [9]. Subjective distraction of 1–2 mm in extension and 1–4 mm in flexion is commonly accepted as balanced. Asano [10] showed that the soft tissue complex around the knee was elastic and consequently extensible and that the joint gap in TKA depended on the strength of the joint distraction force applied (Fig. 11.4).

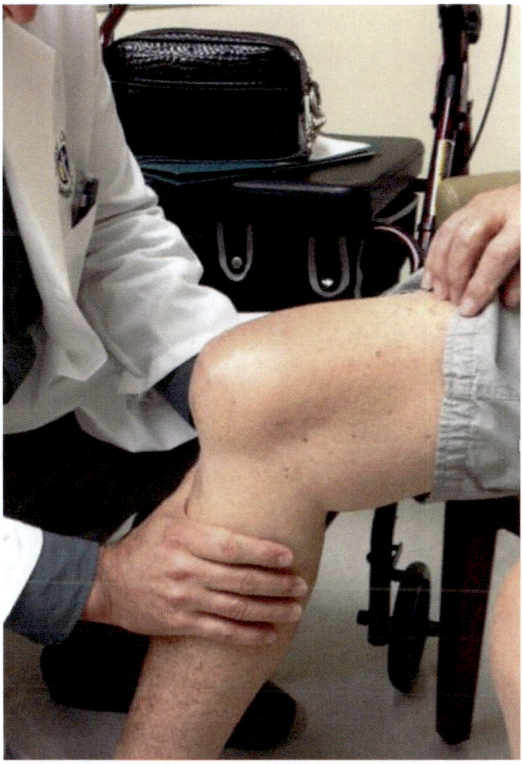

Fig. 11.2 Post-op picture of a posterior drawer exhibiting flexion sag and instability of a TKR

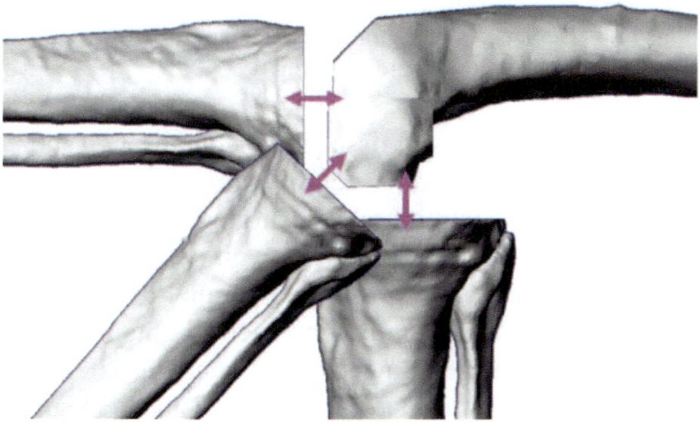

Fig. 11.3 Illustrates the equal gap distances in a knee model at 0°–45°–90°

The goal of TKA is to obtain symmetric and balanced flexion and extension gaps. The question remains as to how to establish this with the best surgical technique. MacDessi [11] reported on the ability of surgeons to detect an unbalanced state. Surgeon defined assessment (SDA) is a poor predictor of the true soft tissue balance when compared to sensor data, particularly in assessing whether a knee is unbalanced. Accuracy of SDA was 63%, 57.5%, and 63.8% at 10°, 45°, and 90°, respectively, when compared to independent sensor data [11]. Traditionally,

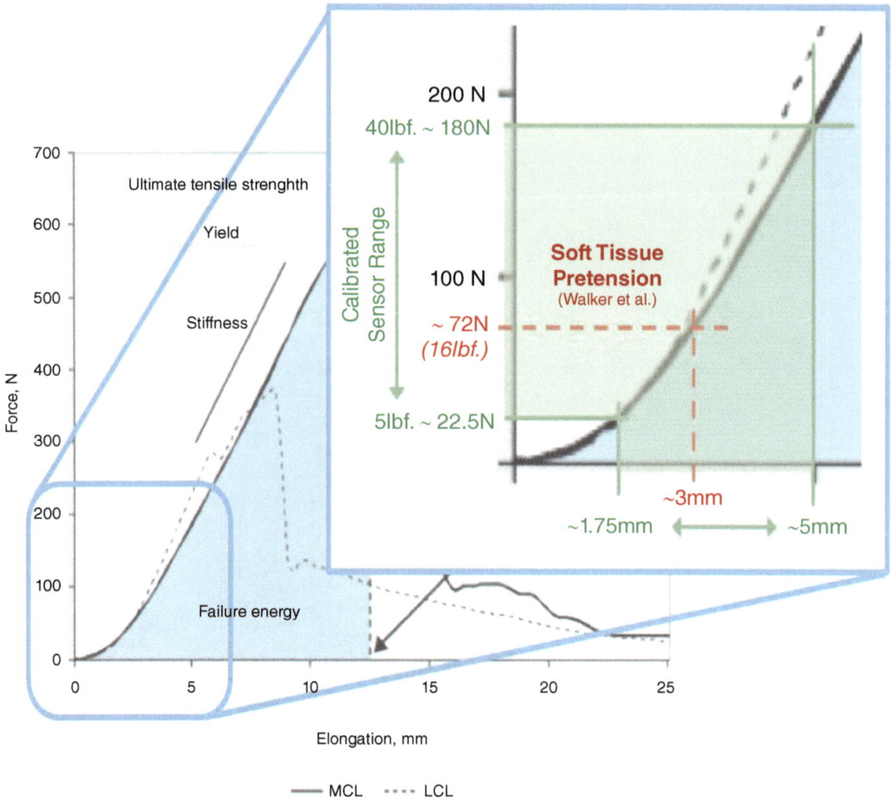

Fig. 11.4 Depicts a stress-strain curve linking forces to mm of ligament distraction and the toe into failure state of a standard ligament

surgeons determine soft tissue balancing through subjective distraction. Factors that can affect the surgeon's determination are "obesity, gender, generalized laxity, degree of joint contracture, and surgical experience" [12].

A gap balancing technique is well described by Dennis et al. [6], in which the femoral component is positioned parallel to the resected proximal tibia with each collateral ligament equally tensioned to obtain a rectangular flexion gap. The balance between the flexion gap (at 90°) and the extension gap (at 0°) can be influenced by both the angle of bone cuts and the tension in surrounding soft tissues [13].

Precise soft tissue balancing combined with accurate bone resections determines rotation of the femoral component. Improper femoral component rotation results in patella femoral instability, anterior knee pain, arthrofibrosis, and flexion gap instability [6]. Gap balancing techniques rely on ligament releases prior to bone cuts. These ligament releases correct fixed deformities and bring the limb into the correct approximate alignment before determination of femoral component rotation. There are basically two gap balancing sequences. One relies on balancing the flexion gap first. The other technique initially balances the knee in extension and later balances the flexion gap to the initially established extension gap [6].

Extension First Technique

Balancing in extension first is considered more reliable, as releases are more precise. After completing the distal femoral cut, the proximal tibia is resected perpendicular to the mechanical axis. Because of the tensioning effect on adjacent ligamentous structures, all osteophytes, including posterior femoral and tibial osteophytes, must then be removed at this point before any soft tissue releases are performed. Following extension gap resection and osteophyte removal, gap symmetry, soft tissue balance, and lower extremity alignment versus the mechanical axis is assessed by placing a spacer block into the extension gap. Ligaments/soft tissues are released to create a rectangular, balanced gap. A tension device is placed in 90° of flexion (Figs. 11.5 and 11.6). A line is made on the posterior femur that creates a rectangular flexion gap of the same thickness as the extension gap. The posterior femoral bone cut is then made regardless of any of the femoral rotational reference lines. This technique creates a rectangular flexion gap with less need of soft tissue/ligament releases. The femoral size is chosen to fit the remaining bone, anterior to posterior. The polyethylene insert size is chosen to maintain the gaps.

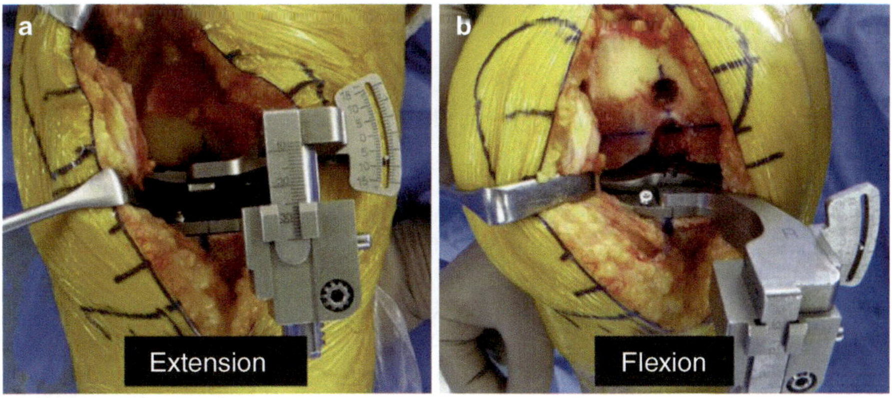

Fig. 11.5 An intra-op picture of a dynamic spacer in the extension and flexion gap

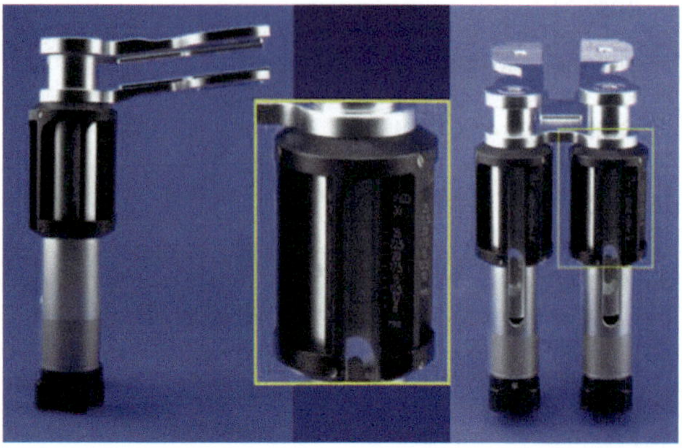

Fig. 11.6 A dynamic manual tensioner (Depuy)

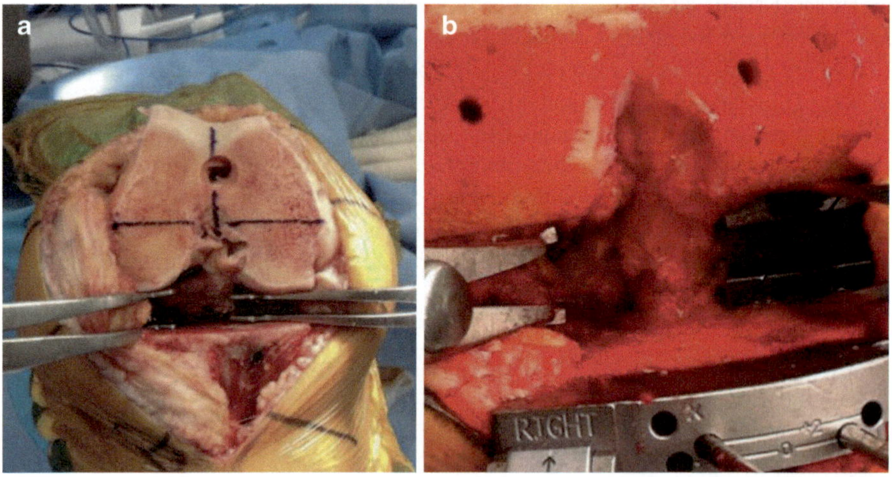

Fig. 11.7 (**a**) Intra-op picture of setting flexion dynamic tension with TEA and Whiteside line depicted. (**b**) Intra-op picture of dynamic tension utilizing lamina spreaders to confirm flexion gaps

Flexion-First Technique

After the initial knee exposure, a perpendicular proximal tibial resection is made relative to the longitudinal axis of the tibia. An accurate proximal tibial cut is crucial because the tibial resection will serve as a base and reference for the femoral bone resections. A varus tibial resection will result in internal rotation of the femoral component when a tensioned rectangular flexion gap is created. Conversely, a valgus tibial resection will lead to excessive external rotation of the femoral component. It is critical to remove all osteophytes before any extensive soft tissue releases or femoral bone resections are performed. When the joint is accurately tensioned in flexion, the tibial cut should align parallel to the transepicondylar axis (TEA) and will be perpendicular to the anteroposterior (AP) axis (Fig. 11.7a, b). Once the joint is accurately tensioned in flexion, anterior and posterior femoral condylar resections are made using an anterior referencing AP cutting block. Spacer blocks can be inserted into the flexion gap to assure appropriate flexion gap symmetry. After accurate balancing in flexion, attention is directed toward the extension gap. With the knee in extension, tensioning devices, set at a similar tension level to flexion gap, establish the extension gap. An intramedullary or extramedullary guide is attached to the tensioning jig and the lower extremity alignment versus the mechanical axis is carefully evaluated. Additional soft tissue balancing can be done to correct alignment. Once a symmetric flexion and extension gap is obtained, the distal femoral cutting jig is applied, and the distal femoral cut is made. Again, a spacer block is inserted into the extension gap to check extension gap symmetry and equality with the flexion gap. Surgeons must recognize, however, that a flexion-first technique for gap balancing is not well indicated for a valgus knee deformity because of the increased risk of internal rotation of the femoral component [6].

Advantages of Gap Balancing

Surgeons have historically utilized either a "measured resection technique" or a "gap balancing technique" to achieve a perfectly balanced TKA [14]. Comparison studies for these two techniques found that patients who underwent TKA surgery utilizing the gap balancing technique reported better reported outcomes [15]. Improved flexion stability can be obtained by using gap balancing techniques to create a rectangular flexion gap. Dennis et al. [6] compared the stability of 40 measured resection TKAs and 20 gap balanced TKAs. The presence and magnitude of femoral condylar lift-off was evaluated for each technique at 0°, 30°, 60°, and 90° of flexion using an automated three-dimensional model fitting kinematic analysis. A gap balancing technique exhibited a much lower incidence of condylar lift-off.

Disadvantages

A precise proximal tibial resection is critical when using a gap balancing technique. A varus tibial resection will result in increased internal rotation of the femoral component when the femoral component is placed parallel to the resected proximal tibia. Correspondingly, a valgus tibial cut will lead to excessive external rotation of the femoral component. Over or under resection of the femoral or tibial bone can lead to a mismatch of flexion and extension gaps. The integrity of the collateral ligaments and precise ligament balancing are critical components of the gap balancing technique. The superficial medial collateral ligament is the primary stabilizer of the medial aspect of the flexion gap. The lateral aspect of the flexion gap is stabilized by the lateral collateral ligament and popliteus tendon. When the superficial MCL is deficient or over released, tensioning of the medial flexion gap will result in an excessive space. This will lead to excessive internal rotation if the femoral component is placed parallel to the resected tibia. When the lateral collateral ligament-popliteus tendon complex is deficient, positioning the femoral component parallel to the resected tibia can result in excessive external rotation.

Babazaadeh [16] reported that the gap balancing technique resulted in a significantly raised joint line compared to measured resection. Gap symmetry was significantly better using gap balancing. Functional outcomes and quality of life were not significantly different at 24 months. Using computer navigation, gap balancing significantly raises the joint line in order to improve gap symmetry. This does not result in a clinical difference in function or quality of life at 24 months. The effects of joint line elevation have been well researched [17]. It can affect knee stability and patellofemoral mechanics [18]. As little as 5 mm of joint line deviation can lead to mid-flexion instability [9]. Joint line change of only 4 mm can also increase PCL strain. This makes joint line position particularly important in cruciate-retaining designs. Griffin [19] noted an increase in external rotation using the gap balancing technique.

Sagittal plane positioning needs to be integrated with coronal displacement techniques. In a study by Kinsey [20], all 30 patients demonstrated posterior tibial translation during flexion ligament tensioning which changed the gap space. They pointed out that this change can significantly alter femoral component sizing during a posterior-stabilized TKA and must be recognized.

Various Alignment Philosophies

The practice of using mechanical limb alignment for total knee arthroplasty arose from the design of the modern condylar knee prosthesis, with the goal of equally distributing stresses across the articulating surfaces of the prosthesis. As new alignment philosophies emerge, the question of joint line obliquity and gap balancing has several factors to contemplate. With the kinematic alignment technique, the restoration of normal joint kinematics is based on three goals: (1) restoring the native tibiofemoral articular surfaces, (2) restoring the native limb and knee alignment, and (3) restoring the native laxity of the knee [21]. With the gap balancing technique, knee balance is primarily achieved through osseous resection and removal. Ligament releases may be necessary prior to completion of the bone resections in order to correct fixed deformities or to restore neutral mechanical alignment before determining component rotation.

Studies have indicated that the majority of native knees fall into an average range of joint surface alignment on the varus-valgus spectrum [22]. In theory, achieving mechanical or neutral alignment (0°) during total knee arthroplasty may not account for the presence of native constitutional varus or valgus. When a total knee arthroplasty is performed with mechanical alignment, patients with constitutional varus or valgus may experience greater strain in the collateral ligaments when they are in tension. This factor may contribute to the proportion of patients who are dissatisfied with the results of total knee arthroplasty.

Various Gap Philosophies

It remains unclear whether gap balance targets in TKA should aim for standardized, equal gaps in flexion and extension or aim to more closely replicate the native knee with greater lateral laxity, particularly in flexion [23]. Many TKA authors advocate for equal flexion and extension gaps to reduce the incidence of stiffness and instability with posterior-stabilized implant designs. In a posterior cruciate-retaining knee, the aim of a balanced flexion gap is commonly seen as more trapezoidal than symmetrical. This is caused as the MCL and PCL are mainly posterior medial flexion stabilizers with increased laxity curve in the posterior lateral soft tissue. Recent studies evaluating cruciate-retaining TKAs have reported improved outcomes with increased flexion gap laxity [24]. This may be attributed to a greater lateral laxity (a trapezoidal flexion gap) occurring in normal knees. The optimal gap distance coupled with appropriate ligament tension is still evolving.

The two philosophies of PCL retaining or sacrificing also define what equal gaps targets are sought. With the PCL retained, the posterolateral gap commonly opens 3–5 mm more that the medial gap. This is part due to the posteromedial vector of the PCL and the isometry of the MC (Fig. 11.8). The posterolateral compartment is

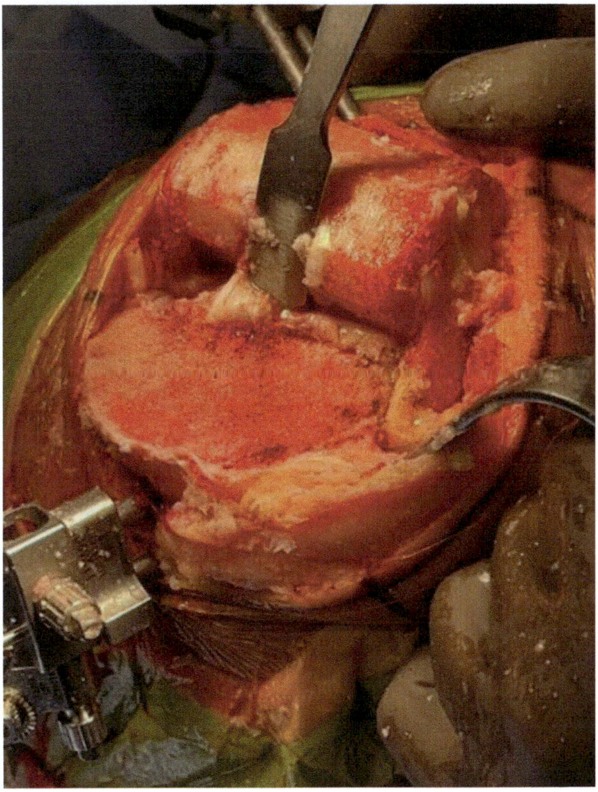

Fig. 11.8 Intra-op picture of the PCL posterior medial-based tibial insertion

constrained by the LCL, popliteus, and capsule which have dynamic properties that allow more laxity and enables posterior lateral rollback in the TKA Shaloub [25] identified several studies [26, 27] supporting the findings of the lateral compartment laxity. Tokuhara [28] demonstrated that the lateral joint gap is significantly laxer than the medial one (6.7 vs 2.1 mm) in normal knees. Okazaki et al. [29] also demonstrated that lateral laxity was significantly greater in both extension and flexion than the medial one in normal knees with varus and valgus stress. Thus, the lateral laxity of the knee joint is physiological, and some authors demonstrated that the lateral laxity led to greater knee flexion angles in cruciate-retaining TKA.

The order of soft tissue release is important to recognize when determining the effect of PCL release on the flexion gap. Shalhoub [25] reported on their data that revealed the importance of partial and complete PCL resection on widening the medial flexion gap when performed as an early step during TKA and after release of the deep MCL. Complete release of the PCL significantly increased the medial, but not lateral, flexion gap. Chow [4] found that patients who underwent sensor-assisted TKA to balance the PCL showed a statistically significant improvement in the Knee Society Score and Oxford Knee Score compared to those who had TKA without sensors.

ACL Preserving Knee Systems

The approach to a fully kinematic ACL preserving knee has been initially addressed with Bi-Uni approach that limits utilization due to patient selection and surgeon expertise (Fig. 11.9).

Historically, TKA designs that attempted ACL preservation were fraught with difficulty in balancing with variable tibial slopes and over tensioning the ACL leading to rupture and instability. Modular poly designs were developed but never gained commercial traction.

Recently, Smith and Nephew launched an ACL preserving knee (XR) that utilizes a linked tibial baseplate with variable poly inserts and a more anatomic femoral implant (Fig. 11.10a, b). Patient selection can be limited as the knee should have

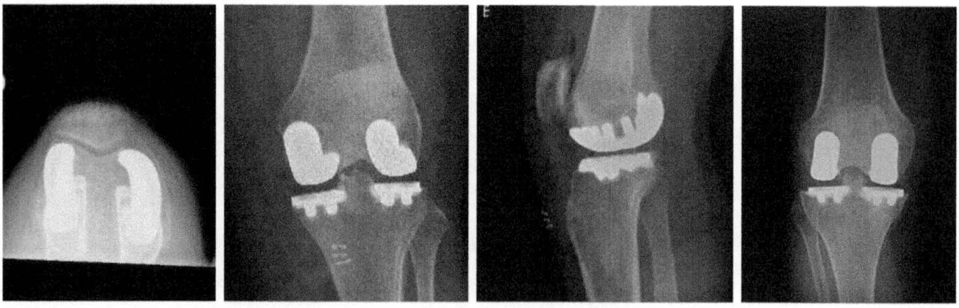

Fig. 11.9 Shows post-op X-rays of a bi-uni implant

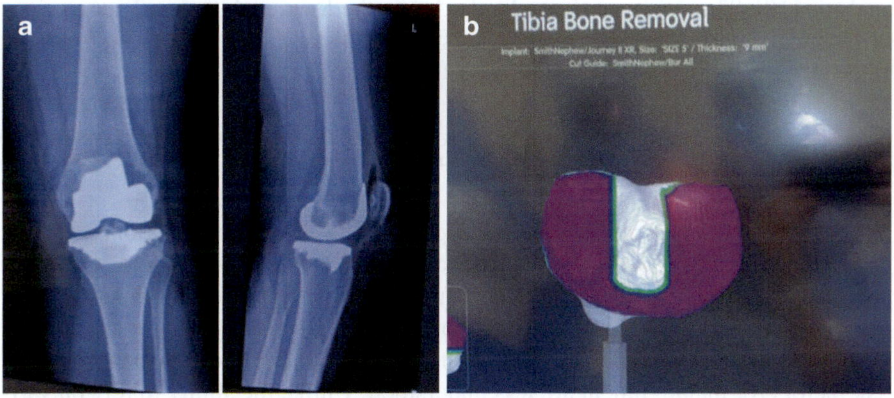

Fig. 11.10 (**a**) Shows a post-op X-ray of XR smith and nephew ACL preserving TKR. (**b**) Reveals the user interface for robotic resection of tibial plateau preserving the ACL

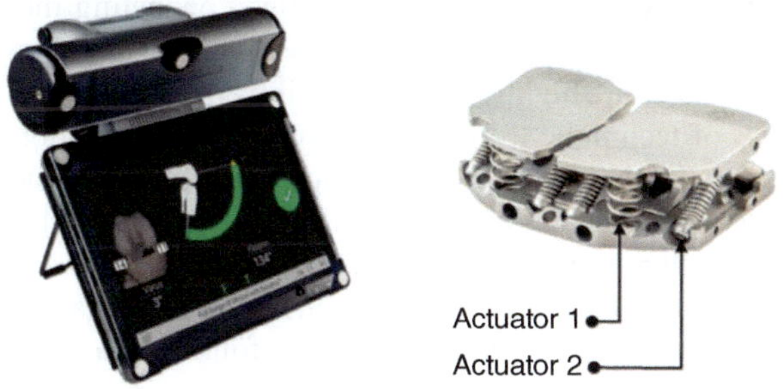

Fig. 11.11 Shows an intra-op distractor to measure gaps between bone cuts

full ROM and correctable coronal alignment. Technical execution can be improved with robotic assistance, as it is necessary to recreate the femoral and tibial joint line obliquity and slope to optimize the ACL-PCL function.

Future technologies include sensorized distraction tools may assist in defining gap kinetics and intercompartmental pressure zones to prevent over tensioning of the cruciate and collateral ligaments prior to any bone resections (Fig. 11.11).

Nielsen et al. [30] found their electronic ligament balancing device was significantly more accurate than the mechanical distraction devices. A mismatch in flexion-extension gaps of up to 6 mm has been reported in approximately 50% of knees using a mechanical device, despite the surgeon's clinical impression that the knee was balanced. Another study found a 20% disagreement in the assessment of "equal gaps" when comparing spacer blocks with distractors [31]. Intraoperative measurements, made after manual balancing was completed, revealed force imbalances averaging 50 lbs. between medial and lateral compartments [32, 33]. Of greater concern was that, despite seemingly appropriate ligament release and intraoperative balancing with a spacer, condylar lift-off was found in 40%, and abnormal tibial rotation in 24% of patients during postoperative fluoroscopic kinematic analysis [19]. These outcomes are likely due to the low resolution and accuracy of mechanical devices that we found in our study [30].

Axial Malrotation Can Lead to Gap Imbalance

In addition to femoral component axial positioning errors, malpositioning of the tibial component has been shown to lead to patellofemoral complications, excessive postoperative pain, and postoperative stiffness, especially for components placed in excessive internal rotation. Tibial axial positioning is not thought to be as sensitive to surgical technique. However, these rotational positioning errors are common, and risk factors for malalignment are less understood. Unlike the ability to rely on various bony landmarks for proper placement of the femoral component, there is no consensus regarding universal tibial bony landmarks guiding placement of the tibial component. Various methods exist, including the tibial crest [34], the tibial tubercle [35], as well as "Akagi's line," a line connecting the medial border of the patellar tendon with the posterior cruciate ligament insertion [36]. However, these bony references are highly variable, risking possible mispositioning of the implant regardless of technique [34]. As more robotic manipulation of the femoral component is utilized to balance the flexion gaps, tibial tray congruency will require smart matching of components at the joint line level and cannot be accomplished with pure axial navigation inputs (Fig. 11.12a, b).

Elkins [37] used CT evaluation after a gap balancing technique, The mean femoral component rotational alignment following a traditional non-navigated gap balanced technique was 0.78° of internal rotation relative to the TEA. This is similar to Aihara et al. [38], who reported a mean of 2.4° of internal rotation for a series of 50 gap balanced knees utilizing a navigation-based technique. Regarding tibial

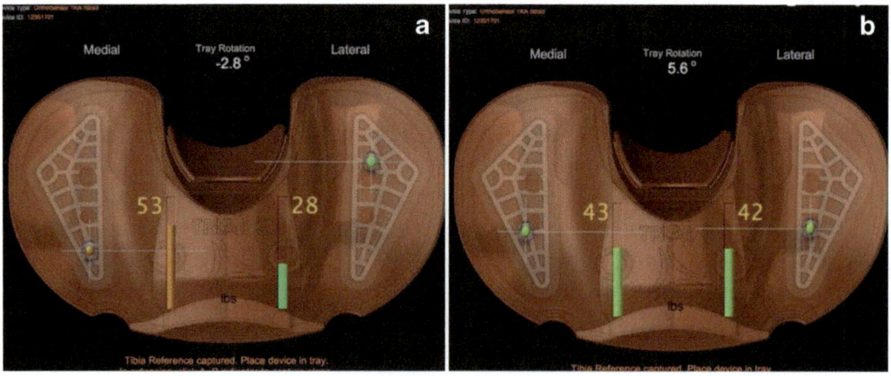

Fig. 11.12 (**a**) Shows the contact points of the femoral component on a sensorized tibial tray—medial pressures of 53 with the tibia internally rotated relative to the femoral component. (**b**) Show a user interface where the tibia has been externally rotated to center the contact points of the femur on the tibial trial and the resultant intercompartmental pressures equalize

alignment, approximately half of the knees assessed exceeded the limit of 18° internal rotation relative to the tibial tubercle. Unlike placement of the femoral cutting guide, it is not immediately apparent how a gap balancing technique may increase or decrease the risk of tibial component malrotation.

Joint Distraction Variability

The native knee laxity was smallest at full extension, then increased significantly until reaching 30° of flexion at which point the gap remained consistent for the remaining arc of flexion [39]. The medial gap was approximately 1 mm smaller than the lateral gap throughout the flexion range. Similar results have been previously reported; however, prior studies quantified laxity only at specific degrees of full extension, midflexion, and deep flexion and not continuously throughout the arc of flexion [39]. The collateral ligaments are tightest at full extension; however, as the knee starts to flex, the distance between the attachment points of the collateral ligaments gets smaller reducing the force applied by these ligaments on the knee joint [39]. The reduction in collateral ligament load and posterior capsule tension, as well as the knee screw home effect, cause the knee laxity to increase up to 30° flexion. The significant increase in the native knee laxity from 0° to 30° of flexion observed in this and in other studies [39] is an under-recognized phenomenon in gap balancing approaches and may imply an anatomic cause for midflexion laxity after TKA. Planning for a zero-millimeter residual gap (i.e., equal gaps) at 0° and 90° resulted in the implanted gaps being the tightest at these flexion angles and the loosest in midflexion. Future studies are needed to evaluate the effect of changing the extension planning angle and the targeted laxity profile on outcomes.

Previous studies showed soft tissue could be easily extended in low soft tissue tension and hardly extended in high tension because of the tension properties of soft tissue complex during TKA [10] and another study demonstrated that larger joint distraction forces led to larger varus ligament balance and larger joint center gap (more trapezoidal gap) because of the difference in soft tissue stiffness between medial and lateral compartments, which could affect the rotation of the femoral posterior condyle resection during gap balancing technique [9, 40]. In gap balancing technique, the applied joint distraction forces during the assessment are different among surgeons, and there is no consensus so far; therefore, the objective and consistent index which is not affected by the joint distraction forces will be ideal for gap balancing technique to avoid the malrotation of the femoral component.

It has been shown that medial instability causes postoperative pain and more abnormal kinematics, and lateral laxity of the knee joint is physiological [28, 29]. Based on these previous findings, excessive medial release was not performed and lateral laxity of approximately 5 mm the extension gap was allowed, essentially making a trapezoidal gap. To perform "medial preserving gap technique" focusing on the medial stability, the difference in the joint center gap and varus ligament balance (the value at flexion minus the value at extension) can be used for creating equal trapezoidal gap in extension and flexion [9, 40].

The rotation of the femoral posterior condyle resection is basically based on the flexion gap. However, the concern of this technique is how much joint distraction forces should be applied during the gap evaluation because the findings of the present study demonstrated that the external rotational angle of the femoral posterior condyle resection would vary depending on the strength of the joint distraction forces during flexion gap evaluation. Moreover, conventional gap balancing technique was on the basis of the rectangular extension gap, but in the present study, the extension and flexion gap were trapezoidal rather than rectangular, which would be due to the difference in soft tissue stiffness between medial and lateral compartments as previously reported [25].

Robotics

Robotics with navigation and pre-operative scans have now brought the ability to define alignment, rotation, and gap distraction prior to bone cuts in certain knee deformities. Surgeons can virtually position TKA components and define gap distances and alignment prior to performing bone resections [23]. These robotic systems, categorized into active, semi-active, and passive types, enhance surgical precision by utilizing pre-operative landmarks or intraoperative registration techniques. The accuracy of the bone cuts enables different tibial resection philosophies to be evaluated. As the gap distraction is relative to two points on the femur and tibia in the coronal plane, care must be taken to interpret the sagittal and rotation interfaces. Roche et al. [41] showed the consistency of 2° of tibial varus resection on decreasing medial joint pressures intra-op and improved 2-year outcomes when compared to MCL pie crusting to achieve balance in the varus knee. Gutske [42] utilized a restricted varus tibial cut of 3° and found the need to perform soft tissue releases was minimized to achieve gap balance utilizing a combined robotic-sensor application. This study demonstrates excellent average 2-year follow-up clinical outcomes with TKAs for varus wear patterns performed with a functional balancing strategy with a restricted 3-degree varus coronal limb and tibial component alignment.

Combined robotic and constant gap distraction technologies may aid in determining optimal patient-specific balance targets, which may reduce the frequency, and the extent of soft tissue releases required to achieve balance and achieve more consistent outcomes in TKA (Fig. 11.13) [25].

Aiming for equal gaps in flexion and extension using a gap balancing technique resulted in a balanced knee in flexion and extension with approximately 2–4 mm of residual laxity in mid flexion. The gaps before femoral resection exhibited the greatest change from 0° to 30° of flexion, with little change, thereafter, suggesting an anatomic cause for increased laxity in midflexion. Computer and robotic-assisted surgical methods that can predict knee implant laxity before making femoral

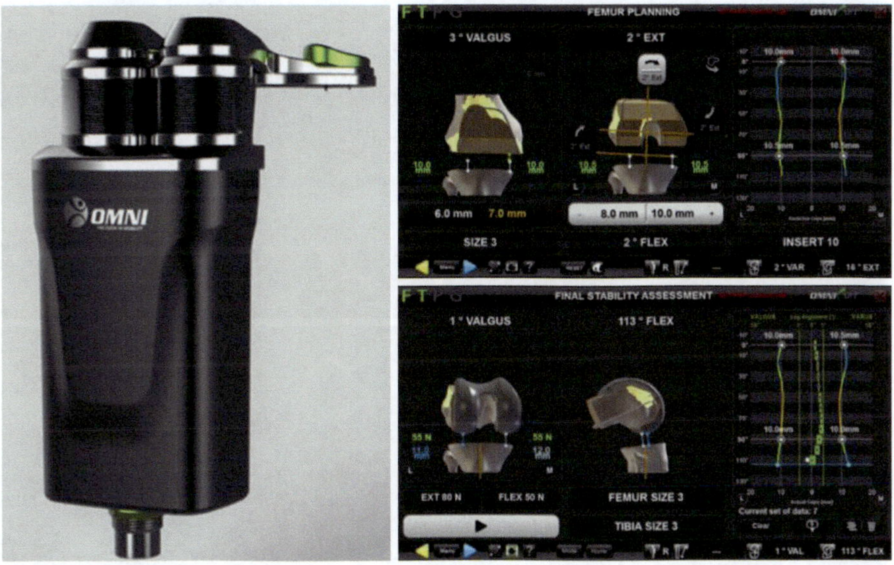

Fig. 11.13 Shows a dynamic constant force distractor and user interface showing gap distances and implant position

resections provide a useful tool for achieving an optimal tradeoff between implant position, alignment, and soft tissue balance (Fig. 11.14). The results from this study provide insight into the native and implant tibiofemoral gaps throughout the flexion range [25].

Integrated sensors give surgeons real-time information about the contact point location and will determine the joint position and the tibiofemoral relationship (Fig. 11.15a, b). This information can then be used to gauge intercompartmental loading throughout the ROM and address any soft tissue abnormalities, as well as aid in achieving target alignment and balance [43, 44].

Implant Designs for TKA

When considering the optimal implant design for TKA, the decision-making process extends beyond the fundamental choice between cruciate-retaining (CR) and posterior-stabilized (PS) designs. While CR and PS implants are the most frequently utilized, advancements in implant technology, such as medial congruent and ultra-congruent modular bearings, have expanded the surgeon's toolkit. These designs reduce the need for traditional cam-and-post mechanisms, offering alternative pathways to achieving knee stability. For experienced surgeons, the challenge lies in selecting the implant design that best aligns with the patient's specific anatomical and functional requirements, considering factors such as ligament integrity, bone

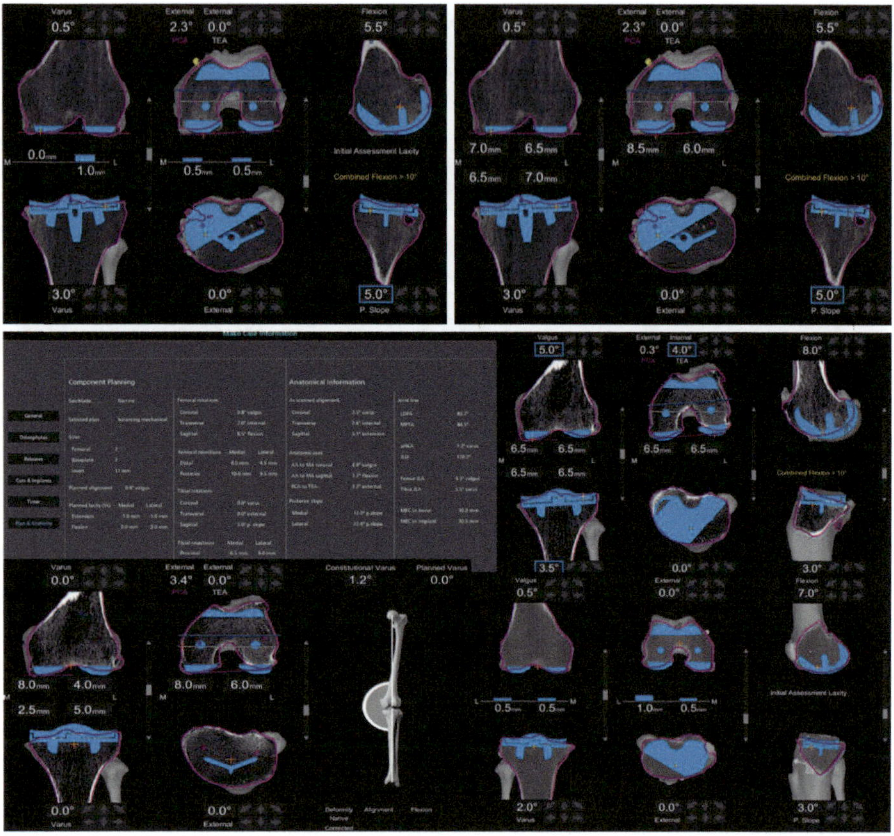

Fig. 11.14 Shows the pre-op information page from the patients CT scan reveals the knee phenotype; femoral joint line angle 4.3° valgus and tibial 5.5° varus. A mechanical starting point and a kinematic starting point on bone resection are plotted. Final implant position to achieve desired gap distance in millimeters is acquired prior to bone resection

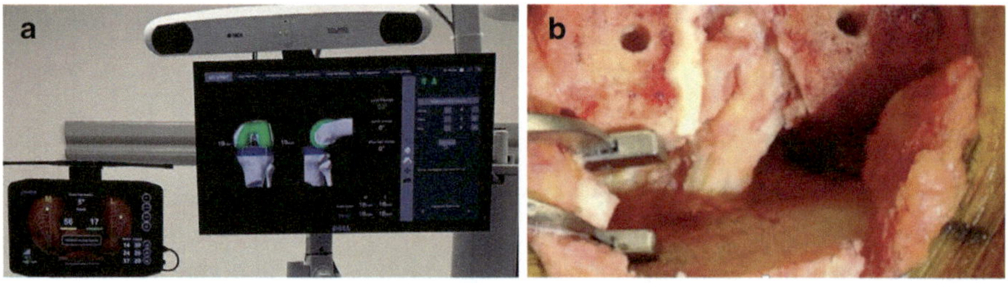

Fig. 11.15 (a) Shows navigation and sensor interfaces. Equal coronal gaps in flexion with the tibial sensor showing excessive medial femoral rollback and an over-tensioned posterior medial compartment consistent with a tight PCL. Bone resection increasing tibial slope or (b); pie crusting of the PCL can assist in obtaining three-dimensional gap balance

quality, and the desired range of motion. Mobile bearing TKRs may be more consistently placed in the gap balancing technique.

Conclusion

The definition of gap balancing is evolving as the targets are becoming more defined. The instrumentation, technology, and techniques are continuing to improve. Tapasvi [45] compared measured resection to the gap balancing technique in a bilateral setting. There were technical differences in the two techniques but the results at 2 years of follow-up were the same.

The theory of equal gaps equate to equal intra-op balance with a more functional post-op outcome is still being studied. Despite the significant advancements in technology, the true targets of alignment and soft tissue tension in TKA are still evolving. The development of technologies capable of monitoring force loads, kinematics, and alignment holds promise for defining personalized targets for various knee phenotypes. As data collection continues to grow, the use of machine learning algorithms to refine these targets will become increasingly important. This underscores the importance of data collection on the development and validation of machine learning tools [46].

References

1. Inui H, Yamagami R, Kono K, Kawaguchi K. What are the causes of failure after total knee arthroplasty? J Joint Surg Res. 2023;1(1):32–40. https://doi.org/10.1016/j.jjoisr.2022.12.002.
2. Bhandari M, Smith J, Miller LE, Block JE. Clinical and economic burden of revision knee arthroplasty. Clin Med Insights Arthritis Musculoskelet Disord. 2012;5:89–94.
3. Lewis PL, Campbell DG, Lorimer MF, Requicha F, Annette W, Robertsson O. Primary total knee arthroplasty revised for instability: a detailed registry analysis. J Arthroplast. 2022;37(2):286–97.
4. Chow JC, Breslauer L. The use of intraoperative sensors significantly increases the patient-reported rate of improvement in primary total knee arthroplasty. Orthopedics. 2017;40(4):e648–51.
5. Insall JN, Binazzi R, Soudry M, Mestriner LA. Total knee arthroplasty. Clin Orthop Relat Res. 1985;(192):13–22.
6. Daines BK, Dennis DA. Gap balancing vs. measured resection technique in total knee arthroplasty. Clin Orthop Surg. 2014;6(1):1–8. https://doi.org/10.4055/cios.2014.6.1.1.
7. Moore RE, Conditt MA, Roche MW, Verstraete MA. How to quantitatively balance a total knee? A surgical algorithm to assure balance and control alignment. Sensors. 2021;21(3):700.
8. Keggi JM, Wakelin EA, Koenig JA, et al. Impact of intra-operative predictive ligament balance on post-operative balance and patient outcome in TKA: a prospective multicenter study. Arch Orthop Trauma Surg. 2021;141(12):2165–74.
9. Nagai K, Muratsu H, Matsumoto T, Miya H, Kuroda R, Kurosaka M. Soft tissue balance changes depending on joint distraction force in total knee arthroplasty. J Arthroplast. 2014;29(3):520–4.

10. Asano H, Muneta T, Hoshino A. Stiffness of soft tissue complex in total knee arthroplasty. Knee Surg Sports Traumatol Arthrosc. 2008;16:51.
11. MacDessi SJ, Gharaibeh MA, Harris IA. How accurately can soft tissue balance be determined in total knee arthroplasty? J Arthroplast. 2019;34(2):290–294.e1. https://doi.org/10.1016/j.arth.2018.10.003.
12. Batailler C, Swan J, Marinier ES, Servien E, Lustig S. Current role of intraoperative sensing technology in total knee arthroplasty. Arch Orthop Trauma Surg. 2021;141(12):2255–65.
13. Parcells B. Balancing TKA. Hip & Knee Book; 2017 Mar 30. https://hipandkneebook.com/tka-technique/2017/3/15/balancing-tka
14. Risitano S, Indelli PF. Is "symmetric" gap balancing still the gold standard in primary total knee arthroplasty? Ann Transl Med. 2017;5(16):325. https://doi.org/10.21037/atm.2017.06.18.
15. He Q, Sun C, Ma J, Guo J. Is gap balancing superior to measured resection technique in total knee arthroplasty? A meta-analysis. Arthroplasty. 2020;2(1):3. https://doi.org/10.1186/s42836-020-0025-1.
16. Babazadeh S, Stoney JD, Lim K, Choong PF. The relevance of ligament balancing in total knee arthroplasty: how important is it? A systematic review of the literature. Orthop Rev. 2009;1(2):e26.
17. Partington PF, Sawhney J, Rorabeck CH, et al. Joint line restoration after revision total knee arthroplasty. Clin Orthop Relat Res. 1999;(367):165–71.
18. Martin JW, Whiteside LA. The influence of joint line position on knee stability after condylar knee arthroplasty. Clin Orthop Relat Res. 1990;(259):146–56.
19. Griffin FM, Insall JN, Scuderi GR. Accuracy of soft tissue balancing in total knee arthroplasty. J Arthroplast. 2000;15:970–3.
20. Kinsey TL, Mahoney OM. Balanced flexion and extension gaps are not always of equal size. J Arthroplast. 2018;33(4):1062–1068.e5. https://doi.org/10.1016/j.arth.2017.10.059.
21. Mercuri JJ, Pepper AM, Werner JA, Vigdorchik JM. Gap balancing, measured resection, and kinematic alignment: how, when, and why? JBJS Rev. 2019;7(3):e2. https://doi.org/10.2106/JBJS.RVW.18.00026.
22. Bellemans J, Colyn W, Vandenneucker H, Victor J. The Chitranjan Ranawat award: is neutral mechanical alignment normal for all patients? The concept of constitutional varus. Clin Orthop Relat Res. 2012;470(1):45–53.
23. Young SW, Clark GW, Esposito CI, Carter M, Walker ML. The effect of minor adjustments to tibial and femoral component position on soft tissue balance in robotic total knee arthroplasty. J Arthroplast. 2023;38(6S):S238–45. https://doi.org/10.1016/j.arth.2023.03.009.
24. Matsumoto T, Takayama K, Muratsu H, et al. Relatively loose flexion gap improves patient-reported clinical scores in cruciate-retaining total knee arthroplasty. J Knee Surg. 2018;31(6):573–9. https://doi.org/10.1055/s-0037-1604446.
25. Shalhoub S, Moschetti WE, Dabuzhsky L, Jevsevar DS, Keggi JM, Plaskos C. Laxity profiles in the native and replaced knee-application to robotic-assisted gap-balancing total knee arthroplasty. J Arthroplast. 2018;33(9):3043–8. https://doi.org/10.1016/j.arth.2018.05.012.
26. Blankevoort L, Huiskes R, de Lange A. The envelope of passive knee joint motion. J Biomech. 1988;21:705–20.
27. Cyr AJ, Shalhoub SS, Fitzwater FG, Ferris LA, Maletsky LP. Mapping of contributions from collateral ligaments to overall knee joint constraint: an experimental cadavericstudy. J Biomech Eng. 2015;137:061006.
28. Tokuhara Y, Kadoya Y, Nakagawa S, Kobayashi A, Takaoka K. The flexion gap in normal knees. An MRI study. J Bone Joint Surg Br. 2004;86:1133–6.
29. Okazaki K, Miura H, Matsuda S, et al. Asymmetry of mediolateral laxity of the normal knee. J Orthop Sci. 2006;11:264–6.
30. Nielsen ES, Hsu A, Patil S, Colwell CW Jr, D'Lima DD. Second-generation electronic ligament balancing for knee arthroplasty: a cadaver study. J Arthroplast. 2018;33(7):2293–300. https://doi.org/10.1016/j.arth.2018.02.057.

31. In Y, Kim SJ, Kim JM, Woo YK, Choi NY, Kang JW. Agreements between different methods of gap balance estimation in cruciate-retaining total knee arthroplasty. Knee Surg Sports Traumatol Arthrosc. 2009;17:60–4.
32. Elmallah RK, Mistry JB, Cherian JJ, et al. Can we really "feel" a balanced total knee arthroplasty? J Arthroplast. 2016;31(9 Suppl):102–5.
33. Scuderi GR, Komistek RD, Dennis DA, Insall JN. The impact of femoral component rotational alignment on condylar lift-off. Clin Orthop Relat Res. 2003;410:148–54.
34. Baldini A, Indelli P, De Luca L, Mariani P, Marcucci M. Rotational alignment of the tibial component in total knee arthroplasty: the anterior tibial cortex is a reliable landmark. Joints. 2013;1:155–60.
35. Bonnin MP, Saffarini M, Mercier PE, Laurent JR, Carrillon Y. Is the anterior tibial tuberosity a reliable rotational landmark for the tibial component in total knee arthroplasty? J Arthroplast. 2011;26:260–7.
36. Akagi M, Oh M, Nonaka T, Tsujimoto H, Asano T, Hamanishi C. An anteroposterior axis of the tibia for total knee arthroplasty. Clin Orthop Relat Res. 2004;420:213–9.
37. Elkins JM, Jennings JM, Johnson RM, Brady AC, Parisi TJ, Dennis DA. Component rotation in well-functioning, gap balanced total knee arthroplasty without navigation. J Arthroplast. 2023;38(6S):S204–8. https://doi.org/10.1016/j.arth.2023.03.033.
38. Aihara AY, Cardoso FN, Debiex P, Castro AM, Luzo MVM, Fernandes ARC. Femoral component axial rotation in the gap-balancing approach to total knee arthroplasty: measurement by computed tomography. J Arthroplast. 2018;33:1222–1230.e2.
39. Roth JD, Howell SM, Hull ML. Native knee Laxities at 0 degrees, 45 degrees, and 90 degrees of flexion and their relationship to the goal of the gap-balancing alignment method of total knee arthroplasty. J Bone Joint Surg Am. 2015;97:1678–84.
40. Nagai K, Muratsu H, Takeoka Y, Tsubosaka M, Kuroda R, Matsumoto T. The influence of joint distraction force on the soft-tissue balance using modified gap-balancing technique in posterior-stabilized total knee arthroplasty. J Arthroplast. 2017;32(10):2995–9. https://doi.org/10.1016/j.arth.2017.04.058.
41. Roche M, Law TY. Correction of coronal deformity and intercompartmental imbalance through bone resection. J Knee Surg. 2023;37(02):104–13. https://doi.org/10.1055/a-2194-0970.
42. Gustke KA, Simon P. A restricted functional balancing technique for total knee arthroplasty with a varus deformity: does a medial soft-tissue release result in a worse outcome? J Arthroplast. 2024;39(8S1):S212–7. https://doi.org/10.1016/j.arth.2024.02.045.
43. Gustke KA, Golladay GJ, Roche MW, Elson LC, Anderson CR. A new method for defining balance: promising short-term clinical outcomes of sensor-guided TKA. J Arthroplast. 2014;29(5):955–60. https://doi.org/10.1016/j.arth.2013.10.020.
44. Moore RE, Conditt MA, Roche MW, Verstraete MA. How to quantitatively balance a total knee? A surgical algorithm to assure balance and control alignment. Sensors (Basel). 2021;21(3):700.
45. Tapasvi SR, Shekhar A, Patil SS, Dipane MV, Chowdhry M, McPherson EJ. Comparison of gap balancing vs measured resection technique in patients undergoing simultaneous bilateral total knee arthroplasty: one technique per knee. J Arthroplast. 2020;35(3):732–40. https://doi.org/10.1016/j.arth.2019.10.002.
46. Karlin EA, Lin CC, Meftah M, Slover JD, Schwarzkopf R. The impact of machine learning on total joint arthroplasty patient outcomes: a systemic review. J Arthroplast. 2023;38(10):2085–95. https://doi.org/10.1016/j.arth.2022.10.039.

Chapter 12
Robotic Technique

Gabrielle N. Swartz, Reza Katanbaf, Sandeep S. Bains, Ronald E. Delanois, and Michael A. Mont

Background

Over the last decade, the utilization of robotic assistance in total knee arthroplasty (TKA) has increased dramatically. It is projected that by 2032, half of all TKAs will be performed with robotic assistance [1]. Though much of this growth has occurred since the introduction of new systems in the mid-2010s, robotic assistance was first used in TKA during the early 2000s. More contemporary systems have sought to add value to the field of joint arthroplasty. Within the last 10 years, eight different manufacturers have received Food and Drug Administration (FDA) clearance for robotic systems performing TKA [2]. These systems aim to improve surgical accuracy, which in turn improves clinical outcomes [3]. In this chapter, we will review the indications, system features, techniques, and literature associated with robotic-assisted TKA.

Indications

Robotic assistance is currently utilized in TKA, unicompartmental knee arthroplasty (UKA), and, more recently, revision TKA [4]. As the indications for robotic-assisted TKA are the same as those of manual TKA, the decision to use robotic assistance typically depends on surgeon preference and experience as well as patient suitability.

G. N. Swartz · R. Katanbaf · S. S. Bains · R. E. Delanois · M. A. Mont (✉)
LifeBridge Health, Sinai Hospital of Baltimore, Rubin Institute for Advanced Orthopedics, Baltimore, MD, USA

A. J. Tria Jr., G. R. Scuderi (eds.), *The Cruciate Ligaments in Total Knee Arthroplasty*, https://doi.org/10.1007/978-3-031-75992-5_12

System Features

Active, Semi-Active, Passive

Robotic surgical systems are typically classified by the level of input that is required by the operating surgeon. Active robotic systems require the least input. Following an initial incision and surgical approach by the surgeon, manual placement of retractors, and positioning of the limb, these systems are able to operate autonomously without real-time input from the surgeon to make predetermined femoral and tibial cuts. The surgeon is able to deactivate the robotic arm at any point during the procedure.

Semi-active systems are predominantly used today. This technology requires the surgeon to guide and operate the robotic arm within the confines of preoperatively determined boundaries. These systems typically utilize haptic feedback (visual, auditory, and tactile) to guide the surgeon. This feedback not only allows for accuracy in component positioning, but for protection against iatrogenic soft-tissue damage.

Passive systems require the most input from the operating surgeon. These systems only provide guidance in the positioning of tools and components, while the surgeon maintains direct, continuous control over the operation. These systems do not provide the same precision and safety features as active and semi-active systems.

Image-Based Versus Imageless

The majority of the robotic systems used in TKA today are image-based (Table 12.1). Depending on the company, these systems utilize preoperative imaging (radiograph, computed tomography (CT) scan, or magnetic resonance imaging (MRI)) to create a three-dimensional model of the knee that is used for surgical planning, component sizing, and intraoperative navigation. While this leads to highly detailed and patient-specific operative planning, the time and cost associated with the additional imaging can be a prohibitive factor.

Imageless systems, on the other hand, rely solely on data collected intraoperatively through the identification of anatomic landmarks and kinematic testing. After the collection of anatomical and kinematic data, an intraoperative surgical plan is made that is customized to the patient's knee. Though these systems remove the need for preoperative imaging, they can result in increased operative time and may require a longer learning curve for the operative physician.

Open Versus Closed

Robotic systems can also be classified as open or closed based on their implant compatibility. Many of today's systems are closed (Table 12.1), meaning they are only compatible with specific vendor implants. Open platforms, however, allow for the use of any implant. While this may cater to surgeon preference, the use of non-specific implants may limit the kinematic data that is available with closed platforms.

Technique

Preparation and Approach

The room and equipment preparation for a robotic-assisted total knee arthroplasty is a crucial part of the procedure. The room must be set up so that the camera and monitor are opposite the surgeon. The foot pedal must be placed on the same side as the surgeon. The robotic arm must be draped in a sterile manner. Once the proper set up has occurred, the surgeon can proceed with their approach of choice to gain exposure to the knee joint.

Registration and Surface Mapping

If using an imageless system, the surgeon should remove any prominent osteophytes prior to registering bony landmarks. However, if using an image-based system, osteophytes cannot be removed as the three-dimensional model was created based on their presence. Next, tracking pins should be placed in the distal femur and proximal tibia. It is important that these pins be visible from the camera, as this is necessary to assess alignment and soft-tissue balance. Once tracking pins and arrays are in place, the surgeon can begin to register landmarks on the bony surface using a probe as directed by the monitor. These landmarks include the medial and lateral malleoli, the center of the tibia, and the intercondylar notch. The hip center is collected by rotating the leg in a circular motion as directed by the monitor. At this point, the knee should be fully extended and flexed to determine neutral alignment. Lastly, a probe is used to map points on the surface of the femoral condyles and tibial plateau.

Table 12.1 Current robotic systems used for TKA

Name	Manufacturer	Introduction year	Platform	Indication	FDA clearance	Type	Technique	Image
T-Solution-One	THINK Surgical Inc., Fremont, CA	2014	Open	THA TKA	THA: 2015 TKA: 2019	Active	Milling	CT
ROSA	Zimmer Biomet, Warsaw, IN	2018	Closed	TKA	2019	Active	Cutting guide	CT
Mako	Stryker, Mahwah, NJ	2005	Closed	UKA PFA TKA THA	2015	Semi-active	Saw	CT
Navio	Smith & Nephew, Memphis, TN	2012	Closed	UKA PFA TKA	2017	Semi-active	Burring, Saw	Image free
OMNIBotic	Corin, Tampa, FL	2004	Closed	TKA	2017	Semi-active	Cutting guide	CT
CORI	Smith & Nephew, Memphis, TN	2020	Closed	UKA TKA	2020	Semi-active	Burring, Saw	Image free
Velys	DePuy Synthes, Westchester, PA	2020	Closed	TKA UKA	2021 2024	Semi-active	Saw	Image free
Sky-Walker	MicroPort NaviBot, Arlington, TN	2022	Closed	TKA	2022	Semi-active	Saw	CT
CASPAR	U.R.S.-ortho GmbH&Co KG, Rastatt, DE	2000	Open	TKA THA	N/A	Active	Milling	CT

Abbreviations: *THA* total hip arthroplasty, *TKA* total knee arthroplasty, *UKA* unicondylar knee arthroplasty, *PFA* patello-femoral arthroplasty, *CT* computerized tomography

For image-based systems, multiple points are collected that are then placed on the preoperative 3D model. For image-based systems, the entire surface of the femoral condyles and tibial plateau must be mapped. This allows for the creation of an intraoperative model.

Intraoperative Planning

For imageless systems, the computer system will determine the suggested sizes of the tibial and femoral components based on the data collected during surface mapping. The depth of femoral and tibial resections will also be determined at this stage. Adjustments in component sizing can be made by the surgeon if they see fit. For image-based systems, the majority of this planning occurs preoperatively though the plan can be adjusted intraoperatively as needed.

The last step of planning is the assessment of the flexion and extension gaps. The knee must be taken through the full range of motion to allow the computer to map out the gaps at 0 and 90 degrees. Some image-based systems perform this step preoperatively based on the three-dimensional model.

Femoral and Tibial Cuts

Once all planning is complete and component sizes are determined, bony cuts can be made. The robotic arm will move the cutting device into place based on the predetermined resection depth. Depending on the system being used, different cutting techniques may be utilized, including traditional sawing, burring, and milling. Once all cuts are made, components can be implanted and trialed as they are in manual TKA. The knee can then be closed in standard fashion.

Clinical Studies

Precision and Component Placement

Perhaps the most highly recognized benefit of robotic-assisted TKA is the precision of component placement and limb alignment. Many authors have demonstrated improved component positioning when compared to manual TKA [5–7]. Mahoney et al. conducted a prospective study comparing 143 patients who underwent robotic-assisted TKA with 86 who underwent manual TKA at four institutions across the United States. Computed tomography scans were performed on all patients at 6 weeks postoperatively to assess several factors related to component placement.

The robotic-assisted TKA cohort demonstrated greater accuracy in tibial component alignment ($P < 0.001$), femoral component rotation ($P = 0.015$), and tibial slope ($P < 0.001$) [5]. Riantho et al. performed a systematic review and meta-analysis of 12 randomized clinical trials with 2591 patients that compared radiographic outcomes between manual and robotic-assisted TKA. The authors found that robotic-assisted TKA was associated with fewer outliers in the hip-knee-ankle angle ($P < 0.0001$), femoral component coronal angle ($P = 0.0006$), femoral component sagittal angle ($P = 0.009$), tibial component coronal angle ($P = 0.05$), and tibial component sagittal angle ($P = 0.01$) when compared to manual TKA [8].

Soft-Tissue Protection

Several studies have explored the impact of robotic assistance on iatrogenic soft-tissue injuries during TKA [9–11]. Hampp et al. performed a cadaver study to compare the soft-tissue damage seen with robotic and manual techniques. In 12 cadavers, a robotic-assisted TKA was performed on one knee while a manual TKA was performed on the other. There were two surgeons who then assessed the knees in a blinded fashion for soft-tissue injuries. Knees that underwent robotic-assisted TKA had significantly less PCL damage than the manual knees ($P < 0.001$) [11].

Clinical Outcomes

There is mixed evidence regarding the impact of robotic assistance on clinical outcomes following TKA. Kayani et al. compared functional outcomes between 40 patients who underwent robotic-assisted TKA and 40 patients who underwent manual TKA by a single surgeon with identical implant designs and rehabilitation protocols. The authors found that robotic-assisted TKA was associated with a shorter time to discharge (77 versus 105 h, $P < 0.001$), reduced pain within the first 3 days ($P < 0.001$), and a decreased number of physiotherapy sessions ($P < 0.001$) [12]. Marchand et al. compared 2-year outcomes between 80 patients who underwent robotic-assisted TKA and 80 patients who underwent manual TKA. The authors reported that at 2 years, patients in the robotic-assisted cohort had higher improvement in mean WOMAC scores ($P = 0.02$), mean physical function ($P = 0.009$), and mean total scores ($P = 0.09$) [13]. However, other authors have reported no differences in clinical outcomes when comparing robotic and manual techniques. A randomized controlled trial of 724 robotic-assisted TKAs and 724 manual TKAs was performed by Kim et al. At an average follow-up of 13 years (minimum 10 years), the cohorts demonstrated no difference in Knee Society Scores, WOMAC scores, range of motion, or UCLA patient activity scores (all $P > 0.05$) [14].

Limitations

Though the utilization of robotic assistance in TKA has increased rapidly over the last decade, there are still some limitations to the technology. Perhaps the most prohibitive is the associated cost. Though hospital and company dependent, the initial cost of purchasing a robotic system can range from $600,000 to $1.5 million. Additional costs include maintenance, preoperative imaging, and consumables [15]. However, some literature has shown that with adequate use, these costs may be offset by decreased episode-of-care costs associated with robotic-assisted TKA. A retrospective review of 4452 patients who underwent TKA by Ong et al. reported lower 90-day ($39,260 versus $41,458, $P = 0.001$) and 1-year ($51,462 versus $54,171, $P = 0.011$) costs for robotic-assisted TKAs when compared to manual [16]. Rajan et al. performed a Markov analysis to determine the cost-effectiveness of robotic-assisted TKA when compared to manual techniques, finding that an institutional case volume of over 24 robotic-assisted TKAs per year resulted in decreased overall costs [17]. Sarel and co-authors recently performed a review of the cost-utility of robotic-arm assisted surgery versus manual surgery by performing a systematic review of all health economic studies that compared CT-based robotic-arm assisted unicompartmental knee arthroplasty, total knee arthroplasty, and total hip arthroplasty with manual techniques [18]. Almost all 21 studies demonstrated a positive effect of CT scan-guided robotic-assisted joint arthroplasty on health economic outcomes. For studies reporting on 90-day episodes of costs, 10 out of 12 found lower costs in the robotic-arm-assisted groups. They concluded that robotic-arm assisted joint arthroplasty patients had shorter lengths of stay and cost savings based on their 90-day episodes of care.

Another commonly cited limitation of robotic TKA is the associated learning curve and increased operative times. A systematic review by Mullaji et al. analyzed operative time in 13 studies with 2112 knees. The operative time ranged from 76 to 156 min in robotic-assisted cases. Of seven cases that compared robotic-assisted TKA to manual TKA, six reported a longer operative time in robotic cases [19]. However, several authors have reported that after the first 15–20 robotic-assisted cases, there is no increase in operative time when compared to manual cases [20–22].

A lack of long-term follow-up data is considered by some to be a major limitation to the widespread implementation of robotic-assisted TKA. As the robotic systems in use today have been released within the last decade, future studies are forthcoming that will elucidate the longer term outcomes associated with modern robotic-assisted TKA.

References

1. Lan YT, Chen YW, Niu R, et al. The trend and future projection of technology-assisted total knee arthroplasty in the United States. Int J Med Robot. 2023;19(1):e2478. https://doi.org/10.1002/rcs.2478.
2. Cantivalli A, Cottino U, Bonasia DE, Rosso F, Rossi R. Robotic systems in knee surgery: current concepts and future perspectives. PRO. 2023;5(4):1257–74. https://doi.org/10.3390/prosthesis5040086.
3. Chen AF, Kazarian GS, Jessop GW, Makhdom A. Robotic technology in orthopaedic surgery. J Bone Joint Surg. 2018;100(22):1984–92. https://doi.org/10.2106/JBJS.17.01397.
4. Ngim HLJ, Van Bavel D, De Steiger R, Tang AWW. Robotic-assisted revision total knee arthroplasty: a novel surgical technique. Arthroplasty. 2023;5(1):5. https://doi.org/10.1186/s42836-022-00160-5.
5. Mahoney O, Kinsey T, Sodhi N, et al. Improved component placement accuracy with robotic-arm assisted total knee arthroplasty. J Knee Surg. 2022;35(3):337–44. https://doi.org/10.1055/s-0040-1715571.
6. Park SE, Lee CT. Comparison of robotic-assisted and conventional manual implantation of a primary total knee arthroplasty. J Arthroplast. 2007;22(7):1054–9. https://doi.org/10.1016/j.arth.2007.05.036.
7. Hampp EL, Chughtai M, Scholl LY, et al. Robotic-arm assisted total knee arthroplasty demonstrated greater accuracy and precision to plan compared with manual techniques. J Knee Surg. 2019;32(3):239–50. https://doi.org/10.1055/s-0038-1641729.
8. Riantho A, Butarbutar JCP, Fidiasrianto K, et al. Radiographic outcomes of robot-assisted versus conventional total knee arthroplasty: a systematic review and meta-analysis of randomized clinical trials. JB JS Open Access. 2023;8(2):e23.00010. https://doi.org/10.2106/JBJS.OA.23.00010.
9. Khlopas A, Chughtai M, Hampp EL, et al. Robotic-arm assisted total knee arthroplasty demonstrated soft tissue protection. Surg Technol Int. 2017;30:441–6.
10. Sultan AA, Piuzzi N, Khlopas A, Chughtai M, Sodhi N, Mont MA. Utilization of robotic-arm assisted total knee arthroplasty for soft tissue protection. Expert Rev Med Devices. 2017;14(12):925–7. https://doi.org/10.1080/17434440.2017.1392237.
11. Hampp EL, Sodhi N, Scholl L, et al. Less iatrogenic soft-tissue damage utilizing robotic-assisted total knee arthroplasty when compared with a manual approach: a blinded assessment. Bone Joint Res. 2019;8(10):495–501. https://doi.org/10.1302/2046-3758.810.BJR-2019-0129.R1.
12. Kayani B, Konan S, Tahmassebi J, Pietrzak JRT, Haddad FS. Robotic-arm assisted total knee arthroplasty is associated with improved early functional recovery and reduced time to hospital discharge compared with conventional jig-based total knee arthroplasty: a prospective cohort study. Bone Joint J. 2018;100-B(7):930–7. https://doi.org/10.1302/0301-620X.100B7.BJJ-2017-1449.R1.
13. Marchand KB, Moody R, Scholl LY, et al. Results of robotic-assisted versus manual total knee arthroplasty at 2-year follow-up. J Knee Surg. 2023;36(2):159–66. https://doi.org/10.1055/s-0041-1731349.
14. Kim YH, Yoon SH, Park JW. Does robotic-assisted TKA result in better outcome scores or long-term survivorship than conventional TKA? A randomized, controlled trial. Clin Orthop Relat Res. 2020;478(2):266–75. https://doi.org/10.1097/CORR.0000000000000916.
15. Kayani B, Konan S, Ayuob A, Onochie E, Al-Jabri T, Haddad FS. Robotic technology in total knee arthroplasty: a systematic review. EFORT Open Rev. 2019;4(10):611–7. https://doi.org/10.1302/2058-5241.4.190022.
16. Ong KL, Coppolecchia A, Chen Z, Watson HN, Jacofsky D, Mont MA. Robotic-arm assisted total knee arthroplasty: cost savings demonstrated at one year. Clinicoecon Outcomes Res. 2022;14:309–18. https://doi.org/10.2147/CEOR.S357112.

17. Rajan PV, Khlopas A, Klika A, Molloy R, Krebs V, Piuzzi NS. The cost-effectiveness of robotic-assisted versus manual total knee arthroplasty: a Markov model-based evaluation. J Am Acad Orthop Surg. 2022;30(4):168–76. https://doi.org/10.5435/JAAOS-D-21-00309.
18. Sarrel K, Hameed D, Dubin J, Mont MA, Jacofsky DJ, Coppolecchia AB. Understanding economic analysis and cost-effectiveness of CT scan-guided, 3-dimensional, robotic-arm assisted lower extremity arthroplasty: a systematic review. J Comp Eff Res. 2024;13(4):e230040. https://doi.org/10.57264/cer-2023-0040.
19. Mullaji AB, Khalifa AA. Is it prime time for robotic-assisted TKAs? A systematic review of current studies. J Orthop. 2022;34:31–9. https://doi.org/10.1016/j.jor.2022.07.016.
20. Sodhi N, Khlopas A, Piuzzi N, et al. The learning curve associated with robotic total knee arthroplasty. J Knee Surg. 2018;31(01):017–21. https://doi.org/10.1055/s-0037-1608809.
21. Chen Z, Bhowmik-Stoker M, Palmer M, et al. Time-based learning curve for robotic-assisted total knee arthroplasty: a multicenter study. J Knee Surg. 2023;36(8):873–7. https://doi.org/10.1055/s-0042-1744193.
22. Tay ML, Carter M, Zeng N, Walker ML, Young SW. Robotic-arm assisted total knee arthroplasty has a learning curve of 16 cases and increased operative time of 12 min. ANZ J Surg. 2022;92(11):2974–9. https://doi.org/10.1111/ans.17975.

Chapter 13
Artificial Intelligence Technique

Ryan Cheng, Tony S. Shen, and David J. Mayman

Introduction

The use of robotics in total knee arthroplasty (TKA) has become increasingly popular since the technology was first introduced to the field in 1988 [1, 2]. Surgical robotics for TKA involves the use of a system that enables surgeons to register each patient's knee to a virtual templating model and track the position of the femur and tibial intraoperatively to assess ligamentous laxity [3]. A robotically enabled instrument can then be used to execute the surgical plan, as determined by the patient's anatomy and ligamentous laxity, which facilitates accurate component placement with optimal soft tissue balance [4].

Different Systems and Their Features

Over the past decades, there have been a variety of semi- and fully autonomous surgical robots developed for TKA, all with different features and tools (Table 13.1). The TSolution One (THINK Surgical Inc., Fremont, CA, USA), formerly known as ROBODOC, is a fully autonomous system that utilizes preoperative computed tomography (CT) scans and allows surgeons to pre-plan resections that achieve the

---

R. Cheng
Adult Reconstruction and Joint Replacement Service, Hospital for Special Surgery, New York, NY, USA

Robert Wood Johnson Medical School, Rutgers University, New Brunswick, NJ, USA

T. S. Shen (✉) · D. J. Mayman
Adult Reconstruction and Joint Replacement Service, Hospital for Special Surgery, New York, NY, USA
e-mail: ShenT@HSS.EDU

A. J. Tria Jr., G. R. Scuderi (eds.), *The Cruciate Ligaments in Total Knee Arthroplasty*, https://doi.org/10.1007/978-3-031-75992-5_13

Table 13.1 Different surgical robots and their features

Robotic system	Company	Type	Pre-operative imaging	Pre-operative planning	Approach
TSolution-One	THINK Surgical Inc. (Fremont, CA, USA)	Fully autonomous	CT scan	Yes	Robot-guided burr
Mako	Stryker Corp. (Kalamazoo, MI, USA)	Semi-autonomous	CT scan	Yes	Surgeon-guided robotic arm with saw
Navio	Smith & Nephew (London, UK)	Semi-autonomous	None	No	Handheld burr
CORI	Smith & Nephew (London, UK)	Semi-autonomous	None	No	Handheld burr
Rosa	Zimmer Biomet Inc. (Warsaw, IN, USA)	Semi-autonomous	Standard X-ray or none	Yes	Robot-assisted cutting jig, handheld saw
VELYS	Depuy Synthes (Warsaw, IN, USA)	Semi-autonomous	None	No	Surgeon-guided robotic arm with saw

target alignment as well as component sizing and placement [5, 6]. Surgeons identify bony landmarks on both the femur and the tibia intraoperatively, enabling the surgical robot to overlay the preoperative surgical plan and imaging onto the registered landmarks. Once the accuracy of the surgical plan is validated, the robot then performs the desired femoral and tibial resections. Though the robot autonomously executes the resections, surgeons are able to manually override the robot and halt the procedure should emergencies arise [5].

Semi-autonomous systems grant surgeons more freedom and control of the femoral and tibial resections and are more commonly used today by the arthroplasty community compared to fully autonomous systems. These platforms involve the registration of the patient's anatomy to a virtual model of the knee, which can then be used to virtually template the position of the femoral and tibial components. Systems can be image-based or imageless. Most systems involve an optical tracking system that allows for intraoperative assessment of ligamentous laxity.

The Mako Robotic-Arm Assisted System (Stryker Corp., Kalamazoo, MI, USA) is an image-based semi-autonomous system that creates a virtual three-dimensional model using a preoperative CT scan. The CT scan allows for direct creation of a three-dimensional model of the patient's anatomy. This system involves a robotic arm and a saw that is active within predetermined boundaries, which may serve to limit soft tissue damage [4].

The CORI Surgical System (Smith & Nephew, London, United Kingdom) is an updated version of the Navio Surgical System (Smith & Nephew, London, United Kingdom). This is an imageless semi-autonomous system that consists of a handheld burr that permits surgeons to perform pre-planned resections with visual feedback [7, 8]. Registration is performed using a point capturing system that matches the shape of the knee against a proprietary database. After virtual templating of the components, a burr is used for bony resection. The burr engages when within the zone of the desired resection.

The Rosa Knee System (Zimmer Biomet Inc., Warsaw, IN, USA) is another semi-autonomous system [8, 9]. The system can be utilized with preoperative radiographs or an imageless option. Registration is completed by capturing key landmarks using the optical tracking system. These points are used as references when assessing ligamentous laxity and measuring resection thickness. A robotic arm is used to position a cutting block through which a handheld saw can be used to perform the resections [9].

The VELYS Robotic-Assisted Solution (Depuy Synthes, Warsaw, IN, USA) is an imageless system that relies on intraoperative bony landmark registrations and soft tissue data to create a surgical plan. The VELYS uses a robotic arm with an oscillating saw that is mounted on the bed-rail to perform resections [10]. The smaller footprint of the system allows for a surgical assistant to provide retraction from multiple angles, which aids with visualization and access while also protecting soft tissues and ligaments.

Alignment Strategies Using a Surgical Robot

Although all robotic systems differ in terms of image use, registration, instrumentation, and footprint, all of these systems involve the combination of real-time assessment of ligamentous laxity with the ability to make adjustments to component positioning prior to making resections. As a result, there has been an increase in the use of non-mechanical alignment strategies that aim to achieve soft tissue balance through small changes in component position. The use of robotic assistance in TKA has been shown to reduce the frequency of soft tissue releases and enables the surgeon to aim for precise targets for limb alignment and component position [11, 12].

Mechanical alignment is an approach in which surgeons position both femoral and tibial components perpendicular to the mechanical axis with the goal of achieving a hip-knee-ankle angle of 180° [7]. Neutral mechanical alignment distributes forces evenly across the bearing surface, allowing for more symmetric wear and delaying complications such as polyethylene wear and tibial component loosening [13, 14]. While mechanical alignment strategies are associated with generally excellent outcomes, critics of mechanical alignment, however, argue that this alignment strategy does not take each patient's unique characteristics into account and may require excessive bony resections and ligament rebalancing to force the knee into neutral alignment, particularly for patients whose pre-osteoarthritic knees were already in varus or valgus [15].

In light of this, a number of "alternative" alignment strategies have been described. Kinematic alignment considers the three-dimensional alignment of the components and strives to recreate the 6–7 degree femoral valgus and 3 degree tibial varus of the typical knee [7, 16]. The philosophy of unrestricted kinematic alignment assumes that the pre-osteoarthritic knee is perfectly balanced; and, therefore, the restoration of the native knee anatomy and joint line obliquity would also restore the native balance of the soft tissue envelope. This alignment strategy has recently been gaining traction as studies have demonstrated that approximately 32% of men and 17% of women have had varus knee alignment since reaching skeletal maturity [15]. For these patients, placing the knee in neutral mechanical alignment would alter the natural joint line and create an unnatural feeling knee.

The functional alignment approach was developed as a technology-enabled strategy that involves a compromise between intraoperative ligamentous laxity and the patient's anatomy to determine optimal component position [16, 17]. In this philosophy, the plane and obliquity of the joint are determined by the natural tension of the soft tissues; and, therefore, soft tissue releases are oftentimes unnecessary. While functional alignment aims to preserve native constitutional laxity and three-dimensional knee alignment, often times, "safe zones" are often used to prevent excessive deformity postoperatively [16]. Optimal targets and safe zones remain an active area of study today.

Cruciate Retaining Implants and Surgical Robotics

Robotic platforms are compatible with multiple implant designs, including cruciate retaining designs. The use of surgical robotics has been associated with good long-term clinical outcomes and implant survivorship with protheses of various constraint levels and designs [18–20].

Two ways in which robotic systems may better facilitate the use of a cruciate retaining implant are enhanced protection against unintentional iatrogenic damage to the PCL and more precise adjustment of the extension and flexion gaps. Hampp et al., for example, conducted a cadaveric study comparing soft tissue injuries between robotic-assisted and manual TKA using cruciate retaining implants and found that robotic-assisted TKA resulted in significantly less damage to the posterior cruciate ligament compared to manually performed procedures [21]. These findings are most relevant for robotic platforms for which the resection instrument is only activated within certain boundaries.

The choice to preserve or sacrifice the PCL has implications for soft tissue balancing, particularly in flexion. Regardless of implant selection, robotic platforms can be used to measure the difference in laxity between the extension and flexion gaps. A surgical robot allows for facile adjustment of component position to optimize sagittal plane balance, particularly that of the femur which may be adjusted in both the anterior-posterior axis and proximal-distal axis to achieve the desired flexion and extension gaps. Van de Graaf et al. demonstrated that when using a robotic-enabled functional alignment approach, the thickness of the distal femoral resections were typically less than the posterior femoral resections in order to balance the flexion and extension gaps. When using a cruciate retaining-type implant, the ability to make these adjustments can be helpful to account for variation in the native tension of the PCL.

Data Captured During Robotic Surgery

Although variation exists between platforms, most robotic systems capture data for component position, ligamentous laxity, and anatomic features such as joint line obliquity and limb alignment (Fig. 13.1). Figure 13.1 is an example of data that is captured on an image-based system, which allows for more precise measurements of patient anatomy. Imageless systems may not only capture as much data on bony anatomy, but also capture data for preoperative deformity, limb alignment, joint line angles, ligamentous laxity, sizing, and planned component position. Today, surgeons analyze and process this data to determine the optimal strategy for any

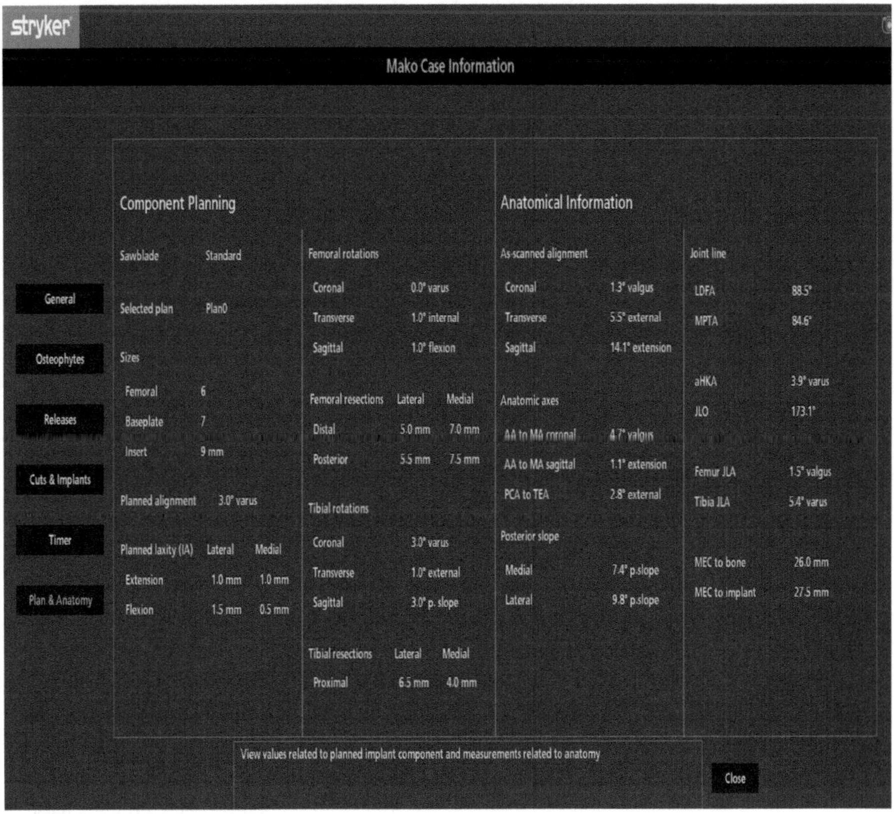

Fig. 13.1 Data captured via the Mako Robotic-Arm Assisted System intraoperatively

individual need. There are variations in philosophy and strategy between different surgeons that are difficult to quantify.

Potential for Artificial Intelligence

In many ways, total knee arthroplasty remains an art for which a surgeon is expected to make multiple judgment calls during surgery to address different situations that may arise. Although the use of robotics has allowed for more objective quantification of ligamentous laxity and provided a precise instrument for component placement, the way in which each surgeon "solves" different problems that arise is a matter of philosophy and clinical judgment. AI may be part of the next evolution of knee replacement techniques. AI involves the use of computing techniques to learn patterns from a large quantity of data inputs. In the same way that surgeons currently process different features of a patient's knee during surgery, AI can be used to quickly determine an ideally positioned knee replacement based on a patient's preoperative and intraoperative characteristics. The development of a decision support tool that automates portions of implant planning may serve to improve reproducibility with knee arthroplasty. There are multiple challenges to the development of such a tool. First, data acquisition needs to be streamlined as most platforms are not designed for large-scale computing research in mind. Second, there is a need for better outcome measurements, whether through patient-reported outcomes or with the use of wearable and other biometric technologies. In the future, it may be possible for an AI system to automatically process a patient's preoperative features, anatomy, deformity, range of motion, ligamentous laxity, bone density, and other parameters to determine an optimal alignment strategy, implant position, and implant type. Robotics lays the groundwork for capturing the data necessary to create such an instrument and much work is needed to achieve this goal.

Conclusion

Over the recent years, there have been a variety of fully and semi-autonomous robotic systems developed for TKA. Robotic-assisted TKA has allowed surgeons a greater degree of surgical precision and reproducibility as well as flexibility with implant selection and alignment strategies. While these robots have helped surgeons to make strides with tensioning ligaments, balancing flexion-extension gaps, and executing surgical plans, AI is not yet advanced enough to independently develop solutions for each knee. Additional research is warranted to examine the link between different surgical strategies and their outcomes and guide AI in the direction of becoming a useful decision-making tool.

References

1. Jakopec M, Harris SJ, Rodriguez y Baena F, Gomes P, Cobb J, Davies BL. The first clinical application of a "hands-on" robotic knee surgery system. Comput Aided Surg. 2001;6(6):329–39. https://doi.org/10.1002/igs.10023.
2. Kurtz S, Ong K, Lau E, Mowat F, Halpern M. Projections of primary and revision hip and knee arthroplasty in the United States from 2005 to 2030. J Bone Joint Surg Am. 2007;89(4):780–5. https://doi.org/10.2106/JBJS.F.00222.
3. Kayani B, Konan S, Ayuob A, Onochie E, Al-Jabri T, Haddad FS. Robotic technology in total knee arthroplasty: a systematic review. EFORT Open Rev. 2019;4(10):611–7. https://doi.org/10.1302/2058-5241.4.190022.
4. Kayani B, Konan S, Pietrzak JRT, Haddad FS. Iatrogenic bone and soft tissue trauma in robotic-arm assisted total knee arthroplasty compared with conventional jig-based Total knee arthroplasty: a prospective cohort study and validation of a new classification system. J Arthroplast. 2018;33(8):2496–501. https://doi.org/10.1016/j.arth.2018.03.042.
5. Liow MHL, Chin PL, Pang HN, Tay DK, Yeo SJ. THINK surgical TSolution-One. SICOT J. 2017;3:63. https://doi.org/10.1051/sicotj/2017052.
6. Vermue H, Batailler C, Monk P, Haddad F, Luyckx T, Lustig S. The evolution of robotic systems for total knee arthroplasty, each system must be assessed for its own value: a systematic review of clinical evidence and meta-analysis. Arch Orthop Trauma Surg. 2023;143(6):3369–81. https://doi.org/10.1007/s00402-022-04632-w.
7. Aflatooni JO, Wininger AE, Park KJ, Incavo SJ. Alignment options and robotics in total knee arthroplasty. Front Surg. 2023;10:1106608. https://doi.org/10.3389/fsurg.2023.1106608.
8. Prakash R, Agrawal Y. Robotic technology in total knee arthroplasty. Br J Hosp Med (Lond). 2023;84(6):1–9. https://doi.org/10.12968/hmed.2022.0491.
9. Batailler C, Hannouche D, Benazzo F, Parratte S. Concepts and techniques of a new robotically assisted technique for total knee arthroplasty: the ROSA knee system. Arch Orthop Trauma Surg. 2021;141(12):2049–58. https://doi.org/10.1007/s00402-021-04048-y.
10. Clatworthy M. Patient-specific TKA with the VELYS™ robotic-assisted solution. Surg Technol Int. 2022;40:315–20. https://doi.org/10.52198/22.STI.40.OS1561.
11. Tian R, Duan X, Kong N, et al. Robotic-assisted total knee arthroplasty is more advantageous for knees with severe deformity: a randomized controlled trial study design. Int J Surg. 2023;109(3):287–96. https://doi.org/10.1097/JS9.0000000000000002.
12. Agarwal N, To K, McDonnell S, Khan W. Clinical and radiological outcomes in robotic-assisted total knee arthroplasty: a systematic review and meta-analysis. J Arthroplast. 2020;35(11):3393–3409.e3392. https://doi.org/10.1016/j.arth.2020.03.005.
13. Abdel MP, Oussedik S, Parratte S, Lustig S, Haddad FS. Coronal alignment in total knee replacement: historical review, contemporary analysis, and future direction. Bone Joint J. 2014;96-B(7):857–62. https://doi.org/10.1302/0301-620X.96B7.33946.
14. Jeffery RS, Morris RW, Denham RA. Coronal alignment after total knee replacement. J Bone Joint Surg Br. 1991;73(5):709 14. https://doi.org/10.1302/0301-620X.73B5.1894655.
15. Bellemans J, Colyn W, Vandenneucker H, Victor J. The Chitranjan Ranawat award: is neutral mechanical alignment normal for all patients? The concept of constitutional varus. Clin Orthop Relat Res. 2012;470(1):45–53. https://doi.org/10.1007/s11999-011-1936-5.
16. Hiranaka T, Suda Y, Saitoh A, et al. Current concept of kinematic alignment total knee arthroplasty and its derivatives. Bone Jt Open. 2022;3(5):390–7. https://doi.org/10.1302/2633-1462.35.BJO-2022-0021.R2.
17. Rivière C, Iranpour F, Auvinet E, et al. Alignment options for total knee arthroplasty: a systematic review. Orthop Traumatol Surg Res. 2017;103(7):1047–56. https://doi.org/10.1016/j.otsr.2017.07.010.
18. Zhang J, Ndou WS, Ng N, et al. Robotic-arm assisted total knee arthroplasty is associated with improved accuracy and patient reported outcomes: a systematic review and meta-

analysis. Knee Surg Sports Traumatol Arthrosc. 2022;30(8):2677–95. https://doi.org/10.1007/s00167-021-06464-4.
19. Pietrzak JRT, Rowan FE, Kayani B, Donaldson MJ, Huq SS, Haddad FS. Preoperative CT-based three-dimensional templating in robot-assisted total knee arthroplasty more accurately predicts implant sizes than two-dimensional templating. J Knee Surg. 2019;32(7):642–8. https://doi.org/10.1055/s-0038-1666829.
20. Bollars P, Janssen D, De Weerdt W, et al. Improved accuracy of implant placement with an imageless handheld robotic system compared to conventional instrumentation in patients undergoing total knee arthroplasty: a prospective randomized controlled trial using CT-based assessment of radiological outcomes. Knee Surg Sports Traumatol Arthrosc. 2023;31(12):5446–52. https://doi.org/10.1007/s00167-023-07590-x.
21. Hampp EL, Sodhi N, Scholl L, et al. Less iatrogenic soft-tissue damage utilizing robotic-assisted total knee arthroplasty when compared with a manual approach: a blinded assessment. Bone Joint Res. 2019;8(10):495–501. https://doi.org/10.1302/2046-3758.810.BJR-2019-0129.R1.

Part V

Rehabilitation Programs

Chapter 14
Variations in Protocols: Physical Therapy, Bracing, Pain Management

Lauren Sacco, Faraz Jamal, and Tony K. George

Introduction

Total knee arthroplasty (TKA) has been performed for over 50 years to correct mobility impairment and pain from knee osteoarthritis. The advent of physiologic total knee arthroplasty began in 1968 with the Stanmore prosthesis and along with it the need to rehabilitate patients after the procedure. Early rehabilitation was emphasized with isometric quadriceps exercises. Articles elaborated weight bearing after regain of quadriceps control, knee flexion after wound healing, and manipulation under anesthesia to improve knee flexion [1].

Rehabilitation Overview

Rehabilitation subcategories included closed kinetic chain exercises integral in proprioceptive feedback and joint stability [2]. Rehabilitation protocols encouraged participation from day one after surgery. The goals include range of motion (ROM) and walking exercises with a crutch or walker. Current Enhanced Recovery After Surgery (ERAS) protocols prioritize early rehabilitation including preoperative patient education, multimodal pain management, targeted anesthesia methodology, minimally invasive interventions, antiemetic therapy, postoperative pain control, and early postoperative rehabilitation [3]. Pre-habilitation prior to TKA includes aquatic exercises, land-based exercise programs, and mind body exercises such as

L. Sacco · F. Jamal
JFK Johnson Rehabilitation Institute, Edison, NJ, USA

T. K. George (✉)
University Orthopaedic Associates, Somerset, NJ, USA

A. J. Tria Jr., G. R. Scuderi (eds.), *The Cruciate Ligaments in Total Knee Arthroplasty*, https://doi.org/10.1007/978-3-031-75992-5_14

Tai Chi and Yoga [4]. Early postoperative rehabilitation prevents several TKA complications. It is well known about 20% of TKA patients remain dissatisfied after TKA and their ability to perform ADL activities [5, 6]. Rehabilitation laxity plays a role in this outcome. Postoperatively, physical therapy can reduce skeletal muscle functional decline.

Deformities of the knee impair movement and limit locomotion. Several supporting structures play crucial roles in knee locomotion. Key muscles, quadriceps, and hamstrings synergistically extend and flex the knee, providing force and counterforce, at different planes of movement. Their weakness impacts knee function even years after surgery. As a key knee extensor, quadriceps muscle's weakness accelerates joint deterioration and eventual function decline and rigorous early quadriceps and patellar strengthening combats weakness from knee osteoarthritis. Quadriceps strength lag is an important indicator for scheduling a TKA [7]. Additionally, it can lose 60% of its strength after a TKA. Studies show preoperative quadriceps weakness impairs postoperative TKA functional recovery, a key indicator of functional ability 1 year after TKA [7]. Partner to the quadriceps is the patella, powering its extension and increasing its lever arm, adding 30% of extension torque in full extension [8] (Fig. 14.1). This necessity has substantiated its preservation in TKA. The

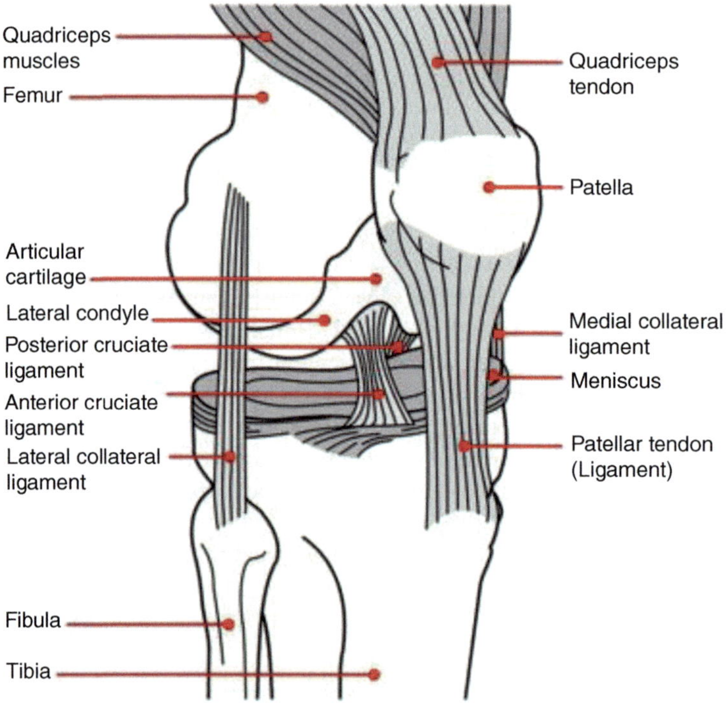

Fig. 14.1 Quadriceps muscle and ligaments of the knee (Reprinted from Human Orthopaedic Biomechanics. Chapter 13: Biomechanics of the knee joint, p. 239–263, by Bernardo Innocenti, 2022 with permission from Elsevier)

hamstring muscles, working antagonistically, provide knee stability against anterior and rotational tibial shear forces with weight bearing. Hamstring weakness increases external rotation, lateral patella tilt, tendon and patellofemoral joint overload and reduced function [9].

Rehabilitation is essential after surgery to decrease gait abnormalities, falls, and other functional impairments. Rehabilitation focuses on three phases: stretching, strengthening, and proprioception. While strict protocols are not universally followed before or after TKA, studies show early rehabilitation, telerehabilitation, outpatient therapy, high intensity and high velocity exercises in the early post-acute surgical period (1–7 days following surgery) are beneficial for patients [10]. Additionally, incorporating therapeutic modalities such as weight bearing biofeedback, neuromuscular electrical stimulation, and balance control can augment traditional rehabilitation [10].

Surgical Approaches

Surgical approaches used to perform TKA are important perioperative considerations affecting rehabilitation. The three most common approaches are the standard medial parapatellar approach, subvastus approach, and midvastus approach. While the medial parapatellar is most commonly used, it is differentiated from the subvastus and midvastus approach incorporating an incision through the quadriceps tendon, which can affect the extensor capabilities of the knee [11]. Compared to the medial parapatellar approach, the subvastus approach improves recovery in the early postoperative rehabilitation phase with quicker return of active straight leg raise, decreased subjective pain day one postoperatively, and greater total range of motion 1 week postoperatively [11].

Rehabilitation Guidelines

Preoperative rehabilitation should contain exercise programs with extensive education to improve patient compliance therefore improving outcomes during the postoperative phase. The preoperative exercise program should be designed to teach patients clear and effective strengthening and flexibility exercises that target current impairments. Targeted areas of concern include but are not limited to knee flexion and extension, active and passive range of motion, quadriceps and hamstring muscle strength, and standing balance. The specific interventions and plan of care should be established following a preoperative examination and evaluation with patient discussion. The preoperative visit may be used as a performance indicator for the postoperative rehabilitation program [12, 13].

As patients transition to the postoperative rehabilitation phase, there is a lack of continuity throughout the literature regarding a clear postoperative rehabilitation plan likely due to the variation in surgical technique, implant design, and the individual patient. Within the postoperative rehabilitation literature there are, however, common components that are recommended for improved functional outcomes and optimal recovery [10, 12]. Essential components of the postoperative rehabilitation program should include general physical activity, motor function training, postoperative range of motion exercises, neuromuscular electrical stimulation, and resistance and variable intensity training.

Motor function training should include balance retraining, walking and movement symmetry as it has been shown that balance retraining with the patient following a joint replacement has led to a significant improvement in walking function. Restoring and optimizing recovery of knee range of motion (ROM) of flexion and extension should begin with a strong focus on knee extension immediately postoperatively. (Fig. 14.2) The knee should be moved through the full range of motion frequently such as once an hour to assist with carryover throughout the day. Building exercise programs that allow the patient to take control of their ROM interventions is essential to optimal outcomes. There is strong evidence that the use of Neuromuscular Electric Stimulation (NMES) after surgery improves quadriceps strength, gait performance, and functional outcomes. Patients who have deficits in

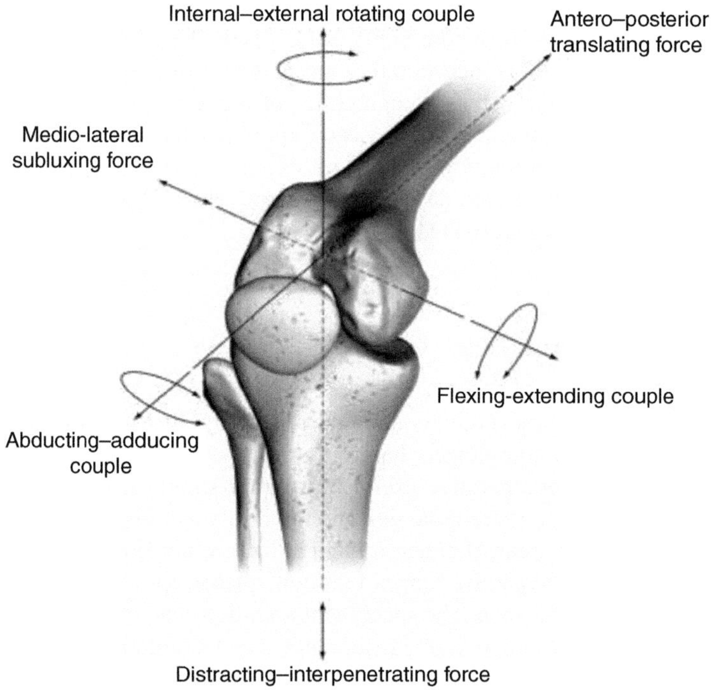

Fig. 14.2 Knee forces and axis of rotation. (Reprinted from Surgical Techniques in Total Knee Arthroplasty and Alternative Procedures, Chapter 2: Biomechanics of the knee, p. 17–35 by Saverio Affatato, 2015 with permission from Elsevier)

their extensor mechanism as demonstrated by an extensor lag or manual muscle testing benefit most from NMES. The stimulation may be used as early as postoperative day 2 and should be used for a minimum of 3 weeks. Early interventions have been shown to improve function, strength, and ROM along with long-term outcomes. Strengthening programs should be performed three times per week in order to see greater improvement in quadriceps muscle strength [10, 12].

Implants

Fixation

There are two options for implant fixation for total knee arthroplasty: cemented and cementless. With a cemented TKA, the patients are full weight bearing or weight bearing as tolerated immediately after surgery with an appropriate assistive device to prevent gait compensations. Most cementless TKAs require restricted weight bearing for 6 weeks to allow for improved osseous integration at the prosthesis-bone interface.

Partial Knee Replacement

A unicompartmental knee replacement (UKA) is a treatment option for patients with more isolated medial or lateral osteoarthritis. There are many benefits to this implant option including faster recovery due to preservation of bone stock and retention of the cruciate and collateral ligaments which leads to a more normalized or native kinematic movement of the knee joint. The implant has been shown to have a significant improvement in knee flexion range of motion compared to a traditional knee replacement implant likely due to the decrease in arthrokinematics changes [14–16]. During the postoperative phase of recovery, it is important to be mindful of the faster recovery for the patient following this procedure. At 3 weeks, knee flexion ROM should be at least 90° with progression to 120° at 6 weeks. Weight machines should be avoided in the first 6 weeks with a focus on active ROM and isometrics to increase muscle activation without stressing the implant. Normalizing gait mechanics and balance retraining should be addressed to assist with transitioning the patient to independent gait without an assistive device. Fillingham et al. found no statistical difference in self-guided home exercise program vs formal outpatient physical therapy [17]. The weight bearing status is determined by the mode of fixation.

PCL Substituting/Stabilized TKA

The posterior cruciate ligament substituting or stabilizing total knee replacement was developed to increase range of motion while decreasing posterior translation of the tibia in relation to the femur. This is accomplished through the use of a femoral cam that would articulate with a central tibial post (Fig. 14.3) which would in turn drive femoral roll back and increase end range of motion. In addition to gaining ROM, this mechanism will also optimize the length tension relationship of the extensor mechanism. This decreases the amount of force required to extend the knee therefore decreasing compressive forces across the patellofemoral joint. During postoperative rehabilitation, there should be a focus on both active and passive range of motion interventions to maximize terminal knee extension as well as knee flexion. Patients should move regularly throughout their full arc of motion to prevent regression while targeting strength of the opposite movement. Progressive resistive exercises of the quadriceps and hamstrings are also essential components to a rehabilitation course of care. This should not only be through exercises in the open chain such as long arc quad or straight leg raises but also through functional movements such as bridging, squatting, step ups, and lunges. These closed kinetic chain exercises will assist with carryover during functional activities such as stair climbing, sit to stand transfers, and floor transfers [18].

The weight bearing status is determined by the mode of fixation.

PCL Retaining TKA

Posterior cruciate ligament retaining total knee arthroplasty designs have been a core option for surgeons for this procedure from its development in the 1970s. The design of the polyethylene liner and implants has evolved over the years to normalize the knee kinematics along with decreasing excessive wearing of the

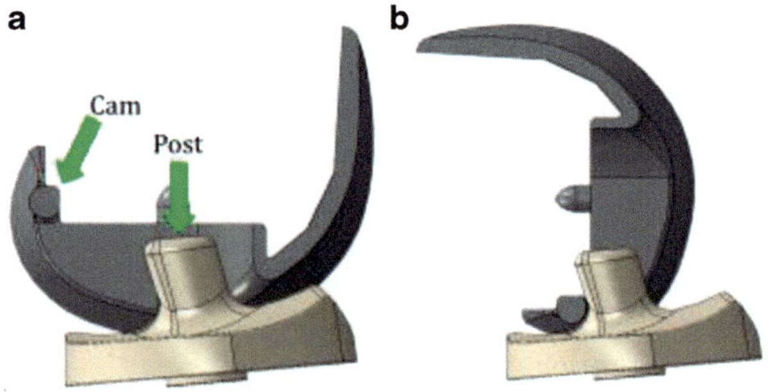

Fig. 14.3 Femoral cam and tibial post mechanism in (**a**) knee extension and (**b**) knee flexion (Reprinted from Human Orthopaedic Biomechanics. Chapter 20: Knee Prosthesis Biomechanics and design, p. 377–407, by Bernardo Innocenti, 2022 with permission from Elsevier)

components. It remains imperative to focus on both active and passive range of motion of knee extension to optimize terminal knee extension as early as possible following the procedure. It is important to deemphasize isolated strengthening of the hamstrings during the first 6–12 weeks. This will decrease posterior tibial translation while protecting the PCL. When hamstring strengthening is initiated small ROM (0–45°) should be used since there is an increased load on the PCL with progressing knee flexion ROM [19]. The progression of closed kinetic chain exercises may begin following a minimum of 6 weeks and limiting knee flexion to 0–45°. Once the patient has passed the 12 weeks with full knee flexion AROM, hamstring progressive resisted exercises may be initiated with a goal of return to function in mind. This may include squatting, lunges, and stair training [19].

The weight bearing status is determined by the mode of fixation.

Bicruciate Retaining TKA

The bicruciate retaining (BCR) total knee arthroplasty preserves the anterior and posterior cruciate ligaments along with the tibial eminence. This technique potentially results in a more native joint kinematics through natural femoral rollback during knee flexion. There is more bone and soft tissue preservation leading to improved recovery times. The anterior cruciate ligament must be intact to proceed with this option which is becoming more common as the average age of a patient seeking to have a TKA is younger [20, 21]. Since the cruciates remain intact, it is important to protect the ligaments during postoperative rehabilitation. Passive ROM should be avoided for the first 6 weeks and ROM should be dependent on AROM with slight assistance. Forced terminal extension can lead to fracture of the bone island and should be avoided. Progression to closed kinetic chain quadriceps strengthening can be initiated at 4 weeks with equal weight bearing. If stability is noted, the patient's active knee extension through full arc of motion is allowed. In addition, promoting protection of the anterior cruciate ligament from future rupture is essential. This is accomplished through a strong focus on eccentric hamstring loading for declaration of the anterior translation of the tibia during closed kinetic chain activities [20–22].

The implant design is usually cemented. However, only partial weight bearing is permitted for the first 6 weeks to protect the bone island and the retained cruciates.

Bicruciate Stabilized TKA

The bicruciate stabilized (BCS) total knee arthroplasty utilizes a dual post cam mechanism to mimic the stability function of the anterior and posterior cruciate ligaments. In addition, the surface design of the implant includes a medial concave and lateral convex design which allows for an amount of rotary pivot shift movement during flexion and extension. The implant is noted to have improved mid flexion stability when compared to the bicruciate retaining implants [21, 23]. There is no limitation on active or passive range of motion postoperatively. It is important to focus on achieving optimal range of motion of full knee extension and flexion as early as possible within the patient's pain tolerance and tissue healing. The ROM should be at least 90–110° by 6 weeks [10, 12].

The weight bearing status is determined by the mode of fixation.

Medial Pivot TKA Design

The knee joint has an asymmetrical arc of motion between the medial and lateral femoral condyles as they articulate with the tibial plateaus. The medial compartment is more stable with decreased excursion during the arc of movement while the lateral femoral condyle rolls and slides posteriorly in an arc motion in relation to the lateral tibial plateau. The resultant movement is pivoting of the lateral compartment around a medial axis of motion. The medial pivot design was developed to mimic this anatomy and kinematics and it can be PCL substituting or retaining. The use of this design has shown positive results with patients in decreased anterior knee pain, improved stair climbing ability and higher patient satisfaction [19, 24, 25].

The PCL sacrificing design allows unrestricted AROM and PROM with full resistive exercises as tolerated. The PCL retaining design has more limitations with full AROM but limited PROM in the first 6 weeks to avoid injury to the retained ligament. This is similar to the PCL sparing TKA design discussed above. The postoperative weight bearing restrictions are implemented based upon the method of implant fixation, cemented or uncemented [19, 24, 25].

Summary

Rehabilitation must be specifically coordinated with the preoperative evaluation, surgical technique, and implant design. This requires close communication between the surgical team and the rehabilitation specialists to arrive at the very best result for the patient.

References

1. Lettin AW, Deliss LJ, Blackburne JS, Scales JT. The Stanmore hinged knee arthroplasty. J Bone Joint Surg Br. 1978;60-B(3):327–32.

2. Lim GR, Kwon EH, Kim DS, et al. The effects of closed kinetic chain exercise and open kinetic chain exercise on the knee position sense in the normal adults. J Int Acad Phys Ther Res. 2010;1(2):126–35.
3. White JJ, Houghton-Clemmey R, Marval P. Enhanced recovery after surgery (ERAS): an orthopaedic perspective. J Perioper Pract. 2013;23(10):228–32.
4. Bannuru RR, Osani MC, Vaysbrot EE, et al. OARSI guidelines for the non-surgical management of knee, hip, and polyarticular osteoarthritis. Osteoarthr Cartil. 2019;27(11):1578–89.
5. Gunaratne R, Pratt DN, Banda J, Fick DP, Khan RJK, Robertson BW. Patient dissatisfaction following total knee arthroplasty: a systematic review of the literature. J Arthroplast. 2017;32(12):3854–60.
6. Nakahara H, Okazaki K, Mizu-Uchi H, et al. Correlations between patient satisfaction and ability to perform daily activities after total knee arthroplasty: why aren't patients satisfied? J Orthop Sci. 2015;20(1):87–92.
7. Mizner RL, Petterson SC, Stevens JE, Axe MJ, Snyder-Mackler L. Preoperative quadriceps strength predicts functional ability one year after total knee arthroplasty. J Rheumatol. 2005;32(8):1533–9.
8. Loudon JK. Biomechanics and pathomechanics of the patellofemoral joint. Int J Sports Phys Ther. 2016;11(6):820–30.
9. Al-Johani AH, Kachanathu SJ, Ramadan Hafez A, et al. Comparative study of hamstring and quadriceps strengthening treatments in the management of knee osteoarthritis. J Phys Ther Sci. 2014;26(6):817–20.
10. Davila Castrodad IM, Recai TM, Abraham MM, et al. Rehabilitation protocols following total knee arthroplasty: a review of study designs and outcome measures. Ann Transl Med. 2019;7(Suppl 7):S255.
11. Berstock JR, Murray JR, Whitehouse MR, Blom AW, Beswick AD. Medial subvastus versus the medial parapatellar approach for total knee replacement: a systematic review and meta-analysis of randomized controlled trials. EFORT Open Rev. 2018;3(3):78–84.
12. Jette DU, Hunter SJ, Burkett L, et al. Physical therapist management of total knee arthroplasty. Phys Ther. 2020;100(9):1603–31.
13. Wang L, Lee M, Zhang Z, Moodie J, Cheng D, Martin J. Does preoperative rehabilitation for patients planning to undergo joint replacement surgery improve outcomes? A systematic review and meta-analysis of randomised controlled trials. BMJ Open. 2016;6(2):e009857.
14. Beard DJ, Davies LJ, Cook JA, et al. The clinical and cost-effectiveness of total versus partial knee replacement in patients with medial compartment osteoarthritis (TOPKAT): 5-year outcomes of a randomised controlled trial. Lancet. 2019;394(10200):746–56.
15. Halawi MJ, Barsoum WK. Unicondylar knee arthroplasty: key concepts. J Clin Orthop Trauma. 2017;8(1):11–3.
16. Parratte S, Ollivier M, Lunebourg A, Abdel MP, Argenson JN. Long-term results of compartmental arthroplasties of the knee: long term results of partial knee arthroplasty. Bone Joint J. 2015;97-B(10 Suppl A):9–15.
17. Fillingham YA, Darrith B, Lonner JH, Culvern C, Crizer M, Della Valle CJ. Formal physical therapy may not be necessary after unicompartmental knee arthroplasty: a randomized clinical trial. J Arthroplast. 2018;33(7S):S93–S99.e3.
18. Sah AP, Higuera JM, Ford MC, Pagnano MW. Alphabet soup of primary total knee arthroplasty liner options-cruciate retaining, posterior stabilized, medial congruent, medial pivot: making sense of the options and what the latest data show. Instr Course Lect. 2024;73:169–81.
19. Senese M, Greenberg E, Todd Lawrence J, Ganley T. Rehabilitation following isolated posterior cruciate ligament reconstruction: a literature review of published protocols. Int J Sports Phys Ther. 2018;13(4):737–51.
20. Arauz P, Klemt C, Limmahakhun S, An S, Kwon YM. Stair climbing and high knee flexion activities in bi-cruciate retaining total knee arthroplasty: in vivo kinematics and articular contact analysis. J Arthroplast. 2019;34(3):570–6.

21. Lutzner J, Firmbach FP, Lutzner C, Dexel J, Kirschner S. Similar stability and range of motion between cruciate-retaining and cruciate-substituting ultracongruent insert total knee arthroplasty. Knee Surg Sports Traumatol Arthrosc. 2015;23(6):1638–43.
22. Cavanaugh JT, Powers M. ACL rehabilitation progression: where are we now? Curr Rev Musculoskelet Med. 2017;10(3):289–96.
23. Kono K, Inui H, Tomita T, et al. Bicruciate-stabilised total knee arthroplasty provides good functional stability during high-flexion weight-bearing activities. Knee Surg Sports Traumatol Arthrosc. 2019;27(7):2096–103.
24. Hodgeson SM, Soeno T, Mears SC, Stambough JB, Barnes CL, Stronach BM. The medial pivot design in total knee arthroplasty. Orthop Clin North Am. 2024;55(1):49–59.
25. Warth LC, Ishmael MK, Deckard ER, Ziemba-Davis M, Meneghini RM. Do medial pivot kinematics correlate with patient-reported outcomes after total knee arthroplasty? J Arthroplast. 2017;32(8):2411–6.

Part VI
Results

Chapter 15
Comparisons of All Designs with Respect to the Cruciate Ligaments

Douglas A. Dennis, Jason A. Bryman, and Richard D. Komistek

Introduction

Kinematic analysis of the knee is the study of motion patterns to assess interaction of the femur relative to the tibia in healthy, nonimplanted knees and various prosthetic knee replacement designs. Numerous surgical techniques and total knee arthroplasty (TKA) designs have been developed to achieve a well-balanced, functional TKA [1]. A comprehensive understanding of the geometric and kinematic profiles of these prostheses is vital for both arthroplasty surgeons and biomedical engineers designing implants. Ideally, the motion patterns of a knee following TKA should closely mimic those of the healthy, nonimplanted knee [2, 3]. Prior to exploring the kinematics of specific TKA implants, one must understand the methods of TKA kinematic analysis, kinematics of the healthy, nonimplanted knee, and the effects of sacrificing the ACL in both healthy, nonimplanted knees and TKAs.

Early investigation of knee kinematics occurred primarily through in vitro cadaveric studies and in vivo gait laboratory analyses [4–6]. Both techniques have significant drawbacks [7–12]. In cadaveric studies, mechanical actuators intended to

D. A. Dennis (✉)
Colorado Joint Replacement, AdventHealth Porter, Denver, CO, USA

Department of Biomedical Engineering, University of Tennessee, Knoxville, TN, USA

Department of Biomedical Engineering, University of Denver, Denver, CO, USA

Department of Orthopaedics, University of Colorado Health School of Medicine, Aurora, CO, USA
e-mail: roseannjohnson@adventhealth.com

J. A. Bryman
Colorado Joint Replacement, AdventHealth Porter, Denver, CO, USA

R. D. Komistek
Department of Biomedical Engineering, University of Tennessee, Knoxville, TN, USA

A. J. Tria Jr., G. R. Scuderi (eds.), *The Cruciate Ligaments in Total Knee Arthroplasty*, https://doi.org/10.1007/978-3-031-75992-5_15

simulate muscle activity often do not duplicate in vivo motion and the ligament properties change, leading to incorrect tensile constraints. Furthermore, the marker systems used in the analysis of gait laboratory systems are imperfect and cannot be corrected even with more markers. Soft tissue artifact and the movement of these markers relative to the bone result in out of plane rotational and translational errors [13, 14]. Building on some of the weaknesses of the now historical cadaveric and gait lab analyses, in vivo video fluoroscopic techniques have emerged as a popular method of kinematic evaluation. Video fluoroscopy uses sequential radiographic images to create a real-time video of dynamic activities, allowing for two-dimensional visualization of the knee joint throughout an entire activity [15, 16] (Fig. 15.1). This offers the distinct advantage of motion analysis of patients under in vivo, weightbearing, dynamic conditions.

The use of weightbearing, video fluoroscopic analysis, which has remained the gold-standard of kinematic analysis since its introduction in the 1990s, has demonstrated numerous abnormal kinematic patterns exist following TKA when compared to the kinematic motion patterns of healthy, nonimplanted knees with intact cruciate ligaments [17–25]. Specifically, abnormal kinematic patterns identified following TKA include paradoxical anteroposterior (AP) femorotibial translation, reverse axial rotation (AR), femoral condylar liftoff (FCLO), and reduced weightbearing knee range of motion (ROM; Tables 15.1, 15.2, and 15.3). AP femorotibial translation describes the sagittal plane movement of the femoral condyle contact points on the tibial plateau during any weightbearing motion activity. The primary activities most commonly analyzed have included gait, weightbearing deep knee bends (WB-DKB), and a step-up maneuver. Axial rotation assesses the rotation of the femur with respect to the tibia throughout range of motion. Lastly, FCLO is defined as separation of the femoral and tibial condylar surfaces during weightbearing activities.

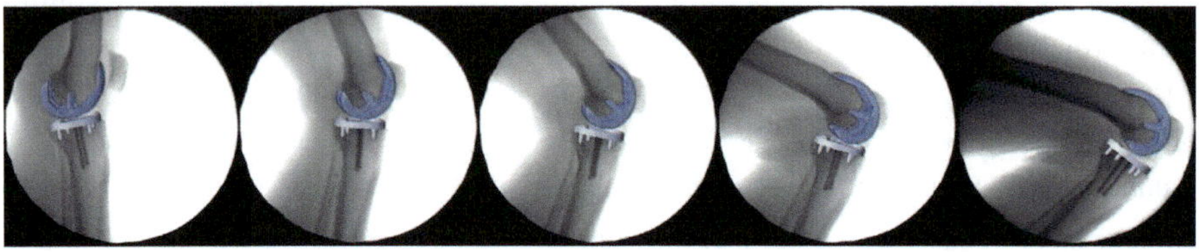

Fig. 15.1 Fluoroscopic images of a patient with a PCR TKA performing a WB-DKB maneuver to maximum weightbearing flexion, in 30-degree increments. Also shown is the corresponding three-dimensional CAD model registered to the two-dimensional fluoroscopic image extracting three-dimensional in vivo kinematics

Table 15.1 Summary of anterior-posterior translation during the stance phase of gait in implanted and nonimplanted knees

Weightbearing gait								
		Posterior rollback (HS-TO)		Average (±SD) movement (HS-TO)		Anterior slide >3.0 mm		Max movement HS-TO, any condyle (mm)[c]
Knee type	# of knees	Lateral (%)	Medial (%)	Lateral (mm)	Medial (mm)	HS-TO, any condyle (%)[a]	Any increment, any condyle (%)[b]	
Normal	10	90	50	−5.8 ± 8.1	−0.4 ± 6.6	30	90	11.9
ACLD	5	60	60	−1.9 ± 4.4	−2.3 ± 6.8	20	40	3.0
PCRF	83	61	46	−1.2 ± 3.2	0.0 ± 2.3	22	52	6.7
PSF	74	61	55	−1.3 ± 3.2	0.5 ± 3.3	23	50	8.1
BCRF	15	53	73	−3.7 ± 7.4	−1.6 ± 7.7	13	40	18.2
PCRM	10	50	40	0.2 ± 5.7	−0.3 ± 4.5	20	50	20.9
PCSM	35	46	46	0.3 ± 2.4	−0.2 ± 3.1	26	51	6.9
PSM	44	52	34	−0.7 ± 2.7	0.5 ± 2.2	11	25	5.4
All TKAs	**261**	**57**	**48**	**−1.0 ± 3.5**	**0.2 ± 3.3**	**19**	**46**	**20.9**
MED UKA	68	—	59	—	−0.3 ± 2.7	10	26	7.7
LAT UKA	7	43	—	1.3 ± 3.9	—	33	17	8.8

Note: This cumulative data originates from many peer-reviewed, published articles from the senior authors. Within the individual papers, all subjects chosen for analysis were considered clinically excellent with knee scores >90 point and without measurable instability or functional disability related to pain

Adapted from Angerame et al. [26]; Published in part: Dennis D et al. [27]; Published in full: Mueller et al. [28]

HS-TO Heel Strike to toe off, *ACLD* Anterior cruciate ligament-deficient knee, *PCRF* Posterior cruciate-retaining TKA, fixed bearing, *PSF* Posterior stabilized TKA, fixed bearing, *BCRF* Bicruciate retaining TKA, fixed bearing, *PCRM* Posterior cruciate-retaining TKA, mobile bearing, *PSM* Posterior stabilized TKA, mobile bearing, *BCSF* Bicruciate stabilized TKA, fixed bearing, *MED UKA* medial unicompartmental knee arthroplasty, *LAT UKA* lateral unicompartmental knee arthroplasty

[a]Refers to the percentage of knees demonstrating anterior slide of either condyle only comparing the increment of heel strike vs. the increment of toe off

[b]Refers to the percentage of knees demonstrating anterior slide of either condyle during any two increments of stance phase (i.e., heel strike vs. 33% of stance phase)

[c]Represents the maximum amount of AP translation (anterior-most contact position vs. the most posterior contact position) observed within each knee type analyzed from heel strike to toe off

Table 15.2 Summary of anterior-posterior translation during a weightbearing, deep knee bend in implanted and nonimplanted knees

Weightbearing, deep knee bend							
		Posterior rollback (0–90°)		Average (±SD) movement (0–90°)		Anterior slide >3.0 mm	
Knee type	# of knees	Lateral (%)	Medial (%)	Lateral (mm)	Medial (mm)	Any condyle (0–90°) (%)	Any increment, any condyle (%)
Normal	104	100	98	−16.4 ± 6.8	−8.9 ± 6.0	2	15
ACLD	5	100	100	−13.3 ± 8.3	−5.9 ± 1.9	0	20
PCRF	43	68	34	−2.4 ± 4.2	0.6 ± 3.7	24	52
PSF	457	71	61	−8.5 ± 8.4	−4.0 ± 5.4	4	27
BCRF	34	91	83	−10.4 ± 5.0	−5.6 ± 5.1	6	32
PCRM	107	68	46	−1.3 ± 3.5	0.4 ± 3.8	25	60
PCSM	76	85	37	−2.1 ± 2.7	0.4 ± 2.6	18	54
PSM	341	59	26	−2.7 ± 4.2	0.6 ± 3.7	16	27
BCSF	95	100	100	−21.9 ± 5.9	−12.5 ± 3.1	0	7
All TKAs	**1453**	**70**	**46**	**−5.8 ± 5.9**	**−1.9 ± 4.0**	**14**	**35**
MED UKA	65	—	63	—	−4.4 ± 4.8	5	31
LAT UKA	3	100	—	−6.3 ± 7.6	—	0	33

Note: This cumulative data originates from many peer-reviewed, published articles from the senior authors. Within the individual papers, all subjects chose for the analyses were considered clinically excellent with knee scores >90 points and without measurable instability or functional disability related to pain

Adapted from Angerame et al. [26]; Published in part: Dennis D et al. [27]; Published in full: Mueller et al. [28]

HS-TO Heel Strike to toe off, *ACLD* Anterior cruciate ligament-deficient knee, *PCRF* Posterior cruciate-retaining TKA, fixed bearing, *PSF* Posterior stabilized TKA, fixed bearing, *BCRF* Bicruciate retaining TKA, fixed bearing, *PCRM* Posterior cruciate-retaining TKA, mobile bearing, *PSM* Posterior stabilized TKA, mobile bearing, *BCSF* Bicruciate stabilized TKA, fixed bearing, *MED UKA* Medial unicompartmental knee arthroplasty, *LAT UKA* lateral unicompartmental knee arthroplasty

Table 15.3 Summary of axial rotation for implanted and nonimplanted knees during a weightbearing deep knee bend

Knee type	Average rotation (0°–90°)	Average maximum normal rotation, any increment (degrees)	Average maximum reverse rotation, any increment (degrees)
Normal	17.8	31.6	−7.3
ACLD	9.8	21.2	−9.8
PCRF TKA	3.9	21.3	−19.0
PSF TKA	5.0	19.1	−18.1
BCRF TKA	5.6	20.9	−14.1
PCRM TKA	3.9	15.6	−11.4
PCSM TKA	3.3	11.4	−5.9
PSM TKA	4.4	27.1	−14.9
BCSF TKA	10.7	22.5	−4.2
All TKAs	4.8	27.1	−19.0
MED UKA	4.3	17.1	−15.3
LAT UKA	−0.7	13.3	−16.1

Note: This cumulative data originates from many peer-reviewed, published articles from the senior authors. Within individual papers, all subjects chosen for analyses were considered clinically excellent with knee scores >90 point and without measurable instability or functional disability related to pain

Adapted from Angerame et al. [26]; Published in part: Dennis D et al. [29]; Published in full: Mueller et al. [28]

ACLD Anterior cruciate ligament-deficient knee, *PCRF* Posterior cruciate-retaining TKA, fixed bearing, *PSF* Posterior stabilized TKA, fixed bearing, *BCRF* Bicruciate retaining TKA, fixed bearing, *PCRM* Posterior cruciate-retaining TKA, mobile bearing, *PSM* Posterior stabilized TKA, mobile bearing, *BCSF* Bicruciate stabilized TKA, fixed bearing, *MED UKA* medial unicompartmental knee arthroplasty, *LAT UKA* lateral unicompartmental knee arthroplasty

Healthy, Nonimplanted Knee Kinematics

AP Translation

Knee Society scores following TKA correlate with patients' perception of increased ROM [30]. Therefore, the AP translation of the femorotibial articulation is paramount in TKA design [31]. In a video fluoroscopic analysis of ten healthy, nonimplanted knees, Dennis et al. assessed the movement of the tibiofemoral contact point throughout the gait cycle [28]. During the stance phase of gait, all except one patient experienced a motion pattern where the lateral condyle moved in the posterior

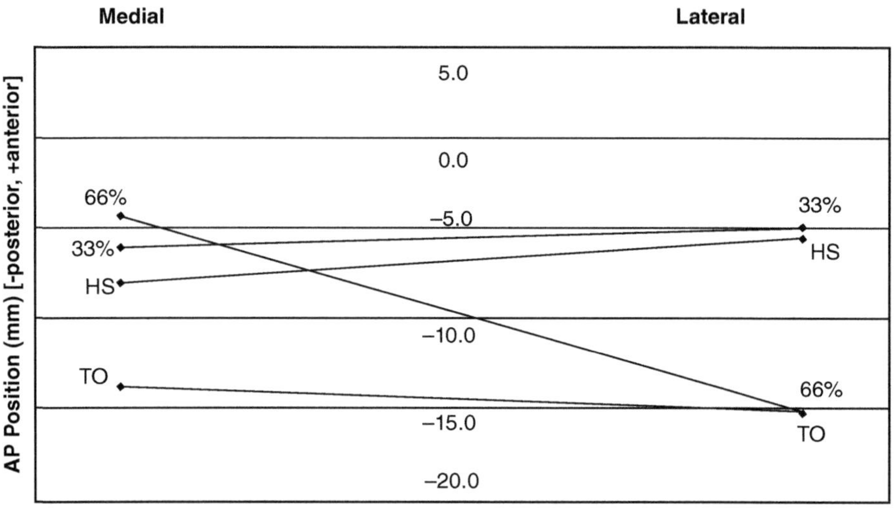

Fig. 15.2 AP translation pattern of the medial and lateral femoral condyles during the stance phase of gait in the healthy, non-implanted knee (HS, heel strike; 33% of stance phase; 66% of stance phase; TO, toe off)

direction more than the medial femoral condyle (MFC), representing a fan-like motion pattern. Although it has been described the normal knee exhibits a medial pivot pattern, the data does not precisely resemble this type of motion as the medial condyle translates in the sagittal plane up to 12 mm during motion cycles. The magnitude of posterior translation during the stance phase of gait averages 5.8 mm laterally vs. 0.4 mm medially (Fig. 15.2). During the entire gait cycle (stance and swing phases), when the direction of knee flexion angle changes from extension to flexion, the lateral condyle translates in the posterior direction. When the angle changes from flexion into extension, the lateral condyle contact point translates anteriorly.

During a WB-DKB using dynamic video fluoroscopy, the magnitude of AP translation is higher as compared to normal gait, which incurs a lesser degree of knee flexion. Mueller et al. [28] have demonstrated that 102 of 104 subjects with a normal knee analyzed under fluoroscopic surveillance while performing a DKB experienced some degree of posterior motion for the MFC, and all 104 experienced posterior motion of the LFC (Fig. 15.3). The medial fan-like kinematic pattern is more consistently present during a WB-DKB as compared to normal gait [29, 32–34].

Freeman et al. has described the normal knee having a medial pivot motion pattern, based on an MRI analysis where the patient was lying on their back and the knee was moved passively, but stationary during each image [35]. The lateral femoral condyle (LFC) predictably moved more posteriorly than the MFC. This is corroborated by the study of Johal et al. [36], in another non-weightbearing MRI analysis that showed that during flexion, the LFC moves posterior while the MFC remains relatively more stationary. The MFC does exhibit some translational movement but is much more constrained than the LFC due to the articulation of a convex

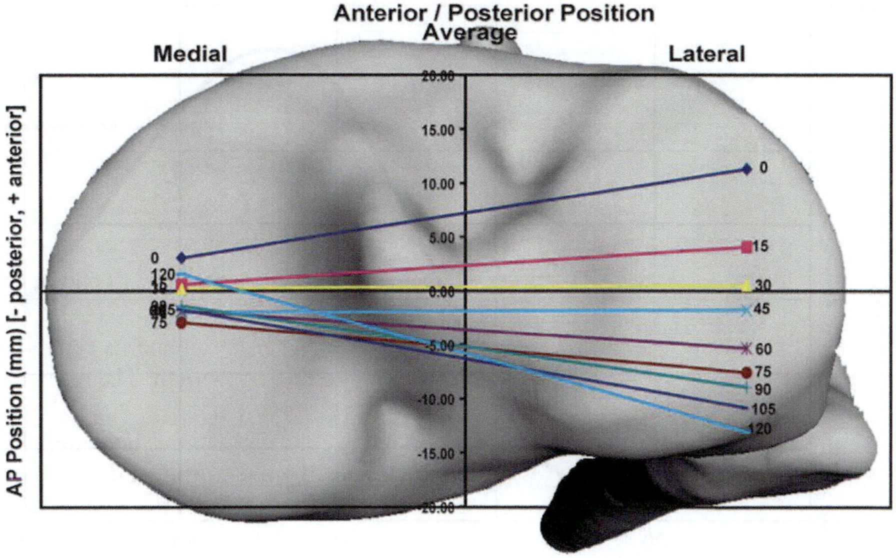

Fig. 15.3 Top view of the fan-like pattern of AP translation of the medial and lateral femoral condyles during a WB-DKB in the healthy, nonimplanted knee. Note that the MFC demonstrates some posterior translation although less than the LFC

MFC with a concave medial tibial plateau, which produces a fan-like distribution of motion [37]. Beyond 120° of flexion during a WB-DKB activity, both condyles move posteriorly to a similar extent.

Axial Rotation

During gait from heel strike to toe off, dynamic, weightbearing fluoroscopic studies have demonstrated that healthy-nonimplanted knees typically experience axial rotation, with the tibia internally rotating in reference to the femur with increasing knee flexion [28] (Fig. 15.4a).

Tibial internal rotation with respect to the femur is also present in the nonimplanted normal knee during higher degrees of knee flexion, such as during a WB-DKB [8, 32, 36, 38]. The magnitudes of axial rotation are greater during a WB-DKB than during normal gait due to the increased flexion incurred during this activity (Fig. 15.4b).

The coupled internal tibia rotation as the femur flexes and external tibial rotation as the femur extends is referred to as the screw-home mechanism [39]. While various explanations exist to explain this axial rotation pattern, common hypotheses include the length and tensioning of the cruciate and collateral ligaments, as well as asymmetry in the geometry of the medial and lateral femoral condyles [39].

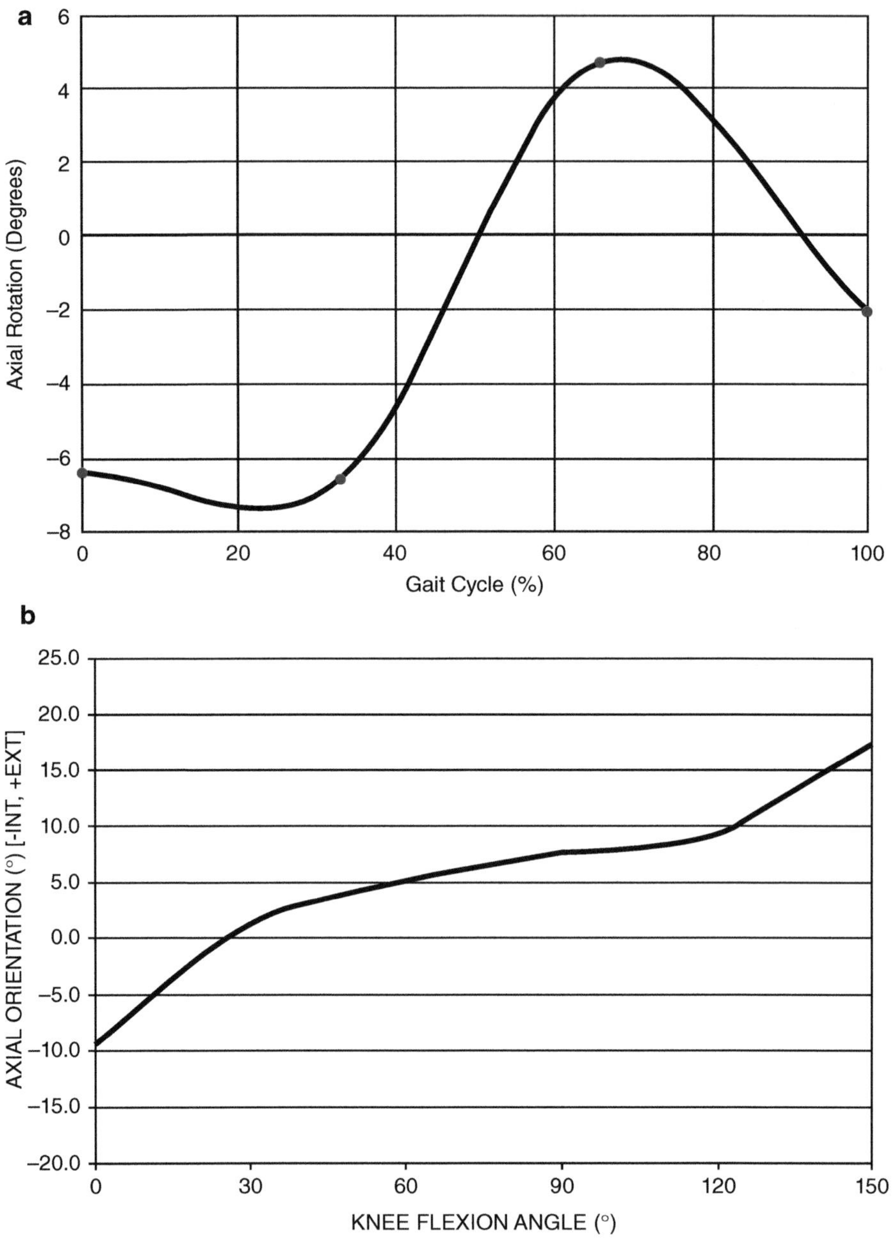

Fig. 15.4 (**a**) Axial rotation pattern of the healthy, nonimplanted knee during gait. (**b**) Axial rotation pattern of the healthy, nonimplanted knee during a WB-DKB

Using both MRI and biplanar fluoroscopic motion analyses, Qi et al. [40] reported in the first 30° of knee flexion, the magnitude of axial rotation is greater and then lessens as flexion proceeds. However, in the stance phase of gait, since the knee flexion angle changes from flexion to extension, both internal and external rotation of the tibia may occur [28]. In fact, many patients experience paradoxical or reverse rotation (in which external rotation of the tibia occurs in reference to the femur) during segments of the stance phase of gait [9, 41–43].

Femoral Condylar Liftoff

FCLO occurs more frequently in the lateral compartment articulation in the healthy, nonimplanted knee [40]. This may occur because of soft tissue impingement, which is compressed between the lateral tibial plateau and femoral condyle, creating a lateral pivot point [40].

ACL-Deficient, Nonimplanted Kinematics

AP Translation

The ACL functions to resist anterior translation of the tibia relative to the femur [8]. Consequently, an ACL-deficient (ACLD) knee has a center of rotation that is posteriorized relative to the healthy, nonimplanted knee [9, 12] (Fig. 15.5). Shear stresses, resulting from the anterior pull of the extensor mechanism on the tibia from 0° to 30° of knee flexion, cause a more posterior femorotibial contact to occur in the absence of the ACL [44–46]. There is a decreased magnitude of anteroposterior translation as well as overall increased variability in kinematic patterns compared to the healthy, nonimplanted knee [39]. Fluoroscopic data confirms since the axis of rotation begins more posterior compared to a knee with intact cruciate ligaments, the MFC has a lesser magnitude of posterior translation in the ACLD knee [8]. Since the ACL function is lost, the lateral condyle contacts the tibia more posterior in extension and minimal change in axial rotation exists, leading to the knee functioning like a malrotated hinge. Lastly, the incidence and magnitude of paradoxical anterior femoral translation observed during progressive knee flexion is greater in ACLD [39]. The differences in AP translation seen between implanted and nonimplanted knees can be attributed to the lack of cruciate ligaments and altered mechanics of the extensor mechanism [44–46]. Shear stresses from the anterior pull of the extensor mechanism on the tibia from 0° to 30° of knee flexion result in a more posterior femorotibial contact to occur due to the absence of the ACL. At greater degrees of flexion (45–60°), the direction of patellar ligament pull on the tibia changes to a posteriorly directed force on the tibia which normally is resisted by the PCL.

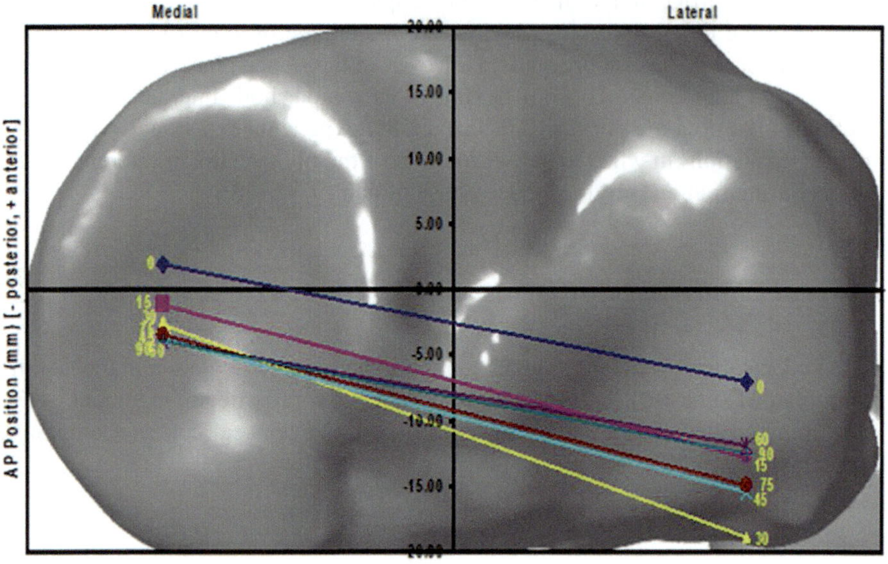

Fig. 15.5 AP translation pattern of the medial and lateral femoral condyles throughout ROM in the ACLD knee. The lateral condyle does not contact anteriorly at full extension like the normal knee, but rather functions like a malrotated hinge and progressive axial rotation does not exist

Anterior femoral translation results in a more anterior axis of flexion which lessens maximum knee flexion. It also decreases the moment arm of the quadriceps and therefore reduces quadriceps efficiency.

Axial Rotation

With the LFC now rotating around a posteriorized MFC, decreased AR occurs in ACLD knees compared to healthy, nonimplanted knees [8, 15, 16, 39, 47]. Mueller et al. in a weightbearing fluoroscopic analysis of 1630 implanted and nonimplanted knees, found that axial rotation magnitudes in ACLD knees (mean 9.8°) are less than that observed in the normal knee (mean 17.8°; Table 15.3) during a WB-DKB [28].

Also, with the lateral condyle positioned more posterior, it cannot rotate in the normal direction, but often incurs reverse rotation because the lateral condyle slides in the anterior direction with increasing knee flexion. In summary, ACL deficiency results in a more posterior center of rotation and axis of flexion, less AR during WB-DKB, and overall, a more variable axial rotational pattern during flexion [39, 47–49].

Femoral Condylar Liftoff

FCLO occurs more frequently in the lateral compartment articulation in the ACL-deficient knee. The ACL acts as a static stabilizer of the lateral femoral condyle, and with an incompetent ACL, the lateral condyle moves more freely in the AP and superior-inferior directions.

PCL Sparing TKA Kinematics

AP Translation

PCL sparing TKAs demonstrate similar kinematic patterns to ACLD, nonimplanted knees throughout the gait cycle [27, 49, 50] (Table 15.1). Cumulative data from the senior authors documents both PCL sparing fixed and mobile bearing designs exhibit minimal AP translation during gait [27, 50]. However, in deeper flexion, such as a DKB maneuver, the contact positions of both PCL sparing designs are more posterior in extension due to the absence of the ACL [51]. Since the ACL is absent, leading to the condyles contacting the tibia more posterior, the only direction the condyles can move is in the anterior direction, opposite of the normal knee. The mean lateral femoral condylar posterior translation with a PCL sparing TKA (−2.4 mm) is significantly less than that observed in the normal knee (−16.4 mm) during a WB-DKB (Table 15.2).

In the normal knee, the lateral condylar contact position is positioned anterior of the medial condylar contact location in extension and translates posteriorly as knee flexion increases. With PCL sparing TKA, the lateral condyle is positioned posterior of the medial condyle in full extension and often paradoxically translates anteriorly with progressive knee flexion. This is opposite of the healthy, nonimplanted knee and likely due to an imbalance between the PCL and an absent ACL. Approximately one of four PCL sparing TKAs experience paradoxical anterior femoral (Fig. 15.6) translation during WB-DKB, despite the initial posterior translation of the lateral femoral condyle relative to the tibia in lesser degrees of flexion. Therefore, PCL sparing TKAs have reduced posterior femoral translation during flexion, and paradoxical anterior femoral translation, if present, is most observed in the first 40° of flexion [52]. Paradoxical anterior femoral translation has been found to occur more frequently in PCL sparing than in other TKA designs (Table 15.2). This can be attributed to inadequate PCL tension in the presence of a posteriorly directed force in deeper flexion exerted by the extensor mechanism and no ACL force to counterbalance the PCL pull [51]. While the extensor mechanism exerts an anterior pull on the tibia from 0 to 30° of flexion, this shifts to a posteriorly directed force in 45–60° of flexion. Without the intact ACL, the PCL acts unopposed, and an alteration of sagittal plane kinematics can occur.

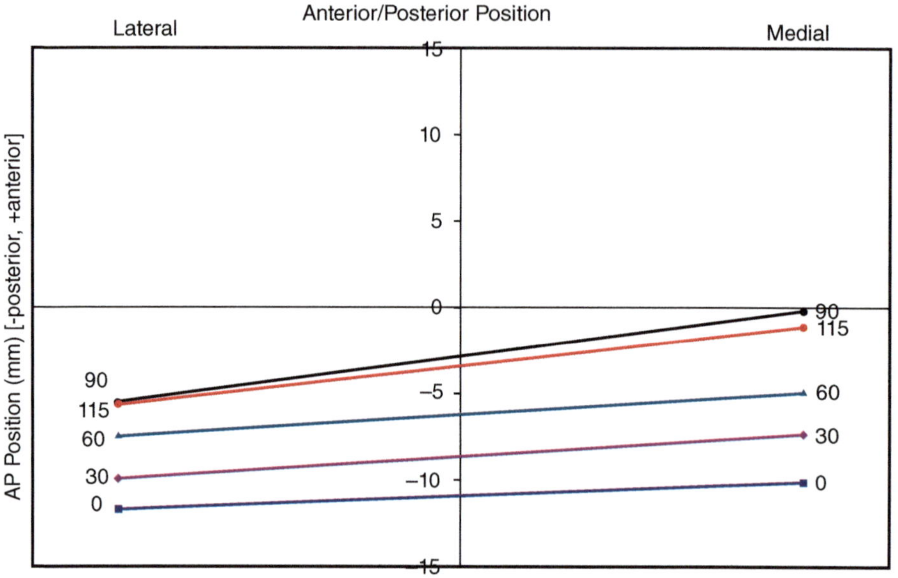

Fig. 15.6 Example of paradoxical anterior femoral translation of a PCL sparing TKA during a WB-DKB

As noted in the nonimplanted ACLD knee, paradoxical anterior femoral translation moves the axis of flexion anteriorly and likely plays a role in reduced weight-bearing knee flexion since posterior structures impinge earlier. It also decreases the moment arm of the extensor mechanism, decreasing quadriceps efficiency. Finally, anterior translation during flexion increases shear forces on the polyethylene liner and risks accelerating polyethylene wear [53]. Paradoxical anterior femoral translation may be limited by certain implant design features in PCL sparing TKAs, including differing J-curves of the medial vs. lateral femoral condyles [54–56] and symmetric femoral component designs which incorporate a gradually reducing femoral radius of curvature (multiple subtle radius of curvature reductions) as opposed to dual radius femoral component designs [57].

Axial Rotation

PCL sparing TKAs exhibit less AR and greater variability than healthy, nonimplanted knees during both gait and WB-DKB [29]. There is also wide variability with respect to maximum normal and reverse rotation [28]. Axial rotation magnitudes during a WB-DKB in PCL sparing TKAs (mean 3.9°) are significantly less than that observed in the normal knee (mean 17.8°; Table 15.3) [28]. Additionally, reverse axial rotation, in which the tibia externally rotates with respect to the femur, has a higher incidence (21%) and higher magnitudes in PCL sparing TKAs than the incidence observed in the normal knee (0%) [29]. Reverse axial rotational patterns are undesirable as it can lead to abnormal patellofemoral function. With tibial external rotation, there is lateralization of the tibial tubercle during deep flexion which can result in patellofemoral instability and tracking issues. Additionally, the reduction in posterior femoral rollback of the lateral femoral condyle may lessen maximal knee flexion.

Femoral Condylar Liftoff

In the implanted knee, asymmetric ligament tension, often associated with femoral component malrotation, likely is the main contributor to FCLO. This has been confirmed in several fluoroscopic-based kinematic studies [20, 22]. For example, if the femoral component is positioned internally rotated relative to the transepicondylar axis, increased bone will be resected from the posterior aspect of the lateral femoral condyle, loosening the lateral flexion gap and enhancing the risk of FCLO laterally. In PCR TKAs, the incidence of FCLO has been observed to be higher laterally than medially. This is believed to be related to the presence of the intact PCL which attaches to the medial femoral condyle and provides a tethering affect to lessen liftoff of the medial femoral condyle. In contrast, the tethering effect of the ACL, which attaches to the lateral femoral condyle, is absent, allowing a higher incidence of lateral FCLO. Therefore, aligning the femoral component to create a symmetric, rectangular flexion gap is essential in decreasing the incidence and magnitude of FCLO in TKA [4, 43]. This can be achieved in both gap-balanced and measured resection techniques. However, Dennis et al. showed that FCLO >1 mm occurred in 45–60% of PCL sparing and substituting TKA patients implanted using measured resection vs. none using a gap-balanced technique [4].

In the senior authors 30-year history of studying TKA kinematics, the incidence of FCLO in fluoroscopic studies performed in the 1990s and early 2000s was common. In the last decade, the incidence and magnitude of FCLO has lessened, likely due to improved surgical instrumentation, ligament balancing techniques and surgeon awareness of this phenomenon.

PCL Substituting TKA Kinematics

PCL Substituting TKA designs utilize a cam-post mechanism that engages in mid-to-later flexion to facilitate PFR, thereby increasing TKA flexion [27, 50]. In most designs, the cam and post do not engage until higher degrees of flexion, resulting in similar kinematic patterns during gait as TKA designs without a cam/post mechanism [50]. Modern PS designs incorporate a thinner sagittal profile of the post, decreased contact stresses and subsequent risk of post wear, while enhancing axial rotation [58].

AP Translation

Neither PCL substituting nor PCL sparing TKA designs duplicate the magnitude of PFR of the healthy, nonimplanted knee during a WB-DKB, but PCL substituting TKAs more closely replicate normal knee kinematics forcing the condyles to move in the posterior direction with increasing knee flexion. The mean lateral femoral condylar translation during a WB-DKB with a PCL substituting TKA (−8.5 mm) is less than that observed in the normal knee (−16.4 mm), but significantly more than a PCL sparing TKA (−2.4 mm) (Table 15.2) [59]. Mueller et al. found that only 4% of 457 PS fixed-bearing TKAs demonstrated paradoxical anterior femoral translation, in contrast to a 24% incidence of paradoxical anterior femoral translation observed in PCL sparing TKA designs [28]. By engagement of the cam-post mechanism, PCL substituting TKAs reliably experience less anterior translation of both the MFC and LFC and greater PFR when compared to PCL sparing designs. This may improve ROM by creating a more posteriorized axis of flexion, which prevents impingement of posterior structures and lessens extensor mechanism tension in deep flexion [60].

Axial Rotation

Throughout the gait cycle, PCL substituting TKAs demonstrate limited AR compared to the healthy, nonimplanted knee, with a higher incidence of reverse rotation [8, 28, 29]. However, in a WB-DKB, PCL substituting TKAs do experience higher mean AR magnitudes (5.0°) than PCL sparing TKAs (3.9°) but substantially less than in normal knees (17.8°) (Table 15.3) [28, 29]. In patients with a PCL substituting TKA, AR centered around the MFC has been shown to lead to higher outcome scores, patient satisfaction, and knee flexion compared to patients with reverse rotation patterns [61]. Since the cam/post mechanism does not engage until later flexion, the lateral condyle is not positioned as far anterior as the normal knee in full extension and during mid-flexion. These TKA designs can experience some condylar sliding, varying based on TKA design. If the posterior aspect of the post is flat, it could lead to a reduction of axial rotation due to a flat cam contacting a flat post. PCL substituting TKA with a rounded posterior cam and post often experience increased axial rotation as the cam can rotate around the post.

Femoral Condylar Liftoff

As previously stated, the incidence of FCLO is similar to that observed in PCL sparing TKAs and is likely more affected by the precision and type of surgical technique. In PCL substituting TKAs, the authors have observed a similar incidence of medial vs. lateral FCLO in contrast to PCL sparing TKAs where the majority of liftoff is observed laterally since the intact PCL helps stabilize the medial femoral condyle.

Bicruciate Substituting TKA Kinematics

Bicruciate substituting (BCS) TKAs utilize a dual cam-post mechanism, attempting to produce kinematics similar to a normal knee with intact anterior and posterior cruciate ligaments. The anterior cam-post mechanism substitutes for the ACL, facilitating anterior contact in extension and lesser degrees of flexion, and a posterior cam-post mechanism to induce posterior condylar rollback in deeper flexion. Additionally, the medial aspect of the polyethylene insert is more conforming with a goal of providing greater AP stability medially and enhancing a medial pivot motion pattern that more closely aligns with the kinematics of the healthy, nonimplanted knee.

AP Translation

It has been reported that BCS TKA reduce ML instability in mid-flexion while improving patient satisfaction [62]. Similar kinematic patterns exist in BCS TKA and the healthy, nonimplanted knee when analyzed fluoroscopically [19]. A randomized controlled trial by Smith et al. has confirmed that BCS TKAs produce more normal sagittal plane kinematics than posterior stabilized designs [63]. In fact, a weightbearing fluoroscopic analysis of 1630 nonimplanted and implanted knees of multiple differing TKA designs shows the mean lateral femoral condylar posterior translation with a BCS TKA (−21.9 mm) is greater than that observed in the normal knee (−16.4 mm) during a WB-DKB [64, 65] (Table 15.2, Fig. 15.7).

Axial Rotation

BCS TKA are designed to limit reverse axial rotation via incorporation of the dual cam-post mechanism with the condyles experiencing anterior contact in full extension more representative of the normal knee. In a weightbearing fluoroscopic kinematic analysis, Grieco et al. [19] observed from 0° to 30° of knee flexion, the BCS subjects exhibited similar patterns of femoral rollback and axial rotation compared to normal knee subjects. From 30° to 60° of knee flexion, BCS subjects experienced negligible anterior-posterior motions and axial rotation while normal knees continued to rollback and externally rotate. Between 60° and 90° the BCS resumed posterior motion and, after 90°, axial rotation increased in a normal-like fashion

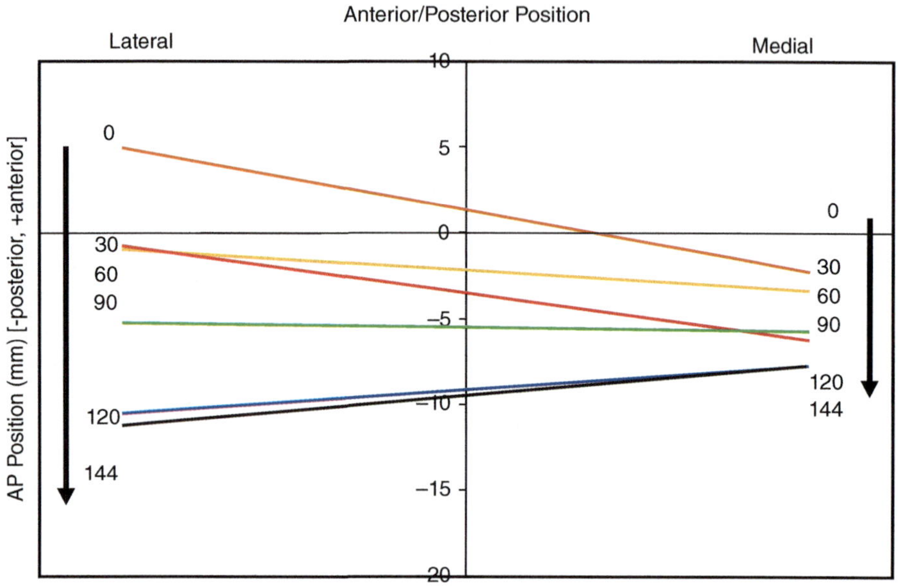

Fig. 15.7 Example of mean AP translation pattern of a bicruciate substituting TKA

(Fig. 15.8). In contrast to most other TKA designs, axial rotation magnitudes in BCS TKAs are greater (mean 10.7°) although less than that observed in the normal knee (mean 17.8°; Table 15.3) [28].

Bicruciate Retaining TKA Kinematics

A bicruciate retaining (BCR) TKA involves preservation of both the ACL and PCL. Historical designs utilized a design rationale that matched the radius of curvature based exclusively on the lateral femoral condyle or the medial femoral condyle. Perhaps because of the symmetric condylar design, kinematic analyses of these implants often demonstrate poor weightbearing flexion [66]. Modern designs with variable radius of curvatures show more favorable kinematic patterns that are more similar to the healthy-nonimplanted knee in both gait (Table 15.1) and a WB-DKB (Table 15.2) [27, 67].

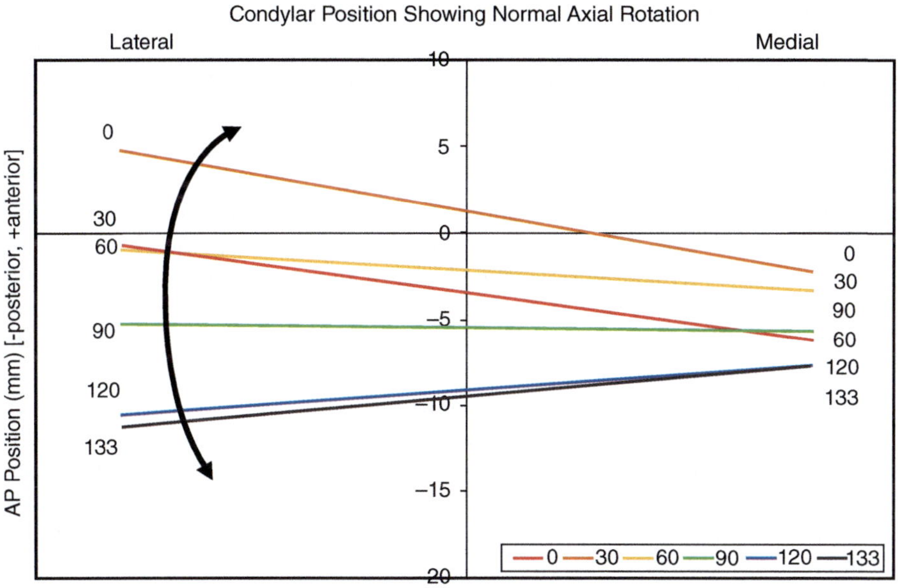

Fig. 15.8 Mean axial rotation patterns of a bicruciate substituting TKA

AP Translation

Retention of both cruciate ligaments and different radius of curvatures for the MFC and LFC allow for superior proprioception compared to the PS TKA design [68]. Specifically, retention of the ACL yields AP laxity that mimics the native knee. In a cadaveric study, Amis et al. found that AP laxity with the PCL sparing TKA was greater than the native knee and BCR TKA, but no difference was found between the BCR TKA and the native knee [69]. The BCR TKA design is at least partially able to successfully restore the kinematic role of the anterior cruciate ligament. BCR TKAs have a pattern of posterior femoral rollback (PFR) that closely mimics the normal knee (Table 15.1) [70]. Mean AP translation during gait of BCS TKAs (−3.7 mm) has been reported to be similar to that observed in the normal knee (−5.9 mm; Table 15.1). During a WB-DKB, mean AP translation of BCR TKAs (−10.4 mm) has been observed to be less than the normal knee cohort (−16.4 mm; Table 15.2).

Axial Rotation

Similar to other TKA designs, BCR TKAs demonstrate less AR than healthy, non-implanted knees during gait and WB-DKB (Table 15.3) [28]. However, Mueller et al. reported a higher magnitude of AR in BCR TKAs compared to ACL-sacrificing TKA designs due to retention of the ACL [28, 29].

Despite a favorable kinematic pattern, implantation of BCR-TKAs is technically demanding given constraints of tibial subluxation without sacrificing the ACL or PCL. Even in modern designs, there are higher than anticipated revision rates, with revision-free survival of 88% at 3 years, significantly lower than existing traditional TKA designs [71]. This may be related to significant anatomic variations in the medial and lateral femoral radii of curvature among patients, which may conflict with the chosen femoral radii of the prosthetic femoral component. Moreover, outcome data shows little difference between BCR and PCR designs [47, 70]. Careful attention must be placed to appropriate balancing of the cruciate ligaments. Kono et al. performed an in vivo kinematic analysis of 15 knees with BCR-TKA fluoroscopically examined while performing a squatting activity [72]. They found that both cruciate ligament tension, especially the PCL tension, was greater than that found in normal knees and emphasized the importance of balanced cruciate ligament tension in both flexion and extension.

Medial Pivot TKA Kinematics

Medial Pivot (MP) TKA describes a spectrum of TKA designs in which increased medial conformity limits medial translation while still allowing knee axial rotation centered about a medial compartment pivot area. These TKA were initially designed based on MRI studies that were conducted with the patient performing quasi-static flexion, where patients first lay on their back and passively flex their knee to various knee flexion angles, then hold their knee still during the MRI scan [35]. Under these passive, quasi-static conditions, the knee motion pattern was described as a "medial pivot." More recent studies, including in vivo high-speed stereo-radiographic kinematic analyses, have shown the actual pivot location varies based on the type of activity being performed and the corresponding degree of knee flexion [73].

It is important to understand the kinematics of all medial pivot TKA designs are not the same. The amount of medial conformity, location of the medial dwell point in the sagittal plane, size matching of the tibial insert with femoral component size (matching vs. up or downsize matching), femoral trochlear designs, and the tracking patterns laterally may differ. Therefore, differing kinematic patterns among designs is to be expected.

AP Translation

In medial pivot TKA designs, unlike PCL substituting designs, there is no tibial posterior stabilizing post or femoral cam. A concave tibial insert with an anterior lip that stabilizes the MFC may allow for better control of AP translation, while allowing for normal LFC motion. Sagittal translation of >7 mm either anteriorly or posteriorly on the medial articulation has been shown to result in subjective feelings of instability [74], and the design rationale behind the MP TKA was to improve this parameter and ultimately outcomes following TKA.

A fluoroscopic analysis by Schmidt et al. has documented that the MP TKA has diminished AP translation of the MFC while the LFC moves posteriorly through flexion [75]. An MP kinematic pattern demonstrates greater excursion of the LFC compared to PCL sparing TKA [76–81].

Axial Rotation

Medial pivot TKAs are designed with a goal of creating an AR pattern that more closely mimics the healthy, nonimplanted knee compared to other TKA designs [75–81]. Warth et al. [33] reported in a cohort of 141 TKAs, including PCL sparing and PCL substituting designs, that only 40% exhibited an MP kinematic pattern; this did not translate into a difference in outcome scores or activity levels. This contrasts the findings of Nishio et al. [61], who reported that an MP pattern of AR led to higher outcome scores, patient satisfaction, and knee flexion compared to patients with reverse AR. The clinical results of the MP design are overall conflicting, with one study showing superior Forgotten Joint Scores at 1 year following surgery [82] and others showing worse outcomes with the MP vs. PCL substituting TKAs [83].

As previously stated, despite the intention of the MP design to improve the kinematics of the implanted knee, the kinematics is design-specific, which may explain the variability in clinical results. Whether to save or sacrifice the PCL also remains a debated technical consideration. In MP designs with less inherent conformity of the medial compartment, reliable AP constraint may only exist in lesser degrees of flexion, leading to sagittal plane instability in higher degrees of flexion and WB-DKB [84].

Mobile Bearing TKA Kinematics

Mobile bearing (MB) designs, in which the polyethylene bearing can freely rotate, were intended to improve axial rotation while decreasing contact stresses and lowering polyethylene wear rates [29]. In vivo, weightbearing fluoroscopic studies demonstrate the MB insert typically tracks with the femoral component [85, 86]. The axial rotation of the MB insert in accordance with the rotating femur maintains a central cam-post contact, which may reduce polyethylene wear of the post in PCL substituting TKA designs [87]. Similarly, this bearing rotation with the femoral component maintains congruency of the articular surfaces. This results in increased contact area and reduced polyethylene contact stresses when axial rotation occurs [86]. In contrast, in fixed-bearing articulations, contact area lessens with a concomitant increase in polyethylene stress during activities which induce axial rotation. A knee simulator analysis under high kinematic conditions (10 mm AP translation; +5° axial rotation), attempting to mimic the high activity level patient, demonstrated substantial wear reduction in a rotating platform mobile bearing design [88]. LaCour et al., in an in vivo three-dimensional kinematic analysis, reported that at 10-year follow-up duration, polyethylene bearing-tibial tray mobility is maintained [89]. Bearing mobility may also facilitate centralization of the extensor mechanism as evidenced by the decreased rate of lateral retinacular release in MB TKA (5.3%) vs. fixed-bearing TKA (14.3%) [90].

With regard to kinematics, both mobile- and fixed-bearing PCL substituting TKAs fail to duplicate the magnitude of PFR of the normal knee during a WB-DKB (Table 15.2). In a weightbearing, fluoroscopic kinematic analysis of 341 PCL substituting MB TKAs, 16% demonstrated anterior femoral translation compared to only 4% of 457 PS fixed-bearing TKAs [28]. The overall pattern of axial rotation during flexion is similar compared to fixed-bearing designs, and less than healthy, nonimplanted knees [29, 91–95]. Lastly, while fluoroscopic studies show most TKAs (multiple designs) rotate <10° during a WB-DKB maneuver, numerous outliers are reported which rotate >20° which is greater than the ideal axial rotation boundaries of fixed-bearing designs. Some theorize mobile bearings would be advantageous in this patient cohort [29].

Knee Range of Motion

Despite kinematic differences, recent studies show no difference in postoperative ROM or outcome scores in PCL sparing vs. PCL substituting designs [96, 97]. However, Dennis et al. have shown while there is no statistical difference in *nonweightbearing* ROM between PCL sparing vs. PCL substituting designs, there is a difference in motion when tested under *weightbearing* conditions [60]. PCL substituting TKAs were found to have an average weightbearing flexion magnitude of 113° vs. 103° in PCL sparing designs, despite preoperative PCL sparing TKA patients having more motion preoperatively. With the decreased posterior femoral rollback seen with PCL sparing designs and increased paradoxical anterior femoral translation seen in deep flexion, there is earlier posterior impingement and a tightened extensor mechanism. This may explain the differences in weightbearing ROM seen between PCL sparing and PCL substituting designs.

Sharma et al. analyzed which kinematic parameters affect ROM following TKA [98]. Two hundred PCL sparing, sacrificing, and substituting TKAs were kinematically evaluated and divided into high (>110°) and low (<95°) weightbearing flexion cohorts. TKAs with higher flexion demonstrated more posterior femoral translation in deep flexion and exhibited a lower incidence of FCLO, suggesting obtaining good ligamentous stability is important to maximize TKA range of motion [98].

Dennis et al. performed an in vivo, weightbearing fluoroscopic kinematic analysis of multiple "high flexion" TKA designs and observed high levels of weightbearing flexion (125°) can be obtained in some, but not all evaluated designs [99]. Multiple evaluations of the same high flexion TKA design performed by different surgeons and involving different patient populations, revealed one study group with high weightbearing flexion and other groups that did not achieve high flexion. This suggests numerous factors other than implant design influence eventual flexion, including the patient, surgical technique, knee kinematics, perioperative complications, and postoperative physiotherapy. There may also be a benefit for inclusion of an anterior cam/post mechanism in TKA such as in the BCS design, where the lateral condyle starts more anterior in extension leading to posterior motion and momentum with increasing knee flexion. LaCour et al. reported that with a BCS TKA, subjects experienced, on average, 132.1 degrees of weightbearing knee flexion [100].

Summary

Study of TKA kinematics is essential as kinematic patterns have been correlated with patient satisfaction, outcome scores, and implant survivorship [34, 101–104]. In comparison to the non-implanted knee, design-specific kinematic variances have been observed. Kinematics also varies based on the type and precision of the surgical technique executed by the operating surgeon. Further analyses that allow for a better understanding of TKA kinematics will lead to continued improvements in technique and prosthetic design.

References

1. Carr BC, Goswami T. Knee implants—review of models and biomechanics. Mater Des. 2009;30:398–413. https://doi.org/10.1016/j.matdes.2008.03.032.
2. Eymard F, Charles-Nelson A, Katsahian S, Chevalier X, Bercovy M. "Forgotten knee" after total knee replacement: a pragmatic study from a single-centre cohort. Joint Bone Spine. 2015;82:177–81.
3. Zeller IM. Parameterization of a next generation in-vivo forward solution physiological model of the human lower limb to simulate and predict demographic and pathology specific knee mechanics [PhD dissertation]. University of Tennessee; 2018.

4. Dennis DA, Komistek RD, Kim RH, Sharma A. Gap balancing versus measured resection technique for total knee replacement. Clin Orthop Relat Res. 2010;468:102–7.
5. Andriacchi TP. Functional analysis of pre- and post-knee surgery. Total knee arthroplasty and ACL reconstruction. J Biomech Eng. 1993;115:575–81.
6. Grood E, Suntry W. A joint coordinate system for the clinical description of three-dimensional motions: application to the knee. J Biomech Eng. 1983;105:136–44.
7. Wren TAL, Do KP, Hara R, Rethlefsen SA. Use of a patella marker to improve tracking of dynamic hip rotation range of motion. Gait Posture. 2008;27:530e4. https://doi.org/10.1016/j.gaitpost.2007.07.006.
8. LaCour MT, Komistek RD. Fluoroscopic analysis of total knee replacement. 6th ed. New York, NY: Elsevier; 2018. p. 307–311.e1. https://doi.org/10.1016/B978-0-323-40046-6.00017-4.
9. Tanaka Y, Nakamura S, Kuriyama S, et al. How exactly can computer simulation predict the kinematics and contact status after TKA? Examination in individualized models. Clin Biomech. 2016;39:65–70. https://doi.org/10.1016/j.clinbiomech.2016.09.006.
10. Vollner F, Pilsl U, Craiovan B, et al. Stability of knee ligament complex of Thiel-embalmed cadaver compared to in vivo knee. J Mech Behav Biomed Mater. 2017;71:392–6. https://doi.org/10.1016/j.jmbbm.2017.04.009.
11. Roth JD, Howell SM, Hull ML. Native knee laxities at 0, 45, and 90 of flexion and their relationship to the goal of the gap-balancing alignment method of total knee arthroplasty. J Bone Joint Surg Am. 2015;97:1678–84. https://doi.org/10.2106/JBJS.N.01256.
12. Marra MA, Vanheule V, Fluit R, et al. A subject-specific musculoskeletal modeling framework to predict in vivo mechanics of total knee arthroplasty. J Biomech Eng. 2015;137:020904. https://doi.org/10.1115/1.4029258.
13. Akbarshahi M, Schache AG, Fernandez JW, et al. Non-invasive assessment of soft-tissue artifact and its effect on knee joint kinematics during functional activity. J Biomech. 2010;43:1292–301.
14. Garling EH, Kaptein BL, Mertens B, et al. Soft-tissue artifact assessment during step-up using fluoroscopy and skin-mounted markers. J Biomech. 2007;40:S18.
15. Mahfouz MR, Hoff WA, Komistek RD, Dennis DA. A robust method for registration of three-dimensional knee implant models to two-dimensional fluoroscopy images. IEEE Trans Med Imaging. 2003;22:1561–74. https://doi.org/10.1109/TMI.2003.820027.
16. Mahfouz MR, Hoff WA, Komistek RD, Dennis DA. Effect of segmentation errors on 3D-to-2D registration of implant models in X-ray images. J Biomech. 2005;38:229–39. https://doi.org/10.1016/j.jbiomech.2004.02.025.
17. LaCour MT, Sharma A, Carr CB, et al. Confirmation of long-term in vivo bearing mobility in eight rotating-platform TKAs. Clin Orthop Relat Res. 2014;472:2766–73.
18. Sharma A, Komistek RD. Contact mechanics of the human knee. In: Norman Scott W, editor. Insall & Scott surgery of the knee. 6th ed. Elsevier; 2017.
19. Grieco TF, Sharma A, Dessinger GM, Cates HE, Komistek RD. In vivo kinematic comparison of a bicruciate stabilized total knee arthroplasty and the normal knee using fluoroscopy. J Arthroplast. 2018;33(2):565–71.
20. Stiehl JB, Dennis DA, Komistek RD, Crane HS. In vivo determination of condylar lift-off and screw-home in a mobile bearing total knee arthroplasty. J Arthroplast. 1999;14:293–9.
21. Haas B, Komistek RD, Dennis DA. In vivo kinematic comparison of posterior cruciate sacrificing and stabilized mobile total bearing knee arthroplasty. Scientific exhibit presented at: 68th Annual Meeting of American Academy of Orthopaedic Surgeons; March 1–4, 2001; San Francisco, CA.
22. Stiehl JB, Dennis DA, Komistek RD, et al. In vivo comparison of posterior cruciate retaining and sacrificing mobile bearing total knee arthroplasty. Am J Knee Surg. 2000;13(1):13–8.
23. Kobori M, Komistek RD, Dennis DA, et al. An in vivo determination of patellar kinematics for fixed and mobile bearing TKA in Japanese patients having either a resurfaced or unresur-

faced patella. Paper presented at: 68th Annual Meeting American Academy of Orthopaedic Surgeons; March 2001; San Francisco.
24. Oakshott R, Komistek RD, Anderson DT, et al. In vivo passive vs weight-bearing knee kinematics for subjects implanted with a mobile bearing that can freely translate and rotate. Internal report. Denver, CO: Rocky Mountain Musculoskeletal Research Laboratory; 2000.
25. Running D, Komistek RD, Haas BD, et al. Determination of in vivo kinematics for subjects having either a traditional or posterior stabilized mobile bearing TKA. Paper presented at: European Society of Biomechanics; August 2000; Dublin, Ireland.
26. Angerame MR, Holst DC, Jennings JM, Komistek RD, Dennis DA. Total knee arthroplasty kinematics. J Arthroplast. 2019;34(10):2502–10. https://doi.org/10.1016/j.arth.2019.05.037.
27. Dennis DA, Komistek RD, Mahfouz MR, Haas BD, Stiehl JB. Coventry award paper: multicenter determination of in vivo kinematics after total knee arthroplasty. Clin Orthop Relat Res. 2003;(416):37–57. https://doi.org/10.1097/01.blo.0000092986.12414.b5.
28. Mueller JKP, Komistek RD, Mahfouz MR, Dennis DA. Fluoroscopic analysis of total knee replacement. In: Insall & Scott surgery of the knee. New York, NY: Elsevier; 2012. https://doi.org/10.1016/B978-1-4377-1503-3.00013-5.e13e1ee13e14.
29. Dennis DA, Komistek RD, Mahfouz MR, Walker SA, Tucker A. A multicenter analysis of axial femorotibial rotation after total knee arthroplasty. Clin Orthop Relat Res. 2004;(428):180–9. https://doi.org/10.1097/01.blo.0000148777.98244.84.
30. Matsuda S, Kawahara S, Okazaki K, Tashiro Y, Iwamoto Y. Postoperative alignment and ROM affect patient satisfaction after TKA. Clin Orthop Relat Res. 2012;471:127–33. https://doi.org/10.1007/s11999-012-2533-y.
31. Devers BN, Conditt MA, Jamieson ML, Driscoll MD, Noble PC, Parsley BS. Does greater knee flexion increase patient function and satisfaction after total knee arthroplasty? J Arthroplast. 2011;26:178–86. https://doi.org/10.1016/J.Arth.2010.02.008.
32. Allen MJ, Hartmann SM, Sacks JM, Calabrese J, Brown PR. Technical feasibility and precision of radiostereometric analysis as an outcome measure in canine cemented total hip replacement. J Orthop Sci. 2004;9:66–75. https://doi.org/10.1007/s00776-003-0743-6.
33. Warth LC, Ishmael MK, Deckard ER, Ziemba-Davis M, Meneghini RM. Do medial pivot kinematics correlate with patient-reported outcomes after total knee arthroplasty? J Arthroplast. 2017;32:2411–6. https://doi.org/10.1016/j.arth.2017.03.019.
34. Meccia B, Komistek RD, Mahfouz M, Dennis D. Abnormal axial rotations in TKA contribute to reduced weightbearing flexion. Clin Orthop Relat Res. 2013;472:248–53. https://doi.org/10.1007/s11999-013-3105-5.
35. Freeman MA, Pinskerova V. The movement of the knee studied by magnetic resonance imaging. Clin Orthop Relat Res. 2003;(410):35–43. https://doi.org/10.1097/01.blo.0000063598.67412.0d.
36. Johal P, Williams A, Wragg P, Hunt D, Gedroyc W. Tibio-femoral movement in the living knee. A study of weight bearing and non-weight bearing knee kinematics using "interventional" MRI. J Biomech. 2005;38:269–76. https://doi.org/10.1016/j.jbiomech.2004.02.008.
37. Cacciola G, Giustra F, Bosco F, et al. Long-term follow-up of medial pivot total knee arthroplasty: a systematic review of the current evidence. PRO. 2023;5(3):622–34. https://doi.org/10.3390/prosthesis5030044.
38. Benoit DL, Ramsey DK, Lamontagne M, Xu L, Wretenberg P, Renstrom P. Effect of skin movement artifact on knee kinematics during gait and cutting motions measured in vivo. Gait Posture. 2006;24:152–64. https://doi.org/10.1016/j.gaitpost.2005.04.012.
39. Dennis DA, Mahfouz MR, Komistek RD, Hoff W. In vivo determination of normal and anterior cruciate ligament-deficient knee kinematics. J Biomech. 2005;38:241–53. https://doi.org/10.1016/j.jbiomech.2004.02.042.
40. Qi W, Hosseini A, Tsai T-Y, Li J-S, Rubash HE, Li G. In vivo kinematics of the knee during weight bearing high flexion. J Biomech. 2013;46:1576–82.
41. Martelli S, Ellis RE, Marcacci M, Zaffagnini S. Total knee arthroplasty kinematics. Computer simulation and intraoperative evaluation. J Arthroplast. 1998;13:145–55.

42. Kang KT, Koh YG, Son J, Kwon OR, Lee JS, Kwon SK. Influence of increased posterior tibial slope in total knee arthroplasty on knee joint biomechanics: a computational simulation study. J Arthroplast. 2018;33(2):572–9. https://doi.org/10.1016/j.arth.2017.09.025.
43. Watanabe M, Kuriyama S, Nakamura S, et al. Varus femoral and tibial coronal alignments result in different kinematics and kinetics after total knee arthroplasty. Knee Surg Sports Traumatol Arthrosc. 2017;25:3459–66. https://doi.org/10.1007/s00167-017-4570-2.
44. Andriacchi TP, Stanwyck TS, Galante JO. Knee biomechanics and total knee replacement. J Arthroplast. 1986;1:211–9.
45. Daniel DM, Stone ML, Barnett P, Sachs R. Use of the quadriceps active test to diagnose posterior cruciate-ligament disruption and measure posterior laxity of the knee. J Bone Joint Surg Am. 1988;70:386–91.
46. van Eijden TM, de Boer W, Weijs WA. The orientation of the distal part of the quadriceps femoris muscle as a function of the knee flexion-extension angle. J Biomech. 1985;18:803–9.
47. Scarvell JM, Smith PN, Refshauge KM, Galloway H, Woods K. Comparison of kinematics in the healthy and ACL injured knee using MRI. J Biomech. 2005;38:255–62. https://doi.org/10.1016/j.jbiomech.2004.02.012.
48. Mahfouz MR, Komistek RD, Dennis DA, Hoff WA. In vivo assessment of the kinematics in normal and anterior cruciate ligament-deficient knees. J Bone Joint Surg Am. 2004;86-A(Suppl. 2):56–61.
49. Komistek RD, Allain J, Anderson DT, Dennis DA, Goutallier D. In vivo kinematics for subjects with and without an anterior cruciate ligament. Clin Orthop Relat Res. 2002;(404):315–25. https://doi.org/10.1097/01.blo.0000026562.55792.90.
50. Dennis DA, Komistek RD, Colwell CE, et al. In vivo anteroposterior femorotibial translation of total knee arthroplasty: a multicenter analysis. Clin Orthop Relat Res. 1998;(356):47–57.
51. Dennis DA, Komistek RD, Hoff WA, Gabriel SM. In vivo knee kinematics derived using an inverse perspective technique. Clin Orthop Relat Res. 1996;(331):107–17.
52. Yue B, Varadarajan KM, Moynihan AL, Liu F, Rubash HE, Li G. Kinematics of medial osteoarthritic knees before and after posterior cruciate ligament retaining total knee arthroplasty. J Orthop Res. 2010;29:40–6. https://doi.org/10.1002/jor.21203.
53. Blunn GW, Walker PS, Joshi A, Hardinge K. The dominance of cyclic sliding in producing wear in total knee replacements. Clin Orthop Relat Res. 1991;(273):253–60.
54. Bertin KC, Komistek RD, Dennis DA, Hoff WA, Anderson DT, Langer T. In vivo determination of posterior femoral rollback for subjects having a NexGen posterior cruciate-retaining total knee arthroplasty. J Arthroplast. 2002;17:1040–8. https://doi.org/10.1054/arth.2002.35793.
55. Takagi H, Asai S, Sato A, Maekawa M, Kawashima H, Kanzaki K. Case series report of navigation-based in vivo knee kinematics in total knee arthroplasty with a gradually reducing femoral radius design. Ann Med Surg (Lond). 2017;17:33–7. https://doi.org/10.1016/j.amsu.2017.03.032.
56. Pfitzner T, Moewis P, Stein P, et al. Modifications of femoral component design in multi-radius total knee arthroplasty lead to higher lateral posterior femoro-tibial translation. Knee Surg Sports Traumatol Arthrosc. 2018;26(6):1645–55. https://doi.org/10.1007/s00167-017-4622-7.
57. Clary CW, Fitzpatrick CK, Maletsky LP, Rullkoetter PJ. The influence of total knee arthroplasty geometry on mid-flexion stability: an experimental and finite element study. J Biomech. 2013;46:1351–7. https://doi.org/10.1016/j.jbiomech.2013.01.025.
58. Catani F, Belvedere C, Ensini A, Feliciangeli A, Giannini S, Leardini A. In-vivo knee kinematics in rotationally unconstrained total knee arthroplasty. J Orthop Res. 2011;29:1484–90. https://doi.org/10.1002/jor.21397.
59. Yoshiya S, Matsui N, Komistek RD, Dennis DA, Mahfouz M, Kurosaka M. In vivo kinematic comparison of posterior cruciate-retaining and posterior stabilized total knee arthroplasties under passive and weight-bearing conditions. J Arthroplast. 2005;20:777–83. https://doi.org/10.1016/j.arth.2004.11.012.

60. Dennis DA, Komistek RD, Stiehl JB, Walker SA, Dennis KN. Range of motion after total knee arthroplasty: the effect of implant design and weight-bearing conditions. J Arthroplast. 1998;13:748–52.
61. Nishio Y, Onodera T, Kasahara Y, Takahashi D, Iwasaki N, Majima T. Intra-operative medial pivot affects deep knee flexion angle and patient-reported outcomes after total knee arthroplasty. J Arthroplast. 2014;29:702–6. https://doi.org/10.1016/j.arth.2013.06.035.
62. Kaneko T, Kono N, Mochizuki Y, Hada M, Toyoda S, Musha Y. Bi-cruciate substituting total knee arthroplasty improved medio-lateral instability in mid-flexion range. J Orthop. 2017;14(1):201–6. https://doi.org/10.1016/j.jor.2016.12.005.
63. Ward TR, Burns AW, Gillespie MJ, Scarvell JM, Smith PN. Bicruciate-stabilised total knee replacements produce more normal sagittal plane kinematics than posterior-stabilised designs. J Bone Joint Surg Br. 2011;93(7):907–13. https://doi.org/10.1302/0301-620X.93B7.26208.
64. Mugnai R, Digennaro V, Ensini A, Leardini A, Catani F. Can TKA design affect the clinical outcome? Comparison between two guided-motion systems. Knee Surg Sports Traumatol Arthrosc. 2013;22:581–9. https://doi.org/10.1007/s00167-013-2509-9.
65. Scarvell JM, Perriman DM, Smith PN, Campbell DG, Bruce WJM, Nivbrant B. Total knee arthroplasty using bicruciate-stabilized or posterior-stabilized knee implants provided comparable outcomes at 2 years: a prospective, multicenter, randomized, controlled, clinical trial of patient outcomes. J Arthroplast. 2017;32:3356–3363.e1. https://doi.org/10.1016/j.arth.2017.05.032.
66. Pelt CE, Sandifer PA, Gililland JM, Anderson MB, Peters CL. Mean three-year survivorship of a new bicruciate-retaining total knee arthroplasty: are revisions still higher than expected? J Arthroplast. 2019;34(9):1957–62. https://doi.org/10.1016/j.arth.2019.04.030.
67. Morooka T-A, Muenchinger M, Canciani J-P, Banks SA. Comparing in vivo kinematics of anterior cruciate-retaining and posterior cruciate-retaining total knee arthroplasty. Knee Surg Sports Traumatol Arthrosc. 2007;15:93–9. https://doi.org/10.1007/s00167-006-0134-6.
68. Baumann F, Bahadin O, Krutsch W, et al. Proprioception after bicruciate-retaining total knee arthroplasty is comparable to unicompartmental knee arthroplasty. Knee Surg Sports Traumatol Arthrosc. 2016;25:1697–704. https://doi.org/10.1007/s00167-016-4121-2.
69. Halewood C, Traynor A, Bellemans J, Victor J, Amis AA. Anteroposterior laxity after bicruciate-retaining total knee arthroplasty is closer to the native knee than ACL-resecting TKA: a biomechanical cadaver study. J Arthroplast. 2015;30(12):2315–9. https://doi.org/10.1016/j.arth.2015.06.021.
70. Osmani FA, Thakkar SC, Collins K, Schwarzkopf R. The utility of bicruciate-retaining total knee arthroplasty. Arthroplast Today. 2017;3:61–6. https://doi.org/10.1016/j.artd.2016.11.004.
71. Schimmel JJ, Defoort KC, Heesterbeek PJ, Wymenga AB, Jacobs WC, van Hellemondt GG. Bicruciate substituting design does not improve maximal flexion in total knee arthroplasty. J Bone Joint Surg Am. 2014;96:e81–8. https://doi.org/10.2106/JBJS.M.00277.
72. Kono K, Tomita T, Yamazaki T, Inui H, Tanaka S, D'Lima DD. In vivo kinematics and cruciate ligament tension are not restored to normal after bicruciate-preserving arthroplasty. J Arthroplast. 2024;S0883-5403(24):00300-0. https://doi.org/10.1016/j.arth.2024.03.060.
73. Hamilton LD, Shelburne KB, Rullkoetter PJ, Barnes CL, Mannen EM. Kinematic performance of medial pivot total knee arthroplasty. J Arthroplast. 2024;39(6):1595–1601.e7. https://doi.org/10.1016/j.arth.2023.11.038.
74. Mochizuki T, Tanifuji O, Sato T, et al. Association between anteroposterior laxity in mid-range flexion and subjective healing of instability after total knee arthroplasty. Knee Surg Sports Traumatol Arthrosc. 2016;25:3543–8. https://doi.org/10.1007/s00167-016-4375-8.
75. Schmidt R, Komistek RD, Blaha JD, Penenberg BL, Maloney WJ. Fluoroscopic analyses of cruciate-retaining and medial pivot knee implants. Clin Orthop Relat Res. 2003;(410):139–47. https://doi.org/10.1097/01.blo.0000063565.90853.a4.

76. Shimmin A, Martinez-Martos S, Owens J, Iorgulescu AD, Banks S. Fluoroscopic motion study confirming the stability of a medial pivot design total knee arthroplasty. Knee. 2015;22:522–6. https://doi.org/10.1016/j.knee.2014.11.011.
77. Wautier D, Thienpont E. Changes in anteroposterior stability and proprioception after different types of knee arthroplasty. Knee Surg Sports Traumatol Arthrosc. 2017;25:1792–800. https://doi.org/10.1007/s00167-016-4038-9.
78. Steinbrück A, Schröder C, Woiczinski M, et al. Femorotibial kinematics and load patterns after total knee arthroplasty: an in vitro comparison of posterior-stabilized versus medial-stabilized design. Clin Biomech. 2016;33:42–8. https://doi.org/10.1016/j.clinbiomech.2016.02.002.
79. Moonot P, Shang M, Railton GT, Field RE, Banks SA. In vivo weight-bearing kinematics with medial rotation knee arthroplasty. Knee. 2010;17:33–7. https://doi.org/10.1016/j.knee.2009.06.009.
80. Moonot P, Mu S, Railton GT, Field RE, Banks SA. Tibiofemoral kinematic analysis of knee flexion for a medial pivot knee. Knee Surg Sports Traumatol Arthrosc. 2009;17:927–34. https://doi.org/10.1007/s00167-009-0777-1.
81. Cho SH, Cho HL, Lee SH, Jin HK. Posterior femoral translation in medial pivot total knee arthroplasty of posterior cruciate ligament retaining type. J Orthop. 2013;10:74–8. https://doi.org/10.1016/j.jor.2013.04.004.
82. Samy DA, Wolfstadt JI, Vaidee I, Backstein DJ. A retrospective comparison of a medial pivot and posterior-stabilized total knee arthroplasty with respect to patient-reported and radiographic outcomes. J Arthroplast. 2018;33(5):1379–83. https://doi.org/10.1016/j.arth.2017.11.049.
83. Kim Y-H, Yoon S-H, Kim J-S. Early outcome of TKA with a medial pivot fixed-bearing prosthesis is worse than with a PFC mobile-bearing prosthesis. Clin Orthop Relat Res. 2008;467:493–503. https://doi.org/10.1007/s11999-008-0221-8.
84. Ueyama H, Kanemoto N, Minoda Y, Nakagawa S, Taniguchi Y, Nakamura H. Association of a wider medial gap (medial laxity) in flexion with self-reported knee instability after medial-pivot total knee arthroplasty. J Bone Joint Surg Am. 2022;104(10):910–8. https://doi.org/10.2106/JBJS.21.01034.
85. Dennis DA, Komistek RD, Mahfouz MR, Outten JT, Sharma A. Mobile-bearing total knee arthroplasty. Clin Orthop Relat Res. 2005;440:88–95. https://doi.org/10.1097/01.blo.0000185464.23505.6e.
86. Komistek RD, Dennis DA, Mahfouz MR, Walker S, Outten J. In vivo polyethylene bearing mobility is maintained in posterior stabilized total knee arthroplasty. Clin Orthop Relat Res. 2004;(428):207–13. https://doi.org/10.1097/01.blo.0000147135.60185.39.
87. Zingde SM, Leszko F, Sharma A, Mahfouz MR, Komistek RD, Dennis DA. In vivo determination of cam-post engagement in fixed and mobile-bearing TKA. Clin Orthop Relat Res. 2014;472(1):254–62. https://doi.org/10.1007/s11999-013-3257-3.
88. McEwen HM, Fisher J, Goldsmith AA, Auger DD, Hardaker C, Stone MH. Wear of fixed bearing and rotating platform mobile bearing knees subjected to high levels of internal and external tibial rotation. J Mater Sci Mater Med. 2001;12(10–12):1049–52. https://doi.org/10.1023/a:1012850224565.
89. LaCour MT, Sharma A, Carr CB, Komistek RD, Dennis DA. Confirmation of long-term in vivo bearing mobility in eight rotating-platform TKAs. Clin Orthop Relat Res. 2014;472(9):2766–73. https://doi.org/10.1007/s11999-014-3642-6.
90. Yang CC, McFadden LA, Dennis DA, Kim RH, Sharma A. Lateral retinacular release rates in mobile-versus fixed-bearing TKA. Clin Orthop Relat Res. 2008;466(11):2656–61. https://doi.org/10.1007/s11999-008-0425-y.
91. Fantozzi S, Catani F, Ensini A, Leardini A, Giannini S. Femoral rollback of cruciate-retaining and posterior-stabilized total knee replacements: in vivo fluoroscopic analysis during activities of daily living. J Orthop Res. 2006;24:2222–9. https://doi.org/10.1002/jor.20306.

92. Wasielewski RC, Komistek RD, Zingde SM, Sheridan KC, Mahfouz MR. Lack of axial rotation in mobile-bearing knee designs. Clin Orthop Relat Res. 2008;466:2662–8. https://doi.org/10.1007/s11999-008-0354-9.
93. Watanabe T, Ishizuki M, Muneta T, Banks SA. Matched comparison of kinematics in knees with mild and severe varus deformity using fixed- and mobile-bearing total knee arthroplasty. Clin Biomech. 2012;27:924–8. https://doi.org/10.1016/j.clinbiomech.2012.07.005.
94. Mahoney OM, Kinsey TL, Banks AZ, Banks SA. Rotational kinematics of a modern fixed-bearing posterior stabilized total knee arthroplasty. J Arthroplast. 2009;24:641–5. https://doi.org/10.1016/j.arth.2008.03.009.
95. Nakamura E, Banks SA, Tanaka A, Sei A, Mizuta H. Three-dimensional tibiofemoral kinematics during deep flexion kneeling in a mobile-bearing total knee arthroplasty. J Arthroplast. 2009;24:1120–4. https://doi.org/10.1016/j.arth.2008.08.008.
96. Bercik MJ, Joshi A, Parvizi J. Posterior cruciate-retaining versus posterior-stabilized total knee arthroplasty. J Arthroplast. 2013;28:439–44. https://doi.org/10.1016/j.arth.2012.08.008.
97. Serna-Berna R, Lizaur-Utrilla A, Vizcaya-Moreno MF, Miralles Munoz FA, Gonzalez-Navarro B, Lopez-Prats FA. Cruciate-retaining versus posterior-stabilized primary total arthroplasty. Clinical outcome comparison with a minimum follow-up of 10 years. J Arthroplast. 2018;33:1–24. https://doi.org/10.1016/j.arth.2018.02.094.
98. Sharma A, Dennis DA, Zingde SM, Mahfouz MR, Komistek RD. Femoral condylar contact points start and remain posterior in high flexing patients. J Arthroplast. 2014;29(5):945–9. https://doi.org/10.1016/j.arth.2013.09.037.
99. Dennis DA, Komistek RD, Scuderi GR, Zingde S. Factors affecting flexion after total knee arthroplasty. Clin Orthop Relat Res. 2007;464:53–60. https://doi.org/10.1097/BLO.0b013e31812f785d.
100. LaCour MT, Dessinger GM, Haas SB, Komistek RD. In vivo weight-bearing kinematics for constrained versus traditional bicruciate stabilized total knee arthroplasty cohorts compared to the normal knee. J Arthroplast. 2024;39(6):1589–94. https://doi.org/10.1016/j.arth.2023.11.033.
101. Stiehl JB, Komistek RD, Dennis DA. Detrimental kinematics of a flat-on-flat total condylar knee arthroplasty. Clin Orthop Relat Res. 1999;(365):139–48.
102. Turcot K, Sagawa Y Jr, Fritschy D, Hoffmeyer P, Suva D, Armand S. How gait and clinical outcomes contribute to patients' satisfaction three months following a total knee arthroplasty. J Arthroplast. 2013;28:1297–300. https://doi.org/10.1016/j.arth.2013.01.031.
103. Bonnefoy-Mazure A, Armand S, Sagawa Y Jr, Suva D, Miozzari H, Turcot K. Knee kinematic and clinical outcomes evolution before, 3 months, and 1 year after total knee arthroplasty. J Arthroplast. 2017;32:793–800. https://doi.org/10.1016/j.arth.2016.03.050.
104. Argenson JN, Parratte S, Ashour A, Komistek RD, Scuderi GR. Patient-reported outcome correlates with knee function after a single-design mobile-bearing TKA. Clin Orthop Relat Res. 2008;466:2669–76. https://doi.org/10.1007/s11999-008-0418-x.

Chapter 16
Future Considerations

Giles R. Scuderi and Alfred J. Tria Jr

Introduction

Over the last 50 years, total knee arthroplasty (TKA) has evolved to be one of the most successful and effective treatments for severe osteoarthritis of the knee. Pioneers, like John N. Insall, Chitranjan Ranawat, Peter Walker, Michael Freeman, and others established the foundation for current modern designs and continue to influence the future directions. Given their impact along with the high success of modern TKA, the volume of TKA has risen over the past decades in the United States, making it one of the most performed orthopedic procedures. The most recent 2040 projections for primary TKA are over 1.2 million cases per year and over 2.9 million in 2060 [1]. This is an estimated increase of 139% in 2040 and 469% in 2060 from our current numbers. With these rising numbers there are efforts to predict the need for TKA using machine learning. Mahmoud et al. in a prospective study using datasets that included patient demographics, medical history, imaging assessments, history of intervention and outcomes was able to devise a predictive and clinically accurate model for predicting the need for TKA [2]. The evolution of artificial intelligence (AI) has the potential to facilitate targeted nonoperative management to modify patient risk, but also identify the ideal time for surgical intervention. The AI predictive models have the potential to empower patients in the surgical decision as we see a shift in the arthroplasty patient population. With improved life expectancy and increasing preference to leading an active like, TKAs are increasing performed in younger and active patients. This shift to a younger population results

G. R. Scuderi
Department of Orthopaedic Surgery, Zucker School of Medicine at Hofstra/Northwell, Hempstead, NY, USA

A. J. Tria Jr (✉)
Department of Orthopedic Surgery (Emeritus), Rutgers-Robert Wood Johnson Medical School, New Brunswick, NJ, USA

A. J. Tria Jr., G. R. Scuderi (eds.), *The Cruciate Ligaments in Total Knee Arthroplasty*, https://doi.org/10.1007/978-3-031-75992-5_16

in greater demands on the knee for a longer duration of time. Younger patients may also have higher expectations in restoration of functional status after TKA with desires to return to more physically demanding activities. TKA has proven to be a predictable and durable procedure, returning patients to both activities of daily living and recreational activities with overall good survivorship. Satisfying patient expectations is the ultimate goal. Despite advances in implant design and surgical technique over the years, up to 20% of patients remain dissatisfied [3, 4]. However, a recent review of the literature found that the average rate of patient dissatisfaction was 10% [5]. What was interesting was that many sociodemographic factors, such as financial status, education, and non-White race, were associated with dissatisfaction, but may not be a direct cause but are associated with an increased risk of poor outcomes through an associated relationship. As an example, the confounding differences with age find that younger patients have a higher expectation of activity following TKA with desires to return to more physically demanding activities, while physiologically older patients have more medical comorbidities and may not be as functionally active. Worse functional outcomes and postoperative complications contribute to patient dissatisfaction and will be the driving force for improvements in TKA design and technique. To further improve patient satisfaction, efforts are needed to further reduce postoperative complications with a critical assessment of the perioperative clinical pathway. Further improvements in implant design, instrumentation, and surgical technique are evolving and are directed towards a more personalized approach, which is expected to be assisted by innovative technology.

Implant Design

The issue of patient dissatisfaction may be reduced by a more individualized patient-specific approach to TKA with more personalized designs and surgical technique. The current inventory of modern implants is providing a wide range of shapes and sizes with more anatomically shaped components. The systems now include closer sizing of the femoral component with 2 mm increments, with standard and narrow options, allowing better fit to the anterior-posterior dimension without overhang. This more personalized fit with off-the-shelf components allows for anatomic referencing while avoiding complications associated with anterior and posterior referencing techniques [6, 7]. The tibial component has seen designs with more anatomic shapes that provide tibial coverage without compromise of the rotational position. The main direction of newer TKA design is to optimize component fit without compromise, improve knee kinematics by restoring the radii of femoral curvature, improve patella tracking with a patella friendly trochlea and restore limb alignment.

There is currently a trending move away from the historical articular design and towards more guided motion knee designs that replicate knee kinematics by the geometry of the femoral tibial articular surface. We have seen from the American Joint Replacement Registry [8] that while PCL substituting (PS) knee designs had been the most popular implant design, PCL retaining (CR) implants are gaining popularity and are the most commonly implanted design. However, the recent AJRR report also noted that there is an increased interest in guided motion knee implant designs, such as the ultracongruent, medial congruent and medial pivot. These newer implant designs may continue to erode on both the PS and CR market share. It appears that the surface geometries, with differential medial and lateral conformities, in these designs influences knee kinematics and motion without the need for the cruciate ligaments or cam-post mechanism. What may be driving the increased interest in guided motion knee designs is that it is coupled with the new interest in alternative alignments in TKA, such as kinematic alignment in contrast to mechanical alignment.

Trends in Alignment

The advent of modern components and advanced technologies has fueled the debate on whether mechanical alignment can be justified in all knees. Currently, a personalized approach to TKA has numerous novel schemes and techniques such as anatomic alignment, unrestricted kinematic alignment, restricted kinematic alignment, inverse restricted kinematic alignment, adjusted mechanical alignment, and functional alignment. The nuances and language of knee alignment is differing and confusing. With each of these personalized alignments, the resection targets and boundaries are individualized and varying without consistency. Some techniques like kinematic alignment pose the risk of reproducing extreme native alignment while restricted kinematic alignment imposes boundaries on implant positioning and ultimate limb alignment. The range of variability between all proposed alignment techniques in targets for the hip knee angle (HKA); femoral and tibial coronal alignment; femoral and tibial sagittal alignment; and femoral axial alignment is wide and varying. There has yet to be an agreed upon personalized technique that has been widely accepted as mechanical alignment [9]. Further research is needed to assess the relevance of these "new" alignment schemes to see if they are really worth the change and which ones are the most relevant for which patients, diagnoses, and degrees of deformity as noted with the coronal plane alignment of the knee (CPAC) classification [10].

Instrumentation

Currently, the most common surgical technique for TKA is conventional manual instrumentation with procedures following a similar plan. However, there has been a shift to innovative technologies to assist in surgical accuracy. Studies have shown that patient anatomy in three dimensions (3D) varies from patient to patient. Advanced imaging and related technologies can better define each patient's specific anatomic features. While computer navigation introduced the concept of a more individualized approach based upon advanced imaging, this has evolved to robotic-assisted surgery. The utility of standard radiographs for preoperative planning has scrutinized as MRI and CT scans have been shown to offer greater detail and allow for a virtual 3D reproduction of the knee. Current robotic systems create a 3D plan based upon intraoperative bone morphology mapping or a preoperative MRI or CT scan. Based upon the 3D reconstruction data collected, the personalized preoperative plan for the individual patient is created. The robotic-assisted surgery also allows an assessment of ligament balancing based upon the bone cuts and implant position. This has the potential to be further enhanced by collecting all the information into a large database and allow artificial intelligence (AI) and machine learning (ML) analysis of the alignment and outcome [11]. With the best aggregated clinical results determined by ML, the computer can be programmed to learn how to make the best recommendation for alignment of each patient, which is then incorporated into the robotic surgical plan. The role of AI will continue to expand with ongoing advances, pushing the boundaries of its capabilities. Incorporating ML has the potential to elevate patient care by identifying the best preoperative patient parameters and postoperative pathways to help drive higher patient satisfaction.

One of the challenges of achieving a satisfactory TKA is ligament balancing. Historically, ligament balance was a qualitative "feel" rather than a quantitative measurement. This "feel is based upon surgeon experience but is influenced by many patient factors including degree of deformity or contracture, generalized ligament laxity, joint stiffness, obesity, and gender. The introduction of intraoperative sensors with the surgical instrumentation provides intraoperative monitoring and objective data to facilitate decision-making regarding implant position and soft tissue releases to improve balance and stability through the full range of motion [12]. Further development of real-time intraoperative sensors incorporated into tensiometers or robotic-assisted surgical system will need to define the normal pressures, as well as the normal ligament tension, within the joint to achieve a well-balanced TKA. This information, along with ML analysis, has the potential to provide a personalized approach to ligament balance for each patient.

Augmented Reality

Augmented reality (AR), an interactive experience, where the knee that resides in the real world is enhanced by computer generated information, is generating increasing interest as a technology that could improve the accuracy and efficiency of TKA [13, 14]. It has been shown that the accuracy of planned bone resection with the assistance of AR matches the preplanned configuration with errors $<1°$ regardless of the target value [14]. This technology also has the potential for soft tissue balance by direct real-time measurement of the strain of the collateral ligaments throughout the range of motion by tracking their movements from their origins and insertions [13]. Intraoperative ligament assessment can be used to establish a patient-specific plan, guiding the surgeon to the best target to achieve proper ligament balance with the potential to improve clinical outcomes. While further research is needed, AR may be the future of innovative technology in TKA instrumentation.

Smart Implants

Though in its infancy, smart implants with embedded sensor technology have the potential to provide the quantitative in vivo data to improve postoperative recovery, reduce postoperative visits, detect early complications, and increase patient satisfaction [15]. The recent introduction of sensor technology within the Persona iQ (Zimmer Biomet, Warsaw, IN) can detect activity and record kinematic data that can characterize a patient's physical recovery and provide diagnostic information. The embedded inertial measurement unit collects step count, walking speed, stride length, cadence, functional range of motion while walking and tibia range of motion. Analysis of the collected data and recovery curves demonstrated that there are patient-specific differences in their early postoperative course with discrete cohorts [16]. Though there is currently limited clinical use of smart implants, it is expected that we will see a growing trend of smart implants as there are refinements in the technology.

Summary

The knowledge and technology from our current experience in TKA is setting the stage for future developments. Enhancements in our understanding of knee anatomy and biomechanics are suggesting ways of improving outcomes and potentially patient satisfaction. Applying this knowledge to implant designs that replicate the anatomy of the knee and kinematics, along with more precise surgical techniques with innovative technology will be the future of TKA. The immersion of augmented reality devices into TKA may help provide enhanced real-world information at the time of surgery, further refining the clinical outcome.

References

1. Shichman I, Roof M, Askew N, et al. Projections and epidemiology of primary hip and knee arthroplasty in Medicare patients to 2040-2060. J Bone Joint Surg Open Acess. 2023;8:e22.00112. https://doi.org/10.2106/JBJS.OA22.00112.
2. Mahmoud K, Alagha MA, Nowinka Z, Jones G. Predicting total knee replacement at 2 and 5 years in osteoarthritis patients using machine learning. BMJ Surg Interv Health Technol. 2023;5:e000141. https://doi.org/10.1136/bmjsit-2022-000141.

3. Noble PC, Conditt MA, Cook KF, Mathis KB. The John Insall Award: patient expectations affect satisfaction with total knee arthroplasty. Clin Orthop Relat Res. 2006;452:35–43.
4. Bourne RB, Chesworth BM, Davis AM, Mahomed NN, Charron KDJ. Patient satisfaction after total knee arthroplasty: who is satisfied and who is not? Clin Orthop Relat Res. 2010;468:57–63.
5. DeFrance MJ, Scuderi GR. Are 20% of patients actually dissatisfied following total knee arthroplasty? A systematic review of the literature. J Arthroplast. 2023;38:594–9.
6. Knapp PW, Scuderi GR. Anatomic referencing restores the anatomy of the distal femur with less compromise. J Knee Surg. 2024;37(2):114–20. https://doi.org/10.1055/a-2186-6087.
7. Campbell BR, Weinberg M, Bischoff J, Scuderi GR. An evaluation of anatomic referencing for femoral component sizing using CT based computer modeling. J Knee Surg. 2024;37:638–41. https://doi.org/10.1055/a-2240-3566.
8. American Joint Replacement Registry annual report 2022.
9. MacDessi SJ, Oussedik S, Abdel MP, Victor J, Pagnano MW, Haddad FS. The language of knee alignment. Updated definitions and considerations for reporting outcomes in total knee arthroplasty. Bone Joint J. 2023;105B(2):102–8.
10. MacDessi SJ, Griffiths-Jones W, Harris IA, Bellemans J, Chen DB. Coronal plane alignment of the knee (CPAK) classification. Bone Joint J. 2021;103-B(2):329–37.
11. Myers TG, Ramkumar PN, Ricciardi BF, Urish KL, Kioper J, Ketonis C. Artificial intelligence, and orthopedics: an introduction for clinicians. J Bone Joint Surg Am. 2020;102(9):830–40.
12. Batailler C, Swan J, Marinier ES, Servien E, Lustig S. New technologies in knee arthroplasty: current concepts. J Clin Med. 2021;10:47. https://doi.org/10.3390/jcm10010047.
13. Fucentese SF, Koch PP. A novel augmented reality based surgical guidance system for total knee arthroplasty. Arch Orthop Trauma Surg. 2021;141:2227–33.
14. Castellarin G, Bori E, Barbieux E, Grandjean VP, Jost G, Innocenti B. Is total knee arthroplasty surgical performance enhanced using augmented reality? A single-center study on 76 consecutive patients. J Arthroplast. 2024;39:332–5.
15. Kelmers E, Szuba A, King SW, et al. Smart knee implants: An overview of current technologies and future possibilities. Indian J Orthop. 2023;57:635–42.
16. Cushner FD, Yergler J, Elashoff BA, Aubin PD, Scuderi GR. Staying ahead of the curve – the case fir recovery curves in total knee arthroplasty. J Arthroplast. 2024; https://doi.org/10.1016/j.arth.2024.07.039.

Correction to: Ligament Gap Balancing Approach

Martin Roche, Tsun Law, Gabrielle Dituri, and Ebony James

Correction to: Chapter 11 in: A. J. Tria Jr., G. R. Scuderi (eds.), *The Cruciate Ligaments in Total Knee Arthroplasty*, https://doi.org/10.1007/978-3-031-75992-5_11

In Chapter 11, "Ligament Gap Balancing Approach," the author's name was incorrectly printed as Gabriella Dituri. This has been corrected to Gabrielle Dituri in Chapter 11 (page 133), Table of Contents, and Contributors List.

The updated version of this chapter can be found at
https://doi.org/10.1007/978-3-031-75992-5_11

A. J. Tria Jr., G. R. Scuderi (eds.), *The Cruciate Ligaments in Total Knee Arthroplasty*, https://doi.org/10.1007/978-3-031-75992-5_17

Index

A. J. Tria Jr., G. R. Scuderi (eds.), *The Cruciate Ligaments in Total Knee Arthroplasty*, https://doi.org/10.1007/978-3-031-75992-5

GPSR Compliance

The European Union's (EU) General Product Safety Regulation (GPSR) is a set of rules that requires consumer products to be safe and our obligations to ensure this.

If you have any concerns about our products, you can contact us on ProductSafety@springernature.com

In case Publisher is established outside the EU, the EU authorized representative is:

Springer Nature Customer Service Center GmbH
Europaplatz 3
69115 Heidelberg, Germany

Batch number: 10726135

Printed by Printforce, the Netherlands